Imaging of Bone and Soft Tissue Tumors

Guest Editor

G. SCOTT STACY, MD

RADIOLOGIC CLINICS OF NORTH AMERICA

www.radiologic.theclinics.com

Consulting Editor
FRANK H. MILLER, MD

November 2011 • Volume 49 • Number 6

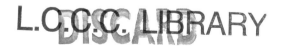

SAUNDERS an imprint of ELSEVIER, Inc.

W.B. SAUNDERS COMPANY
A Division of Elsevier Inc.

1600 John F. Kennedy Boulevard • Suite 1800 • Philadelphia, Pennsylvania 19103-2899

http://www.theclinics.com

RADIOLOGIC CLINICS OF NORTH AMERICA Volume 49, Number 6
November 2011 ISSN 0033-8389, ISBN 13: 978-1-4557-1152-9

Editor: Barton Dudlick
Developmental Editor: Donald E. Mumford

Radiologic Clinics of North America (ISSN 0033-8389) is published bimonthly by Elsevier Inc., 360 Park Avenue South, New York, NY 10010-1710. Months of issue are January, March, May, July, September, and November. Periodicals postage paid at New York, NY and additional mailing offices. Subscription prices are USD 386 per year for US individuals, USD 610 per year for US institutions, USD 185 per year for US students and residents, USD 450 per year for Canadian individuals, USD 766 per year for Canadian institutions, USD 556 per year for international individuals, USD 766 per year for international institutions, and USD 266 per year for Canadian and foreign students/residents. To receive student and resident rate, orders must be accompanied by name of affiliated institution, date of term and the signature of program/residency coordinatior on institution letterhead. Orders will be billed at individual rate until proof of status is received. Foreign air speed delivery is included in all *Clinics* subscription prices. All prices are subject to change without notice. **POSTMASTER:** Send address changes to *Radiologic Clinics of North America*, Elsevier Health Sciences Division, Subscription Customer Service, 3251 Riverport Lane, Maryland Heights, MO63043. **Customer Service: Telephone: 1-800-654-2452** (U.S. and Canada); **1-314-447-8871** (outside U.S. and Canada). **Fax: 1-314-447-8029. E-mail: journalscustomerservice-usa@elsevier.com** (for print support); **journalsonlinesupport-usa@elsevier.com** (for online support).

Reprints. For copies of 100 or more of articles in this publication, please contact the Commercial Reprints Department, Elsevier Inc., 360 Park Avenue South, New York, New York 10010-1710. Tel.: (+1) 212-633-3812; Fax: (+1) 212-462-1935; E-mail: reprints@elsevier.com.

Radiologic Clinics of North America also published in Greek Paschalidis Medical Publications, Athens, Greece.

Radiologic Clinics of North America is covered in *MEDLINE/PubMed (Index Medicus), EMBASE/Excerpta Medica, Current Contents/Life Sciences, Current Contents/Clinical Medicine, RSNA Index to Imaging Literature, BIOSIS, Science Citation Index,* and *ISI/BIOMED.*

Printed in the United States of America.

Contributors

CONSULTING EDITOR

FRANK H. MILLER, MD
Professor of Radiology; Chief, Body Imaging
Section and Fellowship Program and
GI Radiology, Medical Director MRI,
Department of Radiology, Northwestern
University Feinberg School of Medicine,
Chicago, Illinois

GUEST EDITOR

G. SCOTT STACY, MD
Associate Professor of Radiology; Chief,
Section of Musculoskeletal Imaging,
Department of Radiology, University of
Chicago Medical Center, Chicago, Illinois

AUTHORS

TESSA BALACH, MD
Assistant Professor, Department
of Orthopaedic Surgery, New England
Musculoskeletal Institute, University
of Connecticut Health Center, Farmington,
Connecticut

CLARISSA CANELLA, MD
Clínica de Diagnóstico por Imagem; Serviço de
Radiologia da, Universidade Federal do Rio de
Janeiro, Rio de Janeiro, Brasil

FLÁVIA MARTINS COSTA, MD
Clínica de Diagnóstico por Imagem; Serviço de
Radiologia da, Universidade Federal do Rio de
Janeiro, Rio de Janeiro, Brasil

LARRY B. DIXON, MD
Associate Professor of Radiology,
Musculoskeletal Imaging, Department
of Radiology, University of Chicago,
Chicago, Illinois

MICHAEL E. FENTON, MD, CDR (USN)
American Institute for Radiologic Pathology,
Silver Spring, Maryland

HILLARY WARREN GARNER, MD
Assistant Professor of Radiology,
Department of Radiology, Mayo Clinic
Florida, Jacksonville, Florida

EMERSON GASPARETTO, MD, PhD
Clínica de Diagnóstico por Imagem; Serviço de
Radiologia da, Universidade Federal do Rio de
Janeiro, Rio de Janeiro, Brasil

REX C. HAYDON, MD
Associate Professor of Surgery, Section
of Orthopaedic Surgery and Rehabilitation
Medicine, University of Chicago, Chicago,
Illinois

AMBROSE J. HUANG, MD
Instructor of Radiology, Department of
Radiology, Harvard Medical School; Assistant
Radiologist, Massachusetts General Hospital,
Boston, Massachusetts

HAKAN ILASLAN, MD
Staff Radiologist and Assistant Professor
of Radiology, Division of Musculoskeletal
Radiology, Imaging Institute, Cleveland Clinic
Foundation, Cleveland, Ohio

AVNIT KAPUR, MD
Radiology Resident, Department
of Radiology, University of Chicago
Medical Center, Chicago, Illinois

SUSAN V. KATTAPURAM, MD
Associate Professor of Radiology, Department
of Radiology, Harvard Medical School;
Radiologist, Massachusetts General Hospital,
Boston, Massachusetts

SUNG H. KIM, MD
Musculoskeletal Radiology Fellow,
Department of Radiology, University
of Maryland Medical Center, Baltimore,
Maryland

MARK J. KRANSDORF, MD
Professor of Radiology, Department of
Radiology, Mayo Clinic Florida, Jacksonville,
Florida

KAMBIZ MOTAMEDI, MD
Associate Professor of Radiology,
Musculoskeletal Imaging, UCLA Radiology,
David Geffen School of Medicine,
University of California, Los Angeles,
California

MICHAEL E. MULLIGAN, MD
Professor of Radiology and Nuclear
Medicine, Department of Radiology,
University of Maryland School of Medicine,
Baltimore, Maryland

MARK D. MURPHEY, MD
American Institute for Radiologic Pathology,
Silver Spring, Maryland; Department of
Radiology, Walter Reed Army Medical Center,
Washington, DC; Department of Radiology
and Nuclear Medicine, Uniformed Services
University of the Health Sciences,
Bethesda, Maryland

OSCAR M. NAVARRO, MD
Associate Professor, Department of Medical
Imaging, University of Toronto; Head,
Ultrasound Section, Department of Diagnostic
Imaging, The Hospital for Sick Children,
Toronto, Ontario, Canada

R. EVAN NICHOLS, MD
Clinical Instructor, Musculoskeletal
Imaging, Department of Radiology,
University of Chicago, Chicago, Illinois

TERRANCE D. PEABODY, MD
The Simon and Kalt Families Professor
of Surgery; Chief, Section of Orthopaedic
Surgery and Rehabilitation Medicine,
University of Chicago, Chicago, Illinois

JEFFREY J. PETERSON, MD
Professor of Radiology, Department
of Radiology, Mayo Clinic Florida,
Jacksonville, Florida

PRABHAKAR RAJIAH, MBBS, MD, FRCR
Clinical Fellow, Division of Musculoskeletal
Radiology, Imaging Institute, Cleveland
Clinic Foundation, Cleveland, Ohio

JOEL S. SALESKY, MD
American Institute for Radiologic
Pathology, Silver Spring, Maryland

LEANNE L. SEEGER, MD
Professor of Radiology and Chief,
Musculoskeletal Imaging, UCLA Radiology,
David Geffen School of Medicine,
University of California, Los Angeles,
California

STACY E. SMITH, MD
Associate Professor of Radiology and Chair,
Musculoskeletal Radiology, Department of
Radiology, Brigham and Women's Hospital,
Boston, Massachusetts

G. SCOTT STACY, MD
Associate Professor of Radiology;
Chief, Section of Musculoskeletal
Imaging, Department of Radiology,
University of Chicago Medical Center,
Chicago, Illinois

MURALI SUNDARAM, MD, FRCR
Professor of Radiology, Division
of Musculoskeletal Radiology, Imaging
Institute, Cleveland Clinic Foundation,
Cleveland, Ohio

ERIC A. WALKER, MD
Department of Radiology, Milton S. Hershey
Medical Center, Hershey, Pennsylvania;
Department of Radiology and Nuclear
Medicine, Uniformed Services University
of the Health Sciences, Bethesda,
Maryland

Contents

small and superficial lesions. MR imaging can be helpful, particularly in the evaluation of large and deep soft tissue lesions. Correlation of the imaging findings with the clinical information is crucial in the diagnostic work-up. This article reviews the most common causes of soft tissue masses that require imaging in children.

Many benign nonneoplastic entities can mimic bone and soft tissue tumors on imaging examinations. Distinguishing between neoplastic and nonneoplastic entities depends on history and physical examination findings and imaging findings, and is an important early step in the patient's overall workup and treatment plan. This article describes some of the pseudotumors seen on imaging studies in our orthopedic oncology clinic, as well as mimics of bone and soft tissue neoplasms described in the medical literature. Tumor mimics resulting from anatomic and developmental variants, trauma, infection and inflammation, osteonecrosis and myonecrosis, articular and juxta-articular conditions, and miscellaneous causes are discussed.

Percutaneous core needle biopsy and fine-needle aspiration are safe and cost-effective methods and can be important steps in the workup of a bone or soft tissue lesion. These procedures should be performed in collaboration with the orthopedic oncologist who performs the definitive surgery. In the extremities, attention to compartmental anatomy is paramount. With frozen section evaluation at the time of biopsy, the chances of a nondiagnostic specimen necessitating rebiopsy are minimized. The principles underlying the percutaneous approach to various lesions are valuable and can be applied to minimally invasive percutaneous therapy for bone and soft tissue lesions.

Posttreatment imaging is important to ensure early detection of oncological complications, and appropriate timing and frequency is an important consideration, especially in high-risk patients. Focused magnetic resonance (MR) imaging is the preferred modality for detection of local recurrence of soft tissue tumors and is also used in high-risk osteosarcoma. Although posttreatment changes can mimic or obscure local recurrence on MR imaging, a systematic approach and knowledge of the features of recurrence versus therapeutic change allows differentiation in almost all cases. Positron emission tomography/computed tomography is also emerging as an important problem-solving tool in local recurrence and in metastatic surveillance.

Magnetic resonance (MR) imaging is an important modality for the preoperative and posttreatment evaluation of musculoskeletal tumors. In some cases, MR imaging is unable to offer information about the extension of tumoral necrosis and the presence of viable cells. Advanced MR imaging techniques are now used in association with conventional MR imaging to improve the diagnostic accuracy and the evaluation of treatment response. This article discusses each advanced MR imaging technique with regard to the clinical applications of tumor detection and characterization, differentiation of benign from malignant tumors and tumor tissue from nontumor tissue, and assessment of treatment response.

GOAL STATEMENT

The goal of the *Radiologic Clinics of North America* is to keep practicing radiologists and radiology residents up to date with current clinical practice in radiology by providing timely articles reviewing the state of the art in patient care.

ACCREDITATION

The *Radiologic Clinics of North America* is planned and implemented in accordance with the Essential Areas and Policies of the Accreditation Council for Continuing Medical Education (ACCME) through the joint sponsorship of the University of Virginia School of Medicine and Elsevier. The University of Virginia School of Medicine is accredited by the ACCME to provide continuing medical education for physicians.

The University of Virginia School of Medicine designates this enduring material activity for a maximum of 15 *AMA PRA Category 1 Credit*(s)™ for each issue, 90 credits per year. Physicians should only claim credit commensurate with the extent of their participation in the activity.

The American Medical Association has determined that physicians not licensed in the US who participate in this CME enduring material activity are eligible for a maximum of 15 *AMA PRA Category 1 Credit*(s)™ for each issue, 90 credits per year.

Credit can be earned by reading the text material, taking the CME examination online at http://www.theclinics.com/home/cme, and completing the evaluation. After taking the test, you will be required to review any and all incorrect answers. Following completion of the test and evaluation, your credit will be awarded and you may print your certificate.

FACULTY DISCLOSURE/CONFLICT OF INTEREST

The University of Virginia School of Medicine, as an ACCME accredited provider, endorses and strives to comply with the Accreditation Council for Continuing Medical Education (ACCME) Standards of Commercial Support, Commonwealth of Virginia statutes, University of Virginia policies and procedures, and associated federal and private regulations and guidelines on the need for disclosure and monitoring of proprietary and financial interests that may affect the scientific integrity and balance of content delivered in continuing medical education activities under our auspices.

The University of Virginia School of Medicine requires that all CME activities accredited through this institution be developed independently and be scientifically rigorous, balanced and objective in the presentation/discussion of its content, theories and practices.

All authors/editors participating in an accredited CME activity are expected to disclose to the readers relevant financial relationships with commercial entities occurring within the past 12 months (such as grants or research support, employee, consultant, stock holder, member of speakers bureau, etc.). The University of Virginia School of Medicine will employ appropriate mechanisms to resolve potential conflicts of interest to maintain the standards of fair and balanced education to the reader. Questions about specific strategies can be directed to the Office of Continuing Medical Education, University of Virginia School of Medicine, Charlottesville, Virginia.

The faculty and staff of the University of Virginia Office of Continuing Medical Education have no financial affiliations to disclose.

The authors/editors listed below have identified no financial or professional relationships for themselves or their spouse/partner:

Tessa Balach, MD; Clarissa Canella, MD; Flávia Martins Costa, MD; Larry B. Dixon, MD; Barton Dudlick, (Acquisitions Editor); Michael E. Fenton, MD; Hillary Warren Garner, MD; Emerson Gasparetto, MD, PhD; Rex C. Haydon, MD; Ambrose J. Huang, MD; Hakan Ilaslan, MD; Avnit Kapur, MD; Susan V. Kattapuram, MD; Sung H. Kim, MD; Mark J. Kransdorf, MD; Frank H. Miller, MD (Consulting Editor); Kambiz Motamedi, MD; Michael E. Mulligan, MD; Mark D. Murphey, MD; Oscar M. Navarro, MD; R. Evan Nichols, MD; Terrance D. Peabody, MD; Jeffery J. Peterson, MD; Prabhakar Rajiah, MBBS, MD, FRCR; Joel S. Salesky, MD; Leanne L. Seeger, MD; Stacy E. Smith, MD; G. Scott Stacy, MD (Guest Editor); Murali Sundaram, MD, FRCR; and Eric A. Walker, MD.

The authors/editors listed below have identified the following financial or professional relationships for themselves or their spouse/partner:

Klaus D. Hagspiel, MD (Test Author) is an industry funded research/investigator for Siemens Medical Solutions.

Disclosure of Discussion of Non-FDA Approved Uses for Pharmaceutical Products and/or Medical Devices

The University of Virginia School of Medicine, as an ACCME provider, requires that all faculty presenters identify and disclose any off-label uses for pharmaceutical and medical device products. The University of Virginia School of Medicine recommends that each physician fully review all the available data on new products or procedures prior to clinical use.

TO ENROLL

To enroll in the Radiologic Clinics of North America Continuing Medical Education program, call customer service at 1-800-654-2452 or sign up online at http://www.theclinics.com/home/cme. The CME program is available to subscribers for an additional annual fee USD 245.

Radiologic Clinics of North America

THE CLINICS ARE NOW AVAILABLE ONLINE!

Access your subscription at:
www.theclinics.com

Preface
Imaging of Bone and Soft Tissue Tumors

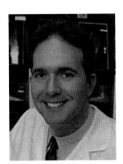

G. Scott Stacy, MD
Guest Editor

The diagnosis of bone and soft tissue neoplasms is often a challenge for physicians. Primary bone and soft tissue malignancies are relatively rare, and hence, most radiologists do not encounter these tumors with enough frequency to allow the development of a sense of familiarity. Orthopedic surgeons and pathologists are typically in a similar predicament and often rely on the radiologist to help determine the true nature of a musculoskeletal tumor, and on occasion to provide appropriate therapy (eg, via percutaneous ablative procedures). The "team approach" to diagnosis and management of bone and soft tissue tumors is paramount to a successful outcome for the patient.

The nomenclature of tumors, particularly soft tissue tumors, is vast and can be confusing, and not infrequently changes based on recent developments in histologic and genetic typing. Furthermore, there are countless "pseudotumors" that mimic bone and soft tissue neoplasms, confounding diagnosis. Many primary bone tumors occur in children, resulting in additional apprehension. As with tumors occurring in other parts of the body, analysis of musculoskeletal neoplasms requires a fundamental knowledge of the different varieties of tumors and tumor-like lesions, as well as a systematic approach to their evaluation.

Imaging is a component of the workup of all bone tumors and most soft tissue tumors, with the exception of some superficial lesions. The radiograph remains the procedure of choice for initial imaging of bone lesions, but advances in imaging modalities during the past few decades have allowed amazing progress in the diagnosis, treatment, and follow-up of musculoskeletal neoplasms; this progress has, in large part, resulted in substantial improvement in the prognosis and survival of patients with musculoskeletal tumors. Not long ago, a soft tissue tumor to a radiologist was just an opacity on the radiograph, assuming it was even visible. Now, cross-sectional imaging allows an accurate prediction of the histolopathologic diagnosis of many soft tissue masses prior to, or in place of, tissue sampling. Newer techniques, such as diffusion-weighted MR imaging and MR spectroscopy, will likely have larger roles in the future diagnosis and follow-up of tumors. Additional applications of molecular imaging and newer therapeutic options, such as high-intensity focused ultrasound ablation, are on the horizon for radiologists in practices with a large musculoskeletal tumor volume.

I am indebted to all of the authors who contributed their time, knowledge, and energy to the articles in this issue. They were carefully selected based on their areas of expertise, and I am grateful for the high quality of the final outcome.

G. Scott Stacy, MD
Section of Musculoskeletal Imaging
Department of Radiology
University of Chicago Medical Center
5841 South Maryland Avenue, MC2026
Chicago, IL 60637, USA

E-mail address:
sstacy@radiology.bsd.uchicago.edu

Radiol Clin N Am 49 (2011) xi
doi:10.1016/j.rcl.2011.07.015

The Clinical Evaluation of Bone Tumors

Tessa Balach, MD[a], G. Scott Stacy, MD[b],
Terrance D. Peabody, MD[c],*

KEYWORDS

- Bone tumor • Benign • Malignant
- Evaluation • Extremity • Sarcoma

Bone tumors are often a source of diagnostic and therapeutic uncertainty. These rare lesions range from benign incidental findings to malignant bone sarcomas. A systematic approach can help clinicians more accurately diagnose these lesions and direct effective treatment.

In the United States in 2010, an estimated 2650 people were diagnosed with a primary malignant tumor of bone, which is an incidence of 0.9/ 100,000 people, compared with an estimated incidence of lung cancer equal to 62.5/100,000 people.[1] Therefore, the likelihood of diagnosing a primary bone malignancy is exceedingly low for most clinicians. Much more common is the diagnosis of bone metastases from carcinoma or myeloma. More than 1.2 million cases of carcinoma are diagnosed in the United States annually.[1] Several investigators have cited incidences of bone metastases from these cancers to be greater than 30% and even as high as 80% in some breast cancer series.[2]

The incidence and prevalence of benign lesions are more difficult to accurately determine. Many benign lesions are asymptomatic and can go undiagnosed, likely resulting in a significant underestimation of the number of these tumors. The estimated prevalence of nonossifying fibroma (NOF; also called fibroxanthoma), believed to be the most common benign skeletal lesion in childhood, is 30% to 40%.[3] Osteoid osteoma accounts for approximately 10% of all benign bone tumors, whereas enchondroma accounts for 12% to 24% of benign bone tumors.[4] Giant cell tumor, a locally aggressive benign bone tumor with a metastatic rate of 3%, accounts for approximately 5% of all bone tumors.[5]

Recognizing benign tumors and differentiating them from malignant ones based on history, examination, and imaging findings is essential to providing effective treatment. In addition, misdiagnosis of bone sarcomas presenting as isolated bone lesions and presumed to be metastatic carcinomas carries significant morbidity.[6,7] It is critical for physicians to understand the algorithm for evaluation of solitary bone lesions to prevent these complications.

An understanding of the systematic approach to bone tumors can help demystify their diagnosis and ensure, when needed, that the patient is properly directed to an orthopaedic oncologist for further evaluation and care.

DIAGNOSIS OF BONE TUMORS

The general outline for approaching a patient with a bone tumor is similar to that of many other

The authors have nothing to disclose.
a Department of Orthopaedic Surgery, New England Musculoskeletal Institute, University of Connecticut Health Center, 263 Farmington Avenue, Farmington, CT 06030-5456, USA
b Section of Musculoskeletal Radiology, Department of Radiology, University of Chicago Medical Center, 5841 South Maryland Avenue, MC 2026, Chicago, IL 60637, USA
c Section of Orthopaedic Surgery and Rehabilitation Medicine, University of Chicago, 5841 South Maryland Avenue, MC 3079, Chicago, IL 60637, USA
* Corresponding author.
E-mail address: tpeabody@surgery.bsd.uchicago.edu

Radiol Clin N Am 49 (2011) 1079–1093
doi:10.1016/j.rcl.2011.07.001

orthopaedic conditions. Patient history and physical examination play a key role in determining whether a lesion is symptomatic and requires treatment, or is incidental, which may indicate a benign or latent process that merits observation alone. The next step is to obtain radiographs, which can be diagnostic in many cases or, at a minimum, suggest whether a lesion is benign or malignant. Further imaging studies can be obtained to aid in diagnosis. Eventually, a biopsy may be necessary to confirm a suspected diagnosis and direct further treatment.

History and Physical Examination

Many patients seen by an orthopaedic oncologist are referred from a primary care physician or general orthopedist for the evaluation of an abnormal radiographic finding. The treating physician should reserve judgment about the radiographic abnormality and determine what disorder caused the patient to present for such imaging in the first place.

Patients usually present to a physician in 1 of 4 possible scenarios: an incidentally noted lesion, a painless bony mass, a painful bone lesion, or a pathologic fracture.[8] The initial step in evaluation of these patients is a complete history and physical examination to determine which of these scenarios applies.

When taking a history, the patient's age is one of the most important factors for generating an accurate differential diagnosis. Diagnostic possibilities for a child are different from those for an adult. Among the lesions seen almost exclusively in children or young adults are NOF, unicameral bone cyst, aneurysmal bone cyst, osteosarcoma, and Ewing sarcoma.[4,8,9] In contrast, in patients more than 40 years of age, metastatic lesions and multiple myeloma are among the most common malignant bone tumors.[4,8,9] Other lesions such as fibrous dysplasia, hemangioma, or infection can occur in patients of any age. Likely diagnoses change significantly depending on the patient's age, making this a key piece of information.

A detailed history should be obtained from the patient to include information about the location of pain, onset and duration of symptoms, timing of symptoms, and alleviating or exacerbating factors. Information about constitutional symptoms, recent changes in weight, a personal history of cancer, and a family history of bone lesions or hereditary musculoskeletal conditions (eg, multiple hereditary exostoses, neurofibromatosis) should be acquired from the patient.

Symptoms that suggest a locally aggressive or malignant tumor are localized bone pain, accompanying local swelling or mass, progressive pain that is not relieved with rest, night pain, recent weight loss, or a personal history of cancer. A patient whose history may suggest a benign lesion presents without pain, symptoms that have resolved since the radiographic evaluation (ie, a resolved contusion), or symptoms that are attributable to a different problem (ie, knee pain from a torn discoid meniscus in a child with a distal femur NOF). A family history of bone tumors may suggest certain heritable conditions, such as multiple hereditary exostoses.

A physical examination to identify signs associated with the patient's complaints allows the physician to determine the cause of the patient's symptoms. Because of the frequency of incidental findings, the physical examination should have 2 specific goals: (1) diagnosis of the problem that caused the patient to present to a physician for evaluation, and (2) evaluation of the area that was identified as having a pathologic lesion on radiographs. The physician should also examine the patient for signs of systemic diseases that may be associated with bone tumors. For example, a patient who presents with bone tumors and café-au-lait spots may carry a diagnosis of McCune-Albright syndrome, which suggests that the bone lesions are fibrous dysplasia. Throughout the examination, the physician is mentally creating and revising a differential diagnosis that either puts the symptoms together with the radiographic findings or attempts to separate them completely.

Of utmost importance is that physical examination findings are correlated with the patient's symptoms and radiographic findings. If the patient's symptoms and signs correlate with diagnostic imaging, the physician can conclude that the lesion may be symptomatic and treatment should be directed according to the diagnosis of this tumor. In contrast, if they do not, the bone lesion is more likely an incidental finding that should be observed while treatment is directed at the symptomatic problem.

There are some cases in which the distinction between these 2 possibilities is not entirely clear. A proximal humerus enchondroma in the face of subacromial impingement and a symptomatic rotator cuff tear is an example of a potential diagnostic dilemma (**Fig. 1**). A benign enchondroma should be a painless incidental finding on routine radiographs in a patient with impingement syndrome. However, an enchondroma that undergoes malignant degeneration can become painful. In this situation, the clinician is faced with the challenge of separating the symptoms of one problem from the other. If a history and physical examination cannot separate the two, a subacromial injection can be administered as a diagnostic

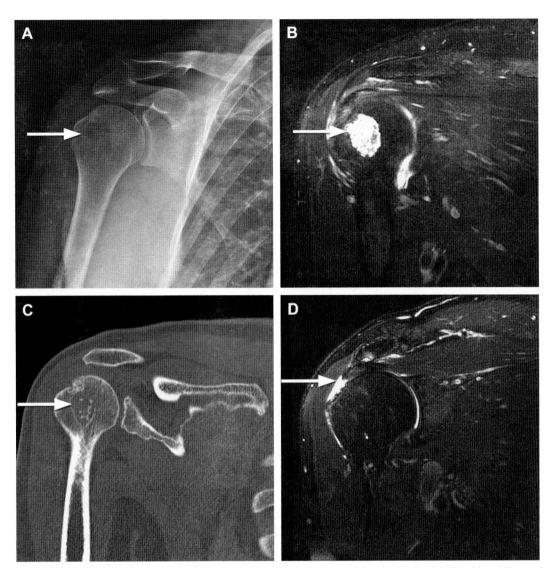

Fig. 1. A 58 year-old man presented to his orthopedist for evaluation of shoulder pain. (*A*) Shoulder radiograph reveals a poorly defined lucent lesion (*arrow*) in the humeral head. (*B*) Fat-suppressed T2-weighted coronal oblique magnetic resonance (MR) image through the posterior aspect of the humeral head reveals a hyperintense lesion (*arrow*) with lobulated margins suggestive of a cartilage neoplasm such as enchondroma. (*C*) Coronal oblique reformatted CT image through the lesion (*arrow*) shows small internal calcifications consistent with a cartilage neoplasm such as enchondroma. Although considered unlikely, the possibility of a malignant cartilage neoplasm was entertained in light of the patient's pain. (*D*) Fat-suppressed T2-weighted coronal oblique MR image through the humeral head more anteriorly than that in (*B*) also shows a full-thickness rotator cuff tear (*arrow*). With an equivocal history and physical examination, a subacromial injection was administered with complete, albeit temporary, resolution of the patient's symptoms confirming the diagnosis of subacromial impingement syndrome and an incidental enchondroma.

tool. Relief of the patient's symptoms after successful injection indicates that the pain is emanating from the impingement syndrome or rotator cuff disorder. However, if the pain is not relieved to any degree with the injection, the clinician should suspect that it may indeed be associated with the bone lesion, which could represent malignant degeneration of a previously benign enchondroma and further evaluation should take place.

A symptomatic lesion neither indicates nor confutes a malignant lesion. However, many benign lesions present as incidental findings, whereas aggressive or malignant lesions that destroy bone may present with bone pain and localizing symptoms.

Radiologic Imaging

There are a variety of imaging techniques for detecting and evaluating bone tumors. The radiograph remains the first line of imaging for initial evaluation of a bone lesion following clinical examination.[10] Radiographs are inexpensive, and the differential diagnosis of most primary bone tumors is generated based on features analyzed on radiographs.[11] In many cases, radiographs provide information that can narrow the differential diagnosis to a small number of possibilities based on lesion location, size, margin, matrix, periosteal reaction, and cortical involvement. An estimation of the lesion's impact on the structural integrity of the bone can also be ascertained. In addition, the ability of the host bone to respond to the lesion, as indicated by the presence or absence of a dense sclerotic zone of transition, cortical destruction, a soft tissue mass or periosteal reaction, can be judged through the review of a radiograph. As a general rule, a bone lesion is classified as either nonaggressive or aggressive from its radiographic characteristics. Radiographs may show features typical of a lesion that does not require additional work-up or treatment. Conversely, they can provide information about a lesion that helps determine appropriate further imaging, such as magnetic resonance (MR) imaging or computed tomography (CT). In some instances, radiographs fail to show the abnormality; a lytic bone lesion, for example, may not be detectable on a conventional radiograph until it has resulted in 30% to 50% loss of mineralization.[12] In these cases, other imaging modalities are required to detect the tumor (**Fig. 2**).

MR imaging is often used as the next modality for patients requiring additional imaging beyond radiographs. It is the most sensitive technique for detecting marrow-based lesions and therefore is the study of choice if the patient has persistent localized symptoms despite normal or indeterminate radiographic findings (see **Fig. 2**).[10] MR imaging, with its superior sensitivity for detecting lesions and depiction of anatomic detail, is generally preferred to radionuclide studies[13] and may offer a diagnosis other than bone tumor (eg, osteonecrosis or radiographically occult fracture) more readily than skeletal scintigraphy. MR imaging also occasionally assists with the histologic diagnosis; for example, in cases of intraosseous lipoma or aneurysmal bone cyst (**Fig. 3**). MR imaging is also superior at showing the extent of marrow and soft tissue involvement compared with skeletal scintigraphy or CT, and is therefore the preferred imaging modality for staging and preoperative evaluation. For suspected primary malignant tumors of bone, the radiologist's report should include a description of the size of the tumor as well as any transcompartmental extension of the tumor, because these features are important for staging. Lymph nodes in the region of the tumor should also be assessed; however, lymphadenopathy accompanying primary bone sarcomas is rare, and a dedicated search for lymph node spread is thus rarely undertaken.

The MR imaging protocol for tumor evaluation depends on the location and radiographic features of the lesion. If a primary bone sarcoma is suspected based on radiographs, then a pulse

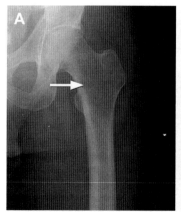
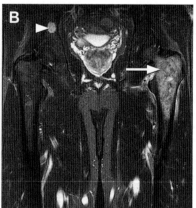

Fig. 2. A 47 year-old male patient with thigh pain. (*A*) Radiograph of the left hip shows a questionable lucent lesion (*arrow*) in the intertrochanteric region of the proximal femur. (*B*) Fat-suppressed T2-weighted coronal MR image reveals a large lesion in the proximal left femur (*arrow*) as well as a second smaller lesion (*arrowhead*) in the right ilium. Staging studies showed a large kidney mass; biopsy confirmed metastatic carcinoma.

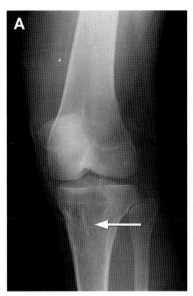
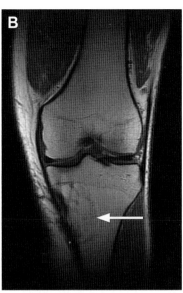

Fig. 3. A 58-year-old man with prominence of the knee. (*A*) Radiograph of the knee reveals a lucent lesion (*arrow*) in the proximal tibia. The differential diagnosis includes both benign (eg, giant cell tumor) and malignant (eg, metastasis) lesions. (*B*) T1-weighted coronal MR image reveals the lesion (*arrow*) to be of fat signal intensity, indicating an intraosseous lipoma. Perceived prominence was caused by an unrelated ossicle in the patellar tendon (not shown).

sequence using a large field of view that includes the entire longitudinal extent of the bone should be considered to search for skip metastases, which can have a significant impact on treatment and survival. Otherwise, the MR imaging sequences should use a surface coil and the smallest field of view possible that includes the entire lesion so that optimal visualization of soft tissue extension, including neurovascular and joint involvement, is achieved. T1-weighted sequences without fat suppression and T2-weighted sequences with and/or without fat suppression performed in the transverse plane and at least 1 orthogonal plane are recommended, at a minimum. Intravenous gadolinium administration can allow better identification of solid tumor amidst necrosis and hemorrhage, which is important in biopsy planning and determination of joint involvement; however, gadolinium is usually not necessary for determining extent of tumor within bone, because the inherent contrast between tumor and normal marrow is often sufficient.[14–16] Special MR imaging techniques, such as dynamic contrast-enhanced MR imaging, MR spectroscopy, and diffusion-weighted MR imaging show potential for differentiating between some benign and malignant tumors, but further investigation is needed.[17–19]

In certain cases, CT is preferable to MR imaging for tumor evaluation. CT is valuable for assessing suspected intralesional mineralization (ie, matrix),

for example in cartilaginous lesions (see **Fig. 1**). It is also preferable for cortically based lesions, such as the central nidus of osteoid osteoma (**Fig. 4**), and for evaluating subtle cortical erosion or penetration.[10] CT can provide additional structural information that can help predict the risk of impending fracture through a lesion. It may also be preferred for lesions arising in flat bones or ribs, and for defining pathologic fractures. Multichannel CT with multiplanar capability is a reasonable substitute for those patients who cannot undergo MR imaging, and it can provide exquisite 3D reformations for volumetric and preoperative assessment.[20] The lung is the most common site of distant metastases from a primary bone sarcoma, and CT is currently the technique of choice for the detection of pulmonary metastases.[21]

Radionuclide bone scan usually does not contribute to the diagnosis of a specific lesion, because many bone tumors, whether benign or malignant, show increased radiotracer uptake. Bone scan is useful for determining multifocality of disease (eg, in a patient with polyostotic fibrous dysplasia), and is the primary imaging examination used to screen for skeletal metastases.[22] Patients who present with a bone lesion on radiographs and who have a known primary tumor or are suspected of having metastatic disease based on data acquired through careful history and physical

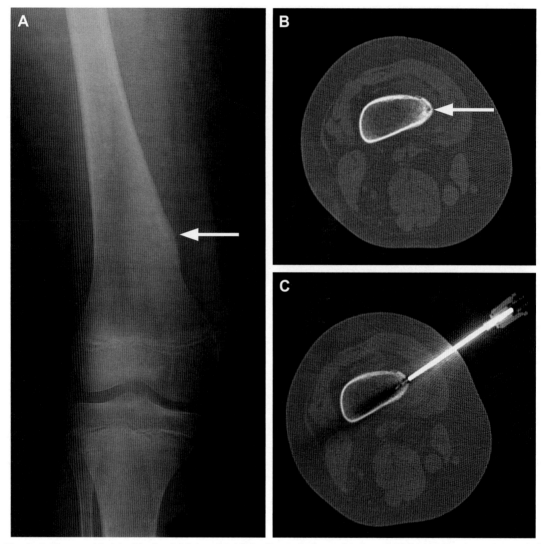

Fig. 4. A 10-year-old girl with distal thigh pain. (*A*) Radiograph shows focal cortical thickening along the medial aspect of the distal femur (*arrow*). (*B*) CT scan of the distal femur shows a small cortically based lucency compatible with osteoid osteoma (*arrow*). (*C*) CT scan during radiofrequency ablation of the osteoid osteoma shows an ablation device within the lesion.

examination may undergo bone scintigraphy to confirm whether there are multiple lesions.[23] The American College of Radiology currently recommends a bone scan for patients with osteosarcoma at presentation for staging, because the presence of a metastatic lesion, although uncommon, could more accurately place the patient in a higher risk category.[22,24,25] Radiographs of the bones showing increased activity on scintigraphy are recommended for lesion characterization (ie, to exclude a benign process); if the radiographs are negative, MR imaging may be appropriate. MR imaging can also assist in differentiating vertebral body collapse caused by osteoporosis from collapse

caused by metastasis, both of which can result in increased activity on bone scan. CT is often preferred for further evaluation of sternal lesions encountered on bone scan.[22] In patients presenting with bone metastases without a known primary tumor, additional imaging is warranted, including CT of the chest and abdomen primarily to search for lung or renal carcinoma; mammography may be considered in women.[26,27] Whole-body MR imaging may be performed instead of skeletal scintigraphy in pregnant patients to search for bone metastases.[22]

The role of positron emission tomography (PET) scanning in the work-up of bone tumors is not yet established.[10] It can be used as a problem-solving tool in certain cases. For example, it can provide an indication of metabolic activity of a lesion, and, with PET/CT fusion images, help guide biopsy to target areas that may result in a higher diagnostic yield. PET is also useful for evaluating metastatic disease. Although it has shown some promise in helping differentiate benign from malignant bone lesions, further research is needed because there is overlap in standard uptake values between benign and malignant tumors, as well as between neoplastic and nonneoplastic conditions.

Biopsy

When to biopsy

A biopsy should be performed (1) to obtain tissue if the diagnosis is uncertain, or (2) to confirm a radiographic diagnosis before the initiation of treatment. Solitary bone lesions in patients more than 50 years of age are biopsied after imaging and staging studies are completed to document a diagnosis of primary bone sarcoma versus metastatic carcinoma, directing further treatment in one direction or another. Radiographs that suggest primary bone sarcoma (eg, osteosarcoma, Ewing sarcoma) in pediatric populations are always biopsied before initiation of chemotherapy. There are situations in which benign conditions such as infection can have a radiographic appearance similar to an aggressive bone sarcoma (**Fig. 5**). Therefore, before treatment begins, diagnosis must be confirmed histologically because therapeutic regimens vary depending on the exact diagnosis.

All local imaging and staging studies should be completed before biopsy. Lesional imaging performed after a biopsy may be more difficult to interpret because reactive changes may impede a clinician's ability to accurately assess the extent of the tumor. Staging studies may influence the differential diagnosis of the lesion or reveal a site of disease that is more easily accessible for biopsy.[9,28–30]

There are some situations in which biopsies should not be performed. Patients with benign latent lesions that can be diagnosed on plain radiographs should not have biopsies (eg, nonossifying fibroma, enchondroma). The risks associated with needle or open biopsies along with the risk of misdiagnosis or overdiagnosis are not warranted in these situations.

How to biopsy

Biopsy should be performed or directed by the surgeon who will ultimately provide definitive surgical care for the patient, because the biopsy technique and approach may have significant prognostic and therapeutic consequences.[6,7] Minimizing contamination of healthy tissue planes is important for the successful treatment of patients with primary bone sarcomas. In image-guided directed needle biopsies, it is essential that the treating surgeon communicate clearly with the radiologist about the approach for the biopsy and direction of needle tract to limit

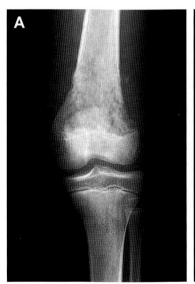 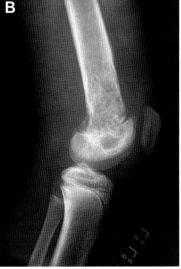

Fig. 5. An 8-year-old boy with knee pain. Anteroposterior (A) and lateral (B) radiographs of the knee show an aggressive-appearing permeative lesion of the distal femoral metaphysis with adjacent soft tissue mineralization initially presumed to represent an osteosarcoma. Staging studies were performed according to standard protocol revealing no additional sites of disease. Biopsy revealed osteomyelitis without malignancy.

contamination of normal tissues and not put the potential surgical plan at risk.[31–33]

The 2 broadest categories of biopsy are open and closed. Open biopsy, performed in the operating room, is the gold standard for diagnosis of a bone tumor. With this technique, a sufficiently large quantity of tissue can be removed for pathologic evaluation. Frozen sections are often obtained to confirm the acquisition of diagnostic tissue. For suspected malignant lesions, biopsy incisions are always longitudinal, as small as possible, and anatomically placed to minimize contamination of normal tissue.[6,7,29] Bone tumors with large soft tissue masses are frequently approached with open biopsy so the neoplastic soft tissue mass is biopsied, as opposed to the reactive bone, which may lead to a misdiagnosis. At the time of the biopsy, tissue should be sent for aerobic, anaerobic, and acid-fast bacterial culture, along with fungal culture, because osteomyelitis may mimic a bone tumor (see **Fig. 5**).

In the setting of a suspected benign but aggressive lesion for which a definitive surgery is planned, an open biopsy can be performed in the same sitting. For example, in a patient with a presumed giant cell tumor who would require curettage, adjuvant treatment, and cementing of the defect, an open biopsy is performed first. If the diagnosis is confirmed with frozen section pathologic analysis, definitive treatment of the lesion can proceed using the same anesthetic. However, if there is any doubt about the diagnosis, the wound is closed and treatment is deferred until a definitive diagnosis can be made.

Although diagnostically considered the gold standard, open biopsy has risks. Compared with needle biopsies, there is increased risk of infection, wound healing problems, tumor cell contamination of normal tissues, hematoma, and pathologic fracture. The complications and consequences of an improperly placed biopsy can be significant and greatly alter a surgical plan.[6,7] An open biopsy should be placed so its tract can be resected en bloc with a malignant tumor. Longitudinal incisions should be used to approach the pathologic tissue for biopsy because they are more easily resected and reconstructed at the time of definitive surgery. Major neurovascular structures should be avoided because their exposure during a biopsy places them in a contaminated tract of tissue that may require resection. In an effort to adhere to these biopsy principles, approaches used for tumor biopsies can be different than standard approaches used for other orthopaedic procedures.

Percutaneous or closed biopsy offers the advantage of being less invasive and theoretically carries a lower risk of tissue contamination with tumor cells. Percutaneous biopsies can be performed with or without image guidance as a fine needle aspiration or core needle biopsy. For bone lesions, CT guidance is frequently used because it allows the physician to visualize the cortical integrity and matrix characteristics of the lesion that may lead him or her to an area of the lesion that is most likely to contain pathologic tissue. CT-guided biopsies of lesions in the spine and pelvis can be much more accurate and safe than open biopsies of these lesions.[34,35]

Percutaneous needle biopsies should approximate the dissection plane to be used by the surgeon for the definitive surgical procedure. Although some have stated that seeding of needle biopsy tracts with sarcoma is rare, suggesting that needle tracts do not need to be resected en bloc with the final specimen, this remains controversial as there are reported cases of recurrence within needle tracks.[36–38] A similar rationale applies to biopsies that violate more than 1 anatomic compartment. In this situation, oncologic principles require resection of tissue from both compartments at the time of resection.

Closed biopsies offer several advantages compared with open biopsies, such as being less invasive, less painful, and less costly[29]; however, they are not without their own set of risks. With good technique and proper planning, multiple studies have shown diagnostic accuracy with needle biopsies of musculoskeletal tumors.[6,29,32,37,39–41] Some of the most significant risks of needle biopsy are not related to the procedure itself (ie, local wound infection); they relate to diagnostic ability. Obtaining insufficient tissue from heterogeneous lesions, underestimation of tumor grade, and making an incorrect diagnosis are risks that, although small, can have a profound effect on a patient's prognosis and treatment. With good technique and proper planning, multiple studies have shown diagnostic accuracy with needle biopsies of musculoskeletal tumors.[6,29,32,37,39–41]

TREATMENT OF BONE TUMORS
Benign Tumors

Not all benign tumors of bone behave the same way; thus their treatment varies based on diagnosis and stage. Enneking[42] developed a staging system for benign tumors that recognizes these differences and divides tumors according to biologic activity, which then directs treatment and ultimately prognosis. The system divides benign lesions into stage 1 (latent benign lesions), stage 2 (active benign lesions), and stage 3 (aggressive benign lesions).[42,43] We approach the treatment of benign lesions according to this staging system.

Latent lesions

Benign latent tumors are usually asymptomatic and discovered incidentally. Although they may slowly progress for long periods of time, they eventually reach a state at which they stabilize and may even spontaneously regress. Lesions in this category include nonossifying fibromas, osteochondromas, and enchondromas. Patients with a diagnosis of a benign, latent lesion should not simply be discharged from care. They should be followed and treated with observation alone.

The skeletally immature patient should be monitored until skeletal maturity is achieved, because the natural history of many of these childhood lesions is regression around the time of skeletal maturity. Our recommended surveillance schedule for these patients is 3 months after first presentation, 6 months later, and then annually thereafter until skeletal maturity. The surveillance interval should be shortened if any progression of the lesion is suspected.

In the adult population, benign lesions should be followed for at least 1 year to document a lack of progression. Similar to the schedule observed in children, interval radiographs are taken 3 months after initial imaging, then every 6 months up to 1 year. Patients can be followed annually thereafter, as clinically indicated. Again, if there is suggestion that the lesion is increasing in size or taking on more aggressive characteristics (eg, cortical destruction, loss of internal matrix), the surveillance interval should be shortened, advanced imaging should be obtained, or biopsy should be considered.

Active and aggressive lesions

The other 2 categories of benign lesions are active and aggressive. Active benign lesions can be mildly symptomatic and often present to a physician as a result. Pathologic fracture through these lesions can occur, although rarely. Biologically, they grow slowly and although they are contained within the bone, these lesions can expand and deform the bone.[42] Lesions in this category include osteoid osteomas, chondromyxoid fibromas, and unicameral bone cysts. Aggressive benign lesions are often symptomatic and can be associated more frequently with pathologic fracture. These lesions can grow rapidly, destroy cortical bone, and form associated soft tissue masses. These aggressive tumors do not metastasize and, thus, are considered benign despite their biologic behavior.[42] Osteoblastoma and giant cell tumor of bone are considered to be aggressive benign tumors. Active and aggressive benign lesions are managed surgically with a variety of techniques and adjuvant therapies.

Radiofrequency ablation (RFA) can be used for the treatment of active benign skeletal tumors, most commonly for the treatment of osteoid osteomas (see **Fig. 4**). The response of these lesions to RFA has been well documented in the literature and offers patients an alternative to prolonged symptomatic treatment with nonsteroidal antiinflammatories and a significantly less invasive alternative to surgical resection.[44–47] RFA for other benign lesions (eg, osteoblastoma, chondroblastoma) has been documented in the literature but not as well elucidated.[48,49] A few reports have suggested the effectiveness of RFA in the treatment of skeletal metastases from metastatic carcinoma.[44,50–52] RFA is typically a safe procedure with a favorable side effect profile. Rarely, skin burns, local infection, necrosis of adjacent tissues, and painful bone infarctions can occur.[44,52] The most significant risk is failure of treatment; however, a second RFA is easily performed in most of these situations.

Larger lesions are treated with open surgical procedures that entail removal of neoplastic tissue and the surrounding reactive zone, followed by reconstruction of the resulting bone loss. Intralesional curettage is the most common treatment

Table 1
Enneking/MSTS staging system for bone sarcomas

Stage	Histologic Grade	Primary Tumor Site	Distant Metastasis
I$_A$	G$_1$	T$_1$	M$_0$
I$_B$	G$_1$	T$_2$	M$_0$
II$_A$	G$_2$	T$_1$	M$_0$
II$_B$	G$_2$	T$_2$	M$_0$
III$_A$	Any G	T$_1$	M$_1$
III$_B$	Any G	T$_2$	M$_1$
Definitions			
Histologic grade	G1: Low grade G2: High grade		
Primary tumor	T1: Intracompartmental T2: Extracompartmental		
Distant metastasis	M0: No distant metastasis M1: Distant metastasis		

Data from Enneking WF. A system of staging musculoskeletal neoplasms. Clin Orthop Relat Res 1986;(204):9–24; and Enneking WF, Spanier SS, Goodman MA. A system for the surgical staging of musculoskeletal sarcoma. Clin Orthop Relat Res 1980;(153):106–20.

of benign active and aggressive lesions such as aneurysmal bone cysts, giant cell tumors, and chondroblastomas. Resection with wide margins is considered excessive in these diseases because the risks and morbidity associated with both the resection and reconstruction are not justified when there is an acceptably low rate of local recurrence and no metastatic potential (with the exception of a small percentage of giant cell tumors). Curettage of the entire tumor from the bone is performed meticulously and, after all visible tumor has been curetted or destroyed. The use of adjuvant treatments varies among institutions and literature exists to support the use of any agent, showing nearly equal recurrence rates among them.[5,53–62] Liquid nitrogen and phenol require a contained defect; the liquid is applied in multiple cycles to the lesion.[5,54,55,57] The argon beam coagulator is another alternative in which an electrical current carried on a stream of argon gas is aimed at the bed of the lesion, resulting in thermal necrosis of a 2-mm thickness of tissue. The coagulator does not require a contained defect because the beam can be directed away from areas where the bone is perforated or areas near critical neurovascular structures that may be injured by the heat from the coagulator.[56,60,61]

The resultant bone void must then be addressed. Structurally, the void needs to be filled and supported to prevent fracture through the lesion. The bone can be filled with any number of products from allograft cancellous bone to absorbable calcium phosphate cements to polymethylmethacrylate cement. In the setting of giant cell tumors in adults, polymethylmethacrylate cement is often used to buttress the weakened subchondral bone and fill the defect left by the curettage of the tumor, in addition to acting as an adjuvant treatment.[56,58] In children, cancellous allograft or absorbable calcium phosphate fillers are used as scaffolds for future host bone ingrowth. Supplemental internal fixation is applied as necessary.

Table 2
AJCC staging system for bone sarcomas

Stage	Primary Tumor	Regional Lymph Nodes	Distant Metastasis	Histologic Grade
IA	T1	N0	M0	G1, G2, GX
IB	T2	N0	M0	G1, G2, GX
	T3	N0	M0	G1, G2, GX
IIA	T1	N0	M0	G3, G4
IIB	T2	N0	M0	G3, G4
III	T3	N0	M0	G3, G4
IVA	Any T	N0	M1a	Any G
IVB	Any T	N1	Any M	Any G
	Any T	Any N	M1b	Any G
Definitions				
Primary tumor		T1: Tumor≤8 cm in greatest dimension T2: Tumor>8 cm in greatest dimension T3: Discontinuous tumors in primary bone		
Regional lymph nodes		NX: Lymph nodes cannot be assessed N0: No regional lymph node metastasis N1: Regional lymph node metastasis		
Distant metastasis		M0: No distant metastasis M1: Distant metastasis 　M1a: Lung 　M1b: Other sites		
Histologic grade		GX: Grade cannot be assessed G1: Well differentiated; low grade G2: Moderately differentiated; low grade G3: Poorly differentiated; high grade G4: Undifferentiated; high grade Ewing sarcoma is G4		

From Edge SB, Byrd DR. AJCC cancer staging manual. 7th edition. New York: Springer; 2010; with permission.

Malignant Tumors

General principles

Malignant bone sarcomas are rare tumors that are often treated with wide surgical resection and chemotherapy. These tumors are staged according the Enneking/Musculoskeletal Tumor Society (MSTS) staging system or the American Joint Committee on Cancer (AJCC) staging system (see Tables 1 and 2).[42,43,63] General principles of bone sarcoma treatment dictate that all disease should be resected if attempting to cure the disease. In the absence of metastatic disease, this necessitates resection of the primary tumor with a wide margin of normal tissue and subsequent reconstruction.

Chemotherapy has a role in the treatment of high-grade bone sarcomas. These tumors are often treated with multiagent neoadjuvant chemotherapy followed by resection and adjuvant chemotherapy. This treatment strategy has had a significant effect on overall survival in patients with a variety of primary bone sarcomas.

With the exception of Ewing sarcoma, most bone sarcomas are not radiosensitive, and data have shown no advantage in local control or overall survival with the addition of radiation therapy to a treatment regimen.[64] Ewing sarcoma deserves special mention because these tumors are both chemosensitive and radiosensitive. This is one of the only bone sarcomas for which radiation therapy is equally effective as wide resection for overall survival.[65–67]

Bone lesions from metastatic carcinoma are approached and treated differently than primary bone sarcomas. In some instances, treatment of the primary cancer has already commenced. In cases in which there are other sites of visceral or bone metastases, impending pathologic fractures are stabilized often without resection of the metastasis. The Mirels classification system provides clinicians with guidance about which lesions are at highest risk for fracture.[68] Although this system is not perfect, it does help guide treatment decisions.[69–71]

When a malignant bone sarcoma is suspected, staging studies should be completed, as previously mentioned, before biopsy. Appropriate staging for these tumors includes radiographs of the entire bone affected, a corresponding MR imaging to evaluate the extent of the lesion and to identify any skip metastases, a CT scan of the chest to evaluate for pulmonary metastatic disease, and a bone scan to evaluate for sites of additional bone tumors.

Resection

Local control of disease in primary sarcomas is achieved with resection of the tumor and a wide

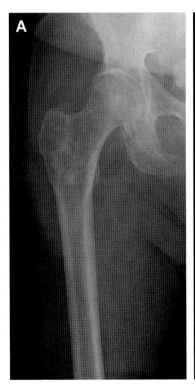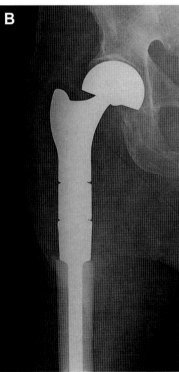

Fig. 6. Preoperative (A) and postoperative (B) radiographs of the proximal femur of a 78-year-old man with a chondrosarcoma. He was treated with wide resection and endoprosthetic reconstruction.

margin of normal tissue. This approach is reserved for curative treatment.

In most cases, resection of bone metastases from carcinoma does not provide a survival advantage and instead these lesions are treated with intralesional procedures such as prophylactic stabilization or intralesional curettage and internal fixation. The one exception to this statement is a solitary bone metastasis from renal carcinoma. Several investigators have shown a survival

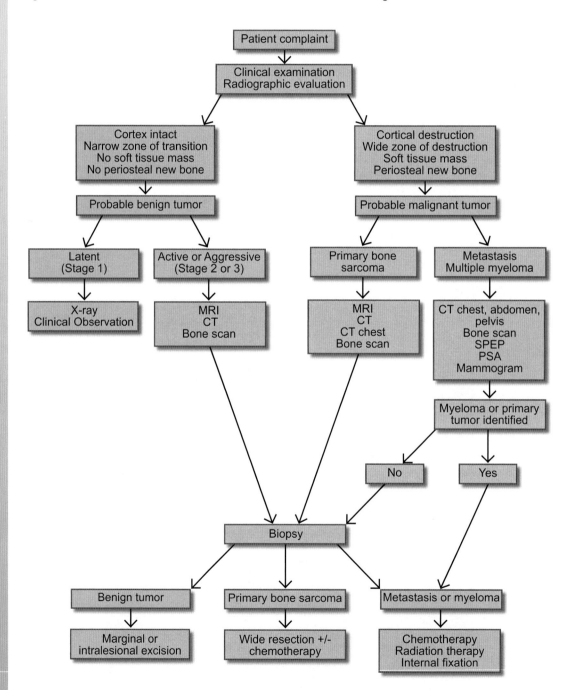

MRI: Magnetic resonance imaging of whole bone involved
CT: Computed tomography of whole bone involved
SPEP: Serum protein electrophoresis
PSA: Prostate specific antigen

Fig. 7. An algorithm for the clinical evaluation of bone tumors.

advantage with wide resection of a solitary bone metastasis in these patients.[72–75]

Reconstruction

Resection with planned limb salvage requires functional reconstruction of the resulting void. In many situations, this reconstruction is achieved with the use of endoprosthetic devices (**Fig. 6**).

FOLLOW-UP OF BONE TUMORS

Bone tumors, whether benign or malignant, should be followed over time. The follow-up period and schedule varies based on diagnosis, patient age, and treatment rendered. Bone tumors are typically followed with radiographs alone.

As previously stated, latent benign lesions in a skeletally immature patient should be observed until skeletal maturity is achieved. The natural history of these lesions is regression or stabilization around the time of skeletal maturity. Our recommended surveillance schedule for these patients is 3 months after first presentation, 6 months later, and annually thereafter until skeletal maturity. The surveillance interval should be shortened if any progression of the lesion is suspected. Latent benign lesions in the skeletally mature patient are followed on a similar schedule for a period of approximately 1–2 years.

Benign active or aggressive lesions that were treated with an intralesional curettage and adjuvant therapy are followed for at least 5 years to evaluate for local recurrence. The surveillance schedule observed at our institution is a clinical examination and radiographic evaluation every 3 months in the first year after surgery, every 4 months during the second year, every 6 months the third year, and annually thereafter. In the setting of giant cell tumor of bone, a chest radiograph is performed to evaluate for pulmonary metastases on the same schedule.

Similarly, malignant lesions that have been resected and reconstructed are followed radiographically. A similar surveillance schedule to that used for aggressive benign tumors is observed, but these patients are followed for at least 10 years, and longer to monitor for endoprosthetic wear or loosening.

SUMMARY

Bone tumors are rare entities that can pose diagnostic challenges. A systematic approach (**Fig. 7**) to these lesions through detailed history and physical examinations, proper imaging modalities, and, if necessary, biopsy is key to effectively treating patients with these conditions.

REFERENCES

1. SEER Cancer stat fact sheets. [SEER Web Site]. 2011. Available at: http://www.seer.cancer.gov/statfacts/index.html. Accessed April 4, 2011.
2. Abeloff MD. Abeloff's clinical oncology. Philadelphia: Churchill Livingstone/Elsevier; 2008.
3. Betsy M, Kupersmith LM, Springfield DS. Metaphyseal fibrous defects. J Am Acad Orthop Surg 2004; 12(2):89–95.
4. Dorfman HC, Czerniak B. Bone tumors. 1st edition. St Louis (Missouri): CV Mosby; 1998.
5. Klenke FM, Wenger DE, Inwards CY, et al. Giant cell tumor of bone: risk factors for recurrence. Clin Orthop Relat Res 2011;469(2):591–9.
6. Mankin HJ, Lange TA, Spanier SS. The hazards of biopsy in patients with malignant primary bone and soft-tissue tumors. J Bone Joint Surg Am 1982;64(8):1121–7.
7. Mankin HJ, Mankin CJ, Simon MA. The hazards of the biopsy, revisited. Members of the Musculoskeletal Tumor Society. J Bone Joint Surg Am 1996; 78(5):656–63.
8. Damron TA. Oncology and basic science. Philadelphia: Lippincott Williams & Wilkins; 2008.
9. Simon MA, Springfield DS. Surgery for bone and soft-tissue tumors. Philadelphia: Lippincott-Raven; 1998.
10. Morrison WB, Zoga AC, Daffner RH, et al. ACR Appropriateness Criteria: Primary Bone Tumors. 2009. Available at: http://www.acr.org/Secondary MainMenuCategories/quality_safety/app_criteria/pdf/ExpertPanelonMusculoskeletalImaging/BoneTumors Doc4.aspx. Accessed March 31, 2011.
11. Sundaram M, McLeod RA. MR imaging of tumor and tumorlike lesions of bone and soft tissue. AJR Am J Roentgenol 1990;155(4):817–24.
12. Ardran GM. Bone destruction not demonstrable by radiography. Br J Radiol 1951;24(278):107–9.
13. Frank JA, Ling A, Patronas NJ, et al. Detection of malignant bone tumors: MR imaging vs scintigraphy. AJR Am J Roentgenol 1990;155(5):1043–8.
14. May DA, Good RB, Smith DK, et al. MR imaging of musculoskeletal tumors and tumor mimickers with intravenous gadolinium: experience with 242 patients. Skeletal Radiol 1997;26(1):2–15.
15. Sundaram M. The use of gadolinium in the MR imaging of bone tumors. Semin Ultrasound CT MR 1997;18(4):307–11.
16. Verstraete KL, Lang P. Bone and soft tissue tumors: the role of contrast agents for MR imaging. Eur J Radiol 2000;34(3):229–46.
17. Geirnaerdt MJ, Hogendoorn PC, Bloem JL, et al. Cartilaginous tumors: fast contrast-enhanced MR imaging. Radiology 2000;214(2):539–46.
18. Wang CK, Li CW, Hsieh TJ, et al. Characterization of bone and soft-tissue tumors with in vivo 1H MR spectroscopy: initial results. Radiology 2004;232(2): 599–605.

19. Costa FM, Ferreira EC, Vianna EM. Diffusion-weighted magnetic resonance imaging for the evaluation of musculoskeletal tumors. Magn Reson Imaging Clin N Am 2001;19(1):159–80.

20. Salamipour H, Jimenez RM, Brec SL, et al. Multidetector row CT in pediatric musculoskeletal imaging. Pediatr Radiol 2005;35(6):555–64.

21. Franzius C, Daldrup-Link HE, Sciuk J, et al. FDG-PET for detection of pulmonary metastases from malignant primary bone tumors: comparison with spiral CT. Ann Oncol 2001;12(4):479–86.

22. Roberts CC, Daffner RH, Weissman BN, et al. ACR appropriateness criteria on metastatic bone disease. J Am Coll Radiol 2006;7(6):400–9.

23. Deely D, Schweitzer M. Imaging evaluation of the patient with suspected bone tumor. In: Taveras JM, Ferrucci JT, editors. Radiology: diagnosis, imaging, intervention, vol. 5. Philadelphia: JB Lippincott; 1998. p. 1–6. Chapter 74.

24. Goldstein H, McNeil BJ, Zufall E, et al. Changing indications for bone scintigraphy in patients with osteosarcoma. Radiology 1980;135(1):177–80.

25. McKillop JH, Etcubanas E, Goris ML. The indications for and limitations of bone scintigraphy in osteogenic sarcoma: a review of 55 patients. Cancer 1981;48(5):1133–8.

26. Rougraff BT, Kneisl JS, Simon MA. Skeletal metastases of unknown origin. A prospective study of a diagnostic strategy. J Bone Joint Surg Am 1993; 75(9):1276–81.

27. Stacy GS, Mahal RS, Peabody TD. Staging of bone tumors: a review with illustrative examples. AJR Am J Roentgenol 2006;186(4):967–76.

28. Heck RK Jr, Peabody TD, Simon MA. Staging of primary malignancies of bone. CA Cancer J Clin 2006;56(6):366–75.

29. Skrzynski MC, Biermann JS, Montag A, et al. Diagnostic accuracy and charge-savings of outpatient core needle biopsy compared with open biopsy of musculoskeletal tumors. J Bone Joint Surg Am 1996;78(5):644–9.

30. Springfield DS. Radiolucent lesions of the extremities. J Am Acad Orthop Surg 1994;2(6):306–16.

31. Anderson MW, Temple HT, Dussault RG, et al. Compartment anatomy: relevance to staging and biopsy of musculoskeletal tumors. AJR Am J Roentgenol 1999;173(6):1663–71.

32. deSantos LA, Murray JA, Ayala AG. The value of percutaneous needle biopsy in the management of primary bone tumors. Cancer 1979;43(2): 735–44.

33. Jelinek JS, Murphey MD, Welker JA, et al. Diagnosis of primary bone tumors with image-guided percutaneous biopsy: experience with 110 tumors. Radiology 2002;223(3):731–7.

34. Heyer CM, Al-Hadari A, Mueller KM, et al. Effectiveness of CT-guided percutaneous biopsies of the spine: an analysis of 202 examinations. Acad Radiol 2008;15(7):901–11.

35. Kornblum MB, Wesolowski DP, Fischgrund JS, et al. Computed tomography-guided biopsy of the spine. A review of 103 patients. Spine (Phila Pa 1976) 1998;23(1):81–5.

36. Kaffenberger BH, Wakely PE Jr, Mayerson JL. Local recurrence rate of fine-needle aspiration biopsy in primary high-grade sarcomas. J Surg Oncol 2010; 101(7):618–21.

37. Kilpatrick SE, Ward WG, Chauvenet AR, et al. The role of fine-needle aspiration biopsy in the initial diagnosis of pediatric bone and soft tissue tumors: an institutional experience. Mod Pathol 1998; 11(10):923–8.

38. Schwartz HS, Spengler DM. Needle tract recurrences after closed biopsy for sarcoma: three cases and review of the literature. Ann Surg Oncol 1997; 4(3):228–36.

39. Adams SC, Potter BK, Pitcher DJ, et al. Office-based core needle biopsy of bone and soft tissue malignancies: an accurate alternative to open biopsy with infrequent complications. Clin Orthop Relat Res 2010;468(10):2774–80.

40. Ayala AG, Zornosa J. Primary bone tumors: percutaneous needle biopsy. Radiologic-pathologic study of 222 biopsies. Radiology 1983;149(3):675–9.

41. Ward WG Sr, Kilpatrick S. Fine needle aspiration biopsy of primary bone tumors. Clin Orthop Relat Res 2000;(373):80–7.

42. Enneking WF. A system of staging musculoskeletal neoplasms. Clin Orthop Relat Res 1986;(204): 9–24.

43. Enneking WF, Spanier SS, Goodman MA. A system for the surgical staging of musculoskeletal sarcoma. Clin Orthop Relat Res 1980;(153):106–20.

44. Volkmer D, Sichlau M, Rapp TB. The use of radiofrequency ablation in the treatment of musculoskeletal tumors. J Am Acad Orthop Surg 2009;17(12): 737–43.

45. Rosenthal DI. Percutaneous radiofrequency treatment of osteoid osteomas. Semin Musculoskelet Radiol 1997;1(2):265–72.

46. Rosenthal DI, Hornicek FJ, Wolfe MW, et al. Percutaneous radiofrequency coagulation of osteoid osteoma compared with operative treatment. J Bone Joint Surg Am 1998;80(6):815–21.

47. Simon MA. Percutaneous radiofrequency coagulation of osteoid osteoma compared with operative treatment. J Bone Joint Surg Am 1999;81(3):437–8.

48. Petsas T, Megas P, Papathanassiou Z. Radiofrequency ablation of two femoral head chondroblastomas. Eur J Radiol 2007;63(1):63–7.

49. Rybak LD, Rosenthal DI, Wittig JC. Chondroblastoma: radiofrequency ablation–alternative to surgical resection in selected cases. Radiology 2009;251(2): 599–604.

50. Kurup AN, Callstrom MR. Ablation of skeletal metastases: current status. J Vasc Interv Radiol 2010; 21(Suppl 8):S242–50.

51. Lane MD, Le HB, Lee S, et al. Combination radiofrequency ablation and cementoplasty for palliative treatment of painful neoplastic bone metastasis: experience with 53 treated lesions in 36 patients. Skeletal Radiol 2011;40(1):25–32.

52. Ruiz Santiago F, Castellano Garcia Mdel M, Guzman Alvarez L, et al. Percutaneous treatment of bone tumors by radiofrequency thermal ablation. Eur J Radiol 2011;77(1):156–63.

53. Algawahmed H, Turcotte R, Farrokhyar F, et al. High-Speed Burring with and without the Use of Surgical Adjuvants in the Intralesional Management of Giant Cell Tumor of Bone: A Systematic Review and Meta-Analysis. Sarcoma 2010;2010. pii: 586090. [Epub ahead of print].

54. Errani C, Ruggieri P, Asenzio MA, et al. Giant cell tumor of the extremity: a review of 349 cases from a single institution. Cancer Treat Rev 2010;36(1):1–7.

55. Kollender Y, Meller I, Bickels J, et al. Role of adjuvant cryosurgery in intralesional treatment of sacral tumors. Cancer 2003;97(11):2830–8.

56. Lewis VO, Wei A, Mendoza T, et al. Argon beam coagulation as an adjuvant for local control of giant cell tumor. Clin Orthop Relat Res 2007;454:192–7.

57. Malawer MM, Bickels J, Meller I, et al. Cryosurgery in the treatment of giant cell tumor. A long-term follow-up study. Clin Orthop Relat Res 1999;(359):176–88.

58. O'Donnell RJ, Springfield DS, Motwani HK, et al. Recurrence of giant-cell tumors of the long bones after curettage and packing with cement. J Bone Joint Surg Am 1994;76(12):1827–33.

59. Owen RJ. Embolization of musculoskeletal tumors. Radiol Clin North Am 2008;46(3):535–43, vi.

60. Cummings JE, Smith RA, Heck RK Jr. Argon beam coagulation as adjuvant treatment after curettage of aneurysmal bone cysts: a preliminary study. Clin Orthop Relat Res 2010;468(1):231–7.

61. Heck RK, Pope WD, Ahn JI, et al. Histologic evaluation of the depth of necrosis produced by argon beam coagulation: implications for use as adjuvant treatment of bone tumors. J Surg Orthop Adv 2009;18(2):69–73.

62. Meller I, Weinbroum A, Bickels J, et al. Fifteen years of bone tumor cryosurgery: a single-center experience of 440 procedures and long-term follow-up. Eur J Surg Oncol 2008;34(8):921–7.

63. Edge SB, Byrd DR. AJCC cancer staging manual. 7th edition. New York: Springer; 2010.

64. Malawer MM, Helman LJ, O'Sullivan B. Sarcomas of bone. In: DeVita VT, Hellman S, Rosenberg SA, editors. Cancer: principles and practice of oncology. 7th edition. Philadelphia; London: Lippincott Williams & Wilkins; 2005. p. 2158, 2 v. (p. lxxv, 2898).

65. Dunst J, Jurgens H, Sauer R, et al. Radiation therapy in Ewing's sarcoma: an update of the CESS 86 trial. Int J Radiat Oncol Biol Phys 1995;32(4):919–30.

66. La TH, Meyers PA, Wexler LH, et al. Radiation therapy for Ewing's sarcoma: results from Memorial Sloan-Kettering in the modern era. Int J Radiat Oncol Biol Phys 2006;64(2):544–50.

67. Weber KL, Sim FH. Ewing's sarcoma: presentation and management. J Orthop Sci 2001;6(4):366–71.

68. Mirels H. Metastatic disease in long bones. A proposed scoring system for diagnosing impending pathologic fractures. Clin Orthop Relat Res 1989;(249):256–64.

69. Biermann JS, Holt GE, Lewis VO, et al. Metastatic bone disease: diagnosis, evaluation, and treatment. J Bone Joint Surg Am 2009;91(6):1518–30.

70. Weber KL, Randall RL, Grossman S, et al. Management of lower-extremity bone metastasis. J Bone Joint Surg Am 2006;88(Suppl 4):11–9.

71. Damron TA, Morgan H, Prakash D, et al. Critical evaluation of Mirels' rating system for impending pathologic fractures. Clin Orthop Relat Res 2003;(415 Suppl):S201–7.

72. Jung ST, Ghert MA, Harrelson JM, et al. Treatment of osseous metastases in patients with renal cell carcinoma. Clin Orthop Relat Res 2003;(409):223–31.

73. Les KA, Nicholas RW, Rougraff B, et al. Local progression after operative treatment of metastatic kidney cancer. Clin Orthop Relat Res 2001;(390):206–11.

74. Lin PP, Mirza AN, Lewis VO, et al. Patient survival after surgery for osseous metastases from renal cell carcinoma. J Bone Joint Surg Am 2007;89(8):1794–801.

75. Takashi M, Takagi Y, Sakata T, et al. Surgical treatment of renal cell carcinoma metastases: prognostic significance. Int Urol Nephrol 1995;27(1):1–8.

Radiographic Analysis of Solitary Bone Lesions

R. Evan Nichols, MD*, Larry B. Dixon, MD

KEYWORDS

• Bone tumor • Solitary • Neoplasm • Radiographic

Solitary bone lesions are a commonly encountered diagnostic dilemma for radiologists. Conventional radiography is frequently the initial imaging study obtained for their evaluation. More and more, however, bone lesions are detected on cross-sectional imaging such as CT scan or MR imaging, in which case correlation with radiographs is often helpful. This article provides an organized approach to analyzing and categorizing solitary bone lesions based on radiographs, with emphasis on developing a reasonable and accurate differential diagnosis and guiding the referring physician if further imaging evaluation is warranted.

After first establishing that a bone lesion is solitary—frequently by bone scintigraphy or CT scan of the chest, abdomen, and pelvis in an attempt to confirm or exclude metastatic disease—specific clinical information provides a good starting point for its assessment. Patient age is readily available to the radiologist reading the study and is one of the most important factors in establishing a differential diagnosis because many bone lesions have a predilection for specific age groups. Although there is considerable overlap between age groups for different tumors, certain lesions can be essentially excluded from the differential diagnosis based on patient age. Patient gender may also be an initial consideration, though generally it does not serve to exclude lesions from the differential diagnosis. Knowledge of the patient's symptoms is also important in the assessment of solitary bone lesions because the mere presence of bone pain in association with specific radiographic findings may affect the decision to biopsy the lesion or to clinically monitor the patient.

After collecting the relevant clinical information, the radiologist can then turn his or her attention to the radiographs. Specific radiographic features of bone tumors have been established from decades of clinical experience. These features provide information that can help narrow the differential diagnosis. These features will be discussed in detail, including lesion location (both in the skeleton and within a specific bone), rate of growth, presence and character of periosteal reaction, tumor matrix, and/or an associated soft tissue mass. With critical evaluation of each of these features, a focused differential diagnosis can be established in most cases. Furthermore, important prognostic information, as well as how the patient is to be managed, may be gleaned from the radiographic analysis.

Although the main purpose of this article is to address solitary lesions of bone, the authors also provide a brief discussion on the radiographic evaluation of soft tissue masses, focusing on features that may provide a specific diagnosis or, more commonly, the lack of specific benign features that should prompt further evaluation with other imaging modalities, such as ultrasound, CT scan, or MR imaging.

CLINICAL CONSIDERATIONS

Decades of orthopedic and radiologic experience have established the age groups in which specific bone tumors occur (**Fig. 1**). Therefore, patient age is the single most important clinical factor radiologists can use to help narrow the differential

The authors have nothing to disclose.

Musculoskeletal Imaging, Department of Radiology, University of Chicago, 5841 South Maryland Avenue, Chicago, IL 60637, USA

* Corresponding author.

E-mail address: renichols@gmail.com

Radiol Clin N Am 49 (2011) 1095–1114

doi:10.1016/j.rcl.2011.07.012

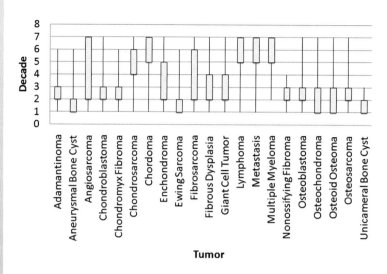

Fig. 1. Age distribution of common bone tumors. (*Data from* Refs.[4,44,45])

diagnosis when encountering a solitary bone lesion. Although there is significant overlap between age groups for specific tumors, the differential diagnosis of lesions seen in the extremes of patient age is relatively limited. For example, with few exceptions, metastatic disease should be the primary consideration when evaluating a bone lesion in a patient greater than 40 years of age, given its vast prevalence when compared with primary bone tumors. Conversely, nonossifying fibroma (also known as fibroxanthoma) should not be considered in this same patient because these lesions "heal in" and typically disappear before age 40.[1,2] Similarly, metastasis should not be the primary consideration when a solitary bone lesion is seen in a 10-year-old patient with no known primary malignancy. In general, solitary bone lesions identified in adult patients have a much higher likelihood of being malignant than those found in pediatric patients.

The gender of the patient is an additional clinical factor that is readily available to the radiologist. Most bone tumors show equal sex predilection or slight male predominance, with the exception of giant cell tumor (1.5:1 female/male), enchondroma (1.5:1 female/male), fibrous dysplasia (1.2:1 female/male), and parosteal osteosarcoma (1.7:1 female/male).[3,4] However, given these relatively slight differences, patient gender fails to eliminate lesions from the differential diagnosis.

Patient race is a demographic factor that is frequently not available to the radiologist when assessing radiographs. It often plays no role in narrowing the differential diagnosis of a solitary bone lesion, with one important exception. Ewing sarcoma occurs overwhelmingly in white patients, accounting for greater than 95% of patients in

some studies, with African Americans accounting for approximately 2% of patients.[5]

The final pieces of clinical information that may help the radiologist analyze a solitary bone lesion are patient symptoms. Most primary bone malignancies result in pain, even in the absence of a pathologic fracture. Therefore, a solitary bone tumor detected on radiographs in the setting of bone pain often warrants further imaging evaluation. Some benign lesions are also painful, such as osteoid osteoma, and the classic history of bone pain at night that responds to nonsteroidal antiinflammatory drug (NSAID) therapy would favor this diagnosis, particularly if a nidus is evident on imaging studies. For example, the mere presence of pain may prompt a biopsy to help distinguish between a benign enchondroma, which is typically not painful, and a chondrosarcoma, which may have a similar radiographic appearance.

LESION LOCATION

With the pertinent clinical information in hand, the next step in analyzing a solitary bone lesion is simply identifying the bone in which the lesion is located. Some lesions have predilections for specific bones (**Fig. 2**) and some bones are sites of origin of a relatively limited number of tumors. Hence, the differential diagnosis can be refined based on the bone of origin. Most adamantinomas, for example, occur in the tibia. A well-defined lucent lesion in the anterior aspect of the body of the calcaneus has a short differential diagnosis of unicameral bone cyst, intraosseous lipoma, and intraosseous ganglion. Most lesions arising in the patella are benign, whereas most lesions arising in the sternum are malignant. The

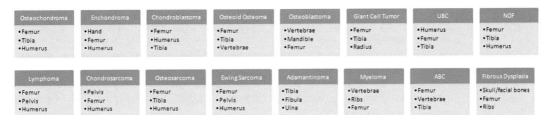

Fig. 2. Top three locations of common bone tumors. (*Data from* Unni KK, Inwards CY. Dahlin's bone tumors. 6th edition. Philadelphia: Lippincott; 2010; and Lokiec F, Wientroub S. Simple bone cyst: etiology, classification, pathology, and treatment modalities. J Pediatr Orthop 1998;7(4):262–73.)

differential diagnosis of a lesion encountered in the mandible is often different from that of a lesion encountered in a rib. Whether the lesion arises in the axial or appendicular skeleton is also important. In the adult, hematopoietically active red marrow is predominantly distributed in the skull, spine, scapulae, sternum, ribs, pelvis, proximal femora, and proximal humeri. Metastatic disease and multiple myeloma preferentially involve these locations initially. As the disease process progresses and the tumor replaces the red marrow spaces, fatty marrow is subsequently reconverted to red marrow, and the tumor can spread more distally within the appendicular skeleton.[6] This will usually be readily apparent radiographically as widespread disease, instead of a solitary bone lesion.

In children, the skeleton is composed of red marrow, which follows an orderly conversion to fatty (yellow) marrow before reaching the adult pattern by approximately age 25. Red marrow conversion generally occurs distally-to-proximally within the skeleton and within a given long bone. It occurs initially within the epiphysis, followed by the diaphysis and distal metaphysis, and finally the proximal metaphysis. As a case-in-point, Ewing sarcoma typically arises in areas of hematopoietically active red marrow, which, in the skeletally immature patient, includes the diaphyses of long bones. Subsequently, the distribution of Ewing sarcoma shifts to the flat bones in patients over the age of 20, following the distribution of red marrow.[4,6]

Detailed analysis of lesion location within a long bone is also critical to narrowing the differential diagnosis (**Fig. 3**). This is, in part, due to the distribution of red marrow (see above discussion) but also relates to the normal physiology of bone remodeling, which predisposes to neoplasia. As is the case in many types of tissues, neoplastic cells commonly arise from sites of rapid cell turnover where, in the process of cell replication, genetic

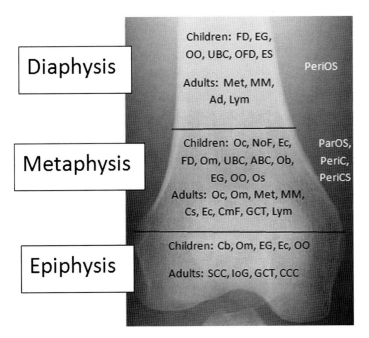

Fig. 3. Location of common bone tumors within long bones. ABC, aneurysmal bone cyst; Ad, adamantinoma; Cb, chondroblastoma; CCC, clear cell chondrosarcoma; CmF, chondromyxoid fibroma; Cs, chondrosarcoma; Ec, enchondroma; EG, eosinophilic granuloma; ES, Ewing sarcoma; FD, fibrous dysplasia; GCT, giant cell tumor; IoG, intraosseous ganglion; Lym, lymphoma; Met, metastasis; MM, multiple myeloma; NoF, nonossifying fibroma; Ob, osteoblastoma; Oc, osteochondroma; OFD, osteofibrous dysplasia; Om, osteomyelitis; OO, osteoid osteoma; Os, osteosarcoma; ParOS, parosteal osteosarcoma; PeriC, periosteal chondroma; PeriCS, periosteal chondrosarcoma; PeriOS, periosteal osteosarcoma; SCC, subchondral cyst; UBC, unicameral bone cyst.

defects occur more often and therefore have a greater chance of overwhelming inherent defense processes such as apoptosis. In bone, this area of increased cellular activity is the metaphysis. Therefore, most primary bone tumors occur in this portion of long bones. For instance, osteosarcoma, the second most common primary malignant neoplasm of bone, arises from mesenchymal cells (most commonly osteoblasts), which normally produces osteoid at the margin of the physis and metaphysis, providing a pathologic basis for the clinical observation that these tumors most commonly involve the metaphysis.[7]

Given the predilection of primary bone tumors to arise from the metaphysis, it is more helpful to commit to memory the comparatively short differential diagnoses of epiphyseal and diaphyseal lesions, than the longer list of metaphyseal lesions. In children, the differential diagnosis of a lytic epiphyseal lesion includes osteomyelitis or abscess and chondroblastoma. Less commonly it includes eosinophilic granuloma, aneurysmal bone cyst, enchondroma, and osteoid osteoma.[8] In adults, the differential diagnosis includes subchondral cyst formation in the setting of osteoarthritis, erosion in the setting of inflammatory or crystalline arthropathy, intraosseous ganglion, giant cell tumor (extending from the metaphysis into the epiphysis). Less commonly it includes clear cell chondrosarcoma.[9] Additional radiographic features, such as the presence of lesional matrix and the nature of the lesion's margins, help further narrow these differential diagnoses (see later discussion).

The differential diagnosis of a diaphyseal lesion in a pediatric patient includes fibrous dysplasia, eosinophilic granuloma, osteoid osteoma (and occasionally osteoblastoma), unicameral bone cyst ("migrated" from the metaphysis), osteofibrous dysplasia (most commonly in the tibia), Ewing sarcoma, and lymphoma. In adults, the list includes metastasis, multiple myeloma, adamantinoma (most commonly in the tibia), and lymphoma.[6,9–11] Although these lists are admittedly simplified, they reinforce the principle that solitary bone lesions detected in adult patients have a much higher likelihood of malignancy than in pediatric patients.

The differential diagnosis of metaphyseal lesions is generally longer than that of epiphyseal or diaphyseal lesions, reflecting the rate of cell turnover at this location. In children, the list includes osteochondroma, nonossifying fibroma, enchondroma, fibrous dysplasia, osteomyelitis, unicameral and aneurysmal bone cysts, eosinophilic granuloma, osteoblastoma, osteoid osteoma, osteosarcoma, and lymphoma. In adults, considerations include osteochondroma, osteomyelitis, metastasis, multiple myeloma, chondrosarcoma, enchondroma, chondromyxoid fibroma, giant cell tumor (extending into the epiphysis), and lymphoma.

The final component of location analysis on radiographs involves determining whether a lesion resides predominantly within the medullary space (central or eccentrically), within the cortex, or juxtacortically. These distinctions may be difficult to appreciate radiographically, and cross-sectional imaging can be helpful in this regard. Lesions arising from the cortex of a long bone are situated peripherally and may result in cortical destruction or proliferation, depending on the lesion type. Examples of cortically-based lesions include osteoid osteoma, which results in proliferation of cortical bone, as well as metastasis (most commonly from a lung primary), osteofibrous dysplasia, and adamantinoma that result in destruction or remodeling of cortical bone.[1,10]

Lesions arising from the medullary space may be situated centrally or peripherally on radiographs, but tend not to result in cortical destruction or proliferation in the early stages of growth. They may cause endosteal scalloping (see later discussion). Classic examples of eccentrically located medullary lesions include giant cell tumor and aneurysmal bone cyst, whereas unicameral bone cyst and enchondroma are typically centrally located (**Fig. 4**).[9]

Juxtacortical lesions arise from the surface of the cortex and have a comparatively short differential diagnosis. Periosteal chondromas arise from the surface of the metaphysis, specifically from the periosteum, and result in saucerization and sclerosis of the adjacent cortex (**Fig. 5**). Periosteal chondrosarcomas may have a similar appearance (although they tend to be larger) and, on cross-sectional imaging, may show extension into the medullary space.[12] Surface osteosarcomas are also included in this group, including parosteal osteosarcoma (most commonly arising from the metaphysis) and periosteal osteosarcoma (most commonly arising from the diaphysis).[7] An osteochondroma may be considered juxtacortical because it is exophytic from the metaphysis; however, it is distinguished from the aforementioned surface lesions by its continuity with the medullary space, as well as its typical orientation away from the adjacent joint.[10]

RATE OF GROWTH

Arguably, the most important role the radiologist plays in the analysis of a solitary bone lesion is determining whether it is an aggressive lesion and, therefore, has a higher likelihood of malignancy, or whether it has a nonaggressive appearance and, therefore, is more likely to be benign. This distinction carries significant weight with

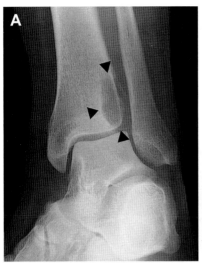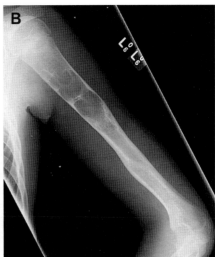

Fig. 4. Eccentric versus central location within the medullary space. (A) Giant cell tumor eccentrically extending to the articular surface of the lateral aspect of the distal tibia (*arrowheads*). (B) Unicameral bone cyst in the central humeral metaphysis extending into the diaphysis.

regard to the management of the patient and is a critical component of the analysis. For example, osteoblastoma and osteosarcoma may be difficult to differentiate histologically; however, when put in context of their different radiographic growth rates, an appropriate clinical approach can be determined (**Fig. 6**).[6]

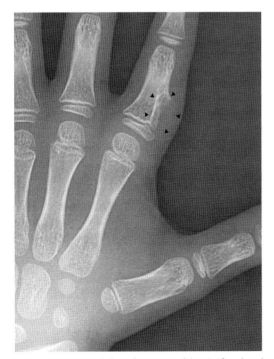

Fig. 5. Juxtacortical chondroma resulting in focal scalloping of the cortex with faint mineralization in the adjacent soft tissues (*arrowheads*).

The aggressiveness of a lesion can be assessed by evaluating the margins and morphology of the associated bone destruction. Perceiving a lytic lesion on radiographs largely depends on contrast with the surrounding bone architecture. Therefore, the character and amount of native bone stock plays an important role in lesion detection. Demineralized bones due to osteopenia or osteoporosis provide less contrast and decrease the likelihood of lesion detection.

Cancellous bone, the lattice-like network of spicules within the medullary space, is concentrated in the epiphysis and metaphysis of long bones, and is largely responsible for the appearance of the trabecular pattern evident on radiographs. A destructive lesion within cancellous bone is more likely to be detected owing to the disruption of the trabecular pattern, consequently providing contrast between the lesion and the adjacent bone. However, it is estimated that 30% to 50% of trabecular bone must be lost before a lesion is detected on a radiograph.[13]

Cortical bone, on the other hand, is composed of longitudinally oriented cylinders of tissue that are most concentrated in the diaphysis of long bones. An intramedullary lesion in the diaphysis may be difficult to detect radiographically owing to the relatively low composition of cancellous trabeculae and subsequent lack of contrast.[13] A lesion may only be detected when it affects the cortical bone, by endosteal scalloping or frank cortical destruction.

The rate of growth of bone lesions, which has been extensively studied and described, greatly affects their radiologic appearance. Growth rate

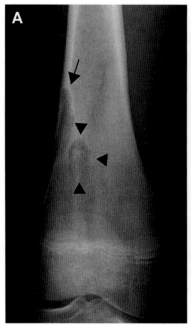
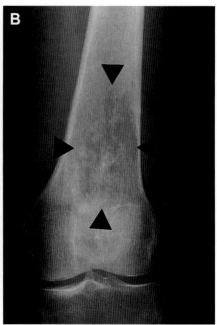

Fig. 6. Rate of growth of osteoblastoma versus osteosarcoma. (*A*) Geographic lytic lesion with faintly mineralized matrix in the distal femoral metaphysis found to be osteoblastoma at biopsy (*arrowheads*). Presumed nonossifying fibroma also seen along the lateral cortex (*arrow*). (*B*) Permeative lytic lesion with faintly mineralized matrix in the distal femoral metaphysis found to be osteosarcoma at biopsy (*arrowheads*).

determines the radiographically evident margin (or lack thereof), the so-called zone of transition, between the lesion and normal native bone. Patterns originally described by Lodwick[14] in the 1960s are still used today (**Fig. 7**), placing lesions

in increasingly aggressive categories that alter the differential diagnosis accordingly.[15] It is important to note that the following patterns frequently coexist within a particular tumor, which may indicate transformation of the lesion toward a more aggressive pattern or the presence of a pathologic fracture resulting in altered biologic activity due to remodeling. Furthermore, there may be little or no radiographic findings to indicate the presence of the most aggressive bone tumors, as the rapidity with which the tumor spreads overwhelms the native bone's biologic response. This has been coined the invisible tumor margin.[13]

LESION PATTERNS
Geographic (Type I)

Lesions described as geographic show comparatively slow rates of growth and are typically less aggressive. These lesions are by definition well-circumscribed with narrow zones of transition, within which all the bone is destroyed.[16] These may be subcategorized based on the radiographic appearance of their margins.

Type IA lesions are geographic with a sclerotic margin. These lesions show the slowest rate of growth and are generally considered benign. The slow rate of growth allows time for osteoblasts to form the reactive sclerotic rim that defines this category of lesions. The rim is thought to play an

Fig. 7. Growth rate and margins of bone tumors. Type IA (geographic with sclerotic margins), type IB (geographic without sclerotic margins), type IC (geographic with poorly defined margins), Moth-eaten (type II), and permeative (type III).

architectural role in transmitting forces around the lesion. Furthermore, pathologic evaluation of these lesions has shown that cells comprising the mass may extend beyond the confines of the sclerotic rim, which plays an important role if surgical resection is warranted.[13]

Lesions that frequently show type IA morphology include subchondral cyst, nonossifying fibroma, unicameral bone cyst, fibrous dysplasia, Brodie abscess, and intraosseous ganglia and lipoma (Fig. 8). Although these lesions may occasionally present without a sclerotic margin, the presence of a sclerotic margin strongly favors benignity and is an important radiographic feature to detect.

The sclerotic rim itself can be closely analyzed to help narrow the differential diagnosis. In benign lesions, such as nonossifying fibroma, the outer margin of the sclerotic rim typically seems sharper than the inner margin. By contrast, inflammatory lesions, such as Brodie abscess, may show a poorly-defined outer margin of sclerosis that seems to fade into the adjacent trabecular pattern, radiographically reflecting the inflammatory response (see Fig. 8B, C).[13]

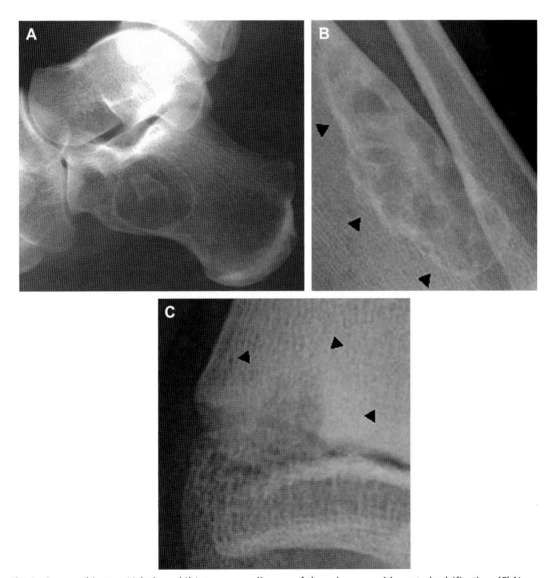

Fig. 8. Geographic type IA lesions. (A) Intraosseous lipoma of the calcaneus with central calcification. (B) Nonossifying fibroma of the distal tibia shows a sharper outer margin of sclerosis compared with the inner margin (*arrowheads*), whereas (C) Brodie abscess shows a sharper inner margin of sclerosis compared with the outer margin (*arrowheads*), suggesting an inflammatory process.

Type IB lesions are geographic but lack a sclerotic margin. Trabeculae in normal unaffected bone may be seen extending to the edge of the lytic lesion (tumor cells rarely extend beyond this margin), unlike the type IA lesions described above. Accordingly, these lesions are best detected in areas of cancellous bone because of the contrast provided by the adjacent trabeculae. If these lesions occur in the diaphysis, where the relative proportion of cancellous bone is lower, they may go undetected or show only endosteal scalloping. Care should be taken to closely analyze the cortical margin of the endosteal scalloping, which will seem sharp if caused by a type IB lesion, commonly a cartilaginous or fibrous tumor. If, however, the margin of the endosteal scalloping is indistinct, a more aggressive lesion must be considered because the medullary component may be difficult to assess owing to the lack of cancellous bone.[13,16,17]

Examples of type IB lesions include benign lesions (eg, giant cell tumor), enchondroma, eosinophilic granuloma, and fibrous dysplasia (**Fig. 9**). However, the classic punched-out lesions of multiple myeloma, as well as some low-grade sarcomas, also meet the type IB criteria. Therefore, consideration of the patient's age and clinical presentation, as discussed previously, can help guide the differential diagnosis.

Type IC lesions are still considered geographic, but the margins are indistinct. This category represents a transition between geographic and the more aggressive moth-eaten pattern and consists of benign and malignant lesions. The poorly defined margins are thought to represent tumor infiltration between adjacent trabeculae, suggesting greater biologic activity.[13] Examples of type 1C lesions are essentially the same as 1B, including giant cell tumor and enchondroma, as well as metastasis and sarcoma (**Fig. 10**).

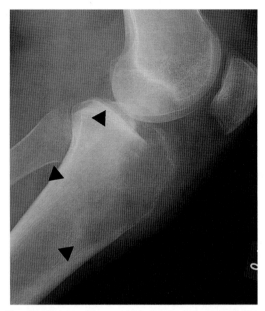

Fig. 10. Geographic type 1C lesion in the proximal tibia found to be Ewing sarcoma at biopsy (*arrowheads*).

Moth-Eaten (Type II)

A more aggressive pattern of bone destruction characterized by multiple small holes of varying sizes is coined moth-eaten owing to its radiographic morphology. The multiple small lucencies combine to form a larger mass with poorly defined margins and a wide zone of transition. The lucent defects are frequently ovoid and parallel the long axis of the bone, measuring 2 to 5 mm in diameter.[13,16] This pattern represents greater biologic activity, with tumor cells infiltrating rapidly among normal cancellous trabeculae and resulting in indistinct endosteal scalloping, in contradistinction to type IB lesions. Pathologically, tumor frequently extends beyond the visible radiographic margins.[16] Examples of moth-eaten lesions include metastasis, multiple myeloma, osteosarcoma, chondrosarcoma, lymphoma, and osteomyelitis; and, occasionally, eosinophilic granuloma and giant cell tumor (**Fig. 11**).[9,16]

Permeative (Type III)

The permeative radiographic pattern is characterized by numerous small (<1 mm) oval lucencies of relatively uniform morphology or lucent bands within cortical bone, indicating the most aggressive pattern of bone destruction. The coalescent mass is poorly defined, with wide zones of transition. This pattern often denotes cortical destruction, and cross-sectional imaging frequently reveals an associated soft tissue mass. However, this pattern may be seen with osteomyelitis, metabolic diseases

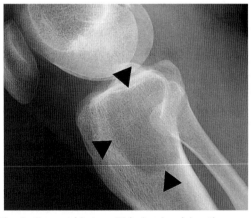

Fig. 9. Geographic type IB lesion involving the proximal tibia found to be giant cell tumor at biopsy (*arrowheads*).

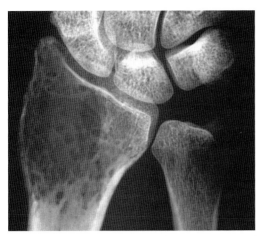

Fig. 11. Type II lesion with areas of moth-eaten osteolysis found to be giant cell tumor at biopsy.

(eg, hyperparathyroidism), and even rapidly progressive osteoporosis, in addition to malignant conditions.[16,17] Examples of malignant lesions causing this pattern include metastasis, multiple myeloma, lymphoma, Ewing sarcoma, osteosarcoma, and high-grade chondrosarcoma (**Fig. 12**).

PERIOSTEAL REACTION

The periosteum of bone is a highly vascular tissue comprised of an outer fibrous layer and an inner cellular (cambium) layer. Perpendicularly oriented collagen fibers, also known as Sharpey fibers, attach the periosteum to the underlying cortex. In adults, the hypocellular fibrous component predominates, reflecting the relatively quiescent biologic activity of the tissue under normal conditions. During normal skeletal maturation and under conditions of injury, the cellular layer enlarges and the two layers separate, and may be distinguished radiographically.[6,18]

Periosteal reactions may be positive, the periosteum is elevated by new bone added to the underlying cortex, or negative, bone is removed (ie, subperiosteal resorption in hyperparathyroidism). The radiographic appearance of such reactions reflects the rapidity with which they occurred and, therefore, the relative biologic activity and aggressiveness of the lesion.[18]

The periosteum is not normally detected on radiographs, as it has the density of soft tissue. Under pathologic conditions, the elevated periosteum will mineralize, making it visible radiographically, a process that takes an estimated 10 to 21 days following the initial inciting event. This process may occur slightly faster in pediatric patients.[18]

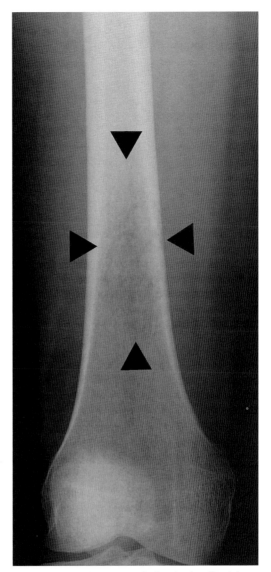

Fig. 12. Permeative type III lesion in the distal femur found to be metastatic colorectal cancer at biopsy (*arrowheads*).

The radiographic appearance of periosteal reaction may be categorized as continuous or interrupted, with multiple subtypes of each. Priolo and Cerase[17] stated that "periosteal reaction is not specific of a particular lesion but indicates biologic activity: the more interrupted and complex the pattern the greater the biologic activity and the more likely aggressive the lesion." Most forms of periosteal reaction have been reported in both benign and malignant lesions. Therefore, this feature should be combined with the features denoting rate of growth, as described above, as well as the tumor matrix, to help steer the differential diagnosis.

Continuous, shell-type periosteal reaction reflects bone remodeling in which endosteal resorption exceeds the rate of periosteal new bone formation, leaving only a thin rim of bone separating the underlying lesion from the adjacent soft tissues. Shell-type reactions may be smooth, seen most commonly with benign lesions, such as giant cell tumor and fibrous dysplasia, or lobulated and ridged, which suggests variable growth rates of the underlying lesion most commonly seen with nonossifying fibroma, but also slow-growing malignancies, such as chondrosarcoma or plasmacytoma.[18] On radiographs, shell-type reactions may be described as adjacent cortical thinning, aneurysmal remodeling, or saucerization of the underlying cortex, descriptors typically used for indolent lesions (**Fig. 13**A).

Another form of continuous periosteal reaction is solid-type reaction, which reflects ossification of multiple layers of periosteal bone in response to a slow-growing lesion.[18] The hallmark of solid-type reaction is stability over time, often unchanged for years. On radiographs, it may be described as adjacent cortical thickening or hyperostosis. Generally reflecting a benign process, a typical example of solid-type reaction is that associated with an osteoid osteoma (see **Fig. 13**B), though it has rarely been seen with malignant lesions.[6]

Undulating periosteal reaction is a variant of the solid-type. This type may become quite thick, greater than 1 cm, and is commonly associated with varicosities, peripheral arterial disease, or chronic lymphedema. Thin (<1 cm) undulating reaction is typically seen on the concave aspect of long bones and may be seen with hypertrophic osteoarthropathy or chronic osteomyelitis.[18,19]

Single-layer lamellar periosteal reaction refers to a single rim of bone separated from the underlying cortex by 1 to 2 mm. The periosteum may be separated from the cortex by edema, dilated periosteal vessels secondary to reactive hyperemia, blood, pus, or tumor. Although classically indicating a benign process such as osteomyelitis, healing or stress fracture, or eosinophilic granuloma (**Fig. 14**A), it has been reported as an uncommon presentation of malignant lesions, such as Ewing sarcoma (see **Fig. 14**B).[5,18,19]

Lamellated periosteal reaction implies the formation of multiple layers of lamellar bone, so-called onion-skinning. Two theories have been proposed to explain this pattern of periosteal reaction. The first suggests repeated insults to the underlying bone, resulting in layer on layer of periosteal reaction reflecting each insult, such as during repeated phases of rapid tumor growth. Arguing against this theory is histologic evidence showing lack of tumor cells between layers of

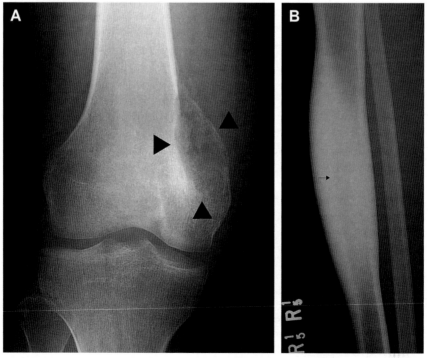

Fig. 13. Shell and solid-type periosteal reactions. (*A*) Remodeling secondary to an aneurysmal bone cyst (*arrowheads*), resulting in typical shell-type periosteal reaction. (*B*) Cortical thickening resulting from an osteoid osteoma, with a faint lucent nidus (*arrow*).

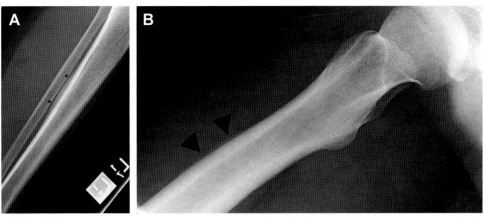

Fig. 14. Single-layer lamellar periosteal reaction. (*A*) Single-layer periosteal reaction in the tibia secondary to eosinophilic granuloma (*arrows*). (*B*) Single-layer periosteal reaction of the proximal femur (*arrowheads*), with no underlying intramedullary lesion detected. Subsequent MR imaging showed a large enhancing intramedullary mass found to be Ewing sarcoma at biopsy.

periosteal reaction, as well as its occurrence in benign processes, such as osteomyelitis and stress fractures.[18] A second theory states that in a persistent pathologic condition, hyperemia may spread beyond the first layer of periosteal reaction, thickening adjacent tissue planes, resulting in modulation of fibroblasts into osteoblasts, which form the next layer.[6] Given the presumed waxing and waning natural history of lesions leading to lamellated-type reaction, it is considered intermediate in terms of aggressiveness of the inciting lesion, having been described with benign and malignant conditions, including Ewing sarcoma and osteosarcoma (**Fig. 15**).[5,9,18]

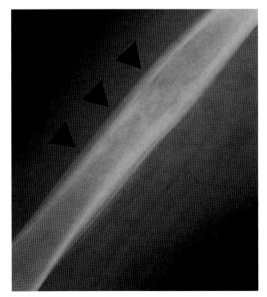

Fig. 15. Onion-skinning periosteal reaction associated with osteosarcoma (*arrowheads*).

Spiculated periosteal reaction typically indicates a more aggressive lesion. Sharpey fibers connecting the periosteum to the underlying cortex become stretched by cellular invasion, inciting osteoblasts to form bone along their tracts, resulting in the so-called hair-on-end appearance of thin linear opacities perpendicular to the cortex on radiographs.[6] The spicules tend to be longest at the epicenter of the lesion, and progressively shorten toward its margins. The classic example of this reaction is thalassemia and other chronic anemias in the calvarium, where the spicules are uniform and thin. However, it has been described more commonly in malignant lesions, such as Ewing sarcoma, osteosarcoma, and metastases, where the spicules are irregular and thicker (**Fig. 16**).[6,18]

Interrupted periosteal reaction implies disruption of the periosteal layers by tumor infiltration, generally implying the presence of an aggressive lesion. Two mechanisms explain this radiographic appearance. Simple space occupation by tumor cells displaces osteoblasts required to form periosteal bone. Alternatively, the presence of some tumor cells stimulates osteoclastic activity to remove periosteal bone. It is by one of these two mechanisms that radiologists perceive cortical destruction. However, it is important to recognize that not all tumor extension beyond the cortex is radiographically evident because tumor cells may infiltrate through dilated Volkmann canals and haversian spaces, resulting in radiographically occult transcortical spread.[18]

Interrupted periosteal reactions may be single-layer lamellar, lamellated, or spiculated, suggesting extension of an aggressive lesion through these preexisting forms of reaction. Because continuous

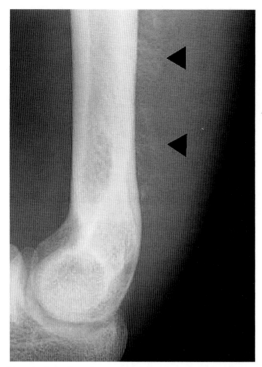

Fig. 16. Spiculated periosteal reaction associated with Ewing sarcoma (*arrowheads*).

lamellated reaction implies a waxing-and-waning pathologic condition, disruption of this pattern may simply represent a relatively aggressive phase in the natural history of the lesion. The prototype of interrupted periosteal reaction is Codman triangle, also known as Codman angle. Originally described by Ribbert in 1914, Codman further associated its presence with transperiosteal extension of a lesion.[20] Its radiographic appearance results from elevation of the periosteum by an underlying space-occupying process that forms an angle where it joins the underlying cortex, with apparent abrupt termination of the periosteum due to cortical disruption by the mechanisms described previously. Although widely considered an indicator of an underlying malignant lesion, often a primary sarcoma of bone (**Fig. 17**), Codman triangles have been reported in several benign conditions, including osteomyelitis and subperiosteal hematoma.[9,18]

Arguably, the most aggressive form of periosteal reaction is the sunburst pattern in which the linear opacities extend radially from the underlying bone instead of perpendicularly, as seen with spiculated reaction. The radiating opacities may actually reflect a combination of reactive periosteal bone formation and osteoid matrix formed by the tumor itself, as in the case of osteosarcoma, a typical culprit (**Fig. 18**A). Ragsdale and colleagues[18]

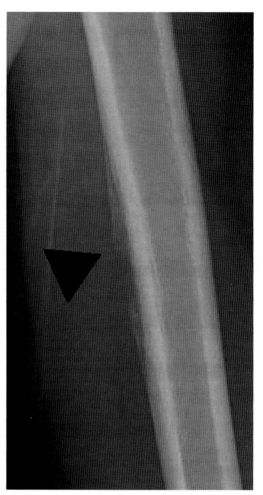

Fig. 17. Codman triangle seen in a patient with Ewing sarcoma (*arrowhead*).

stated, "it is highly suggestive of, but not pathognomonic for, osteosarcoma" because it has also been reported with blastic metastases, such as prostate (see **Fig. 18**B) and breast cancer, as well as in pediatric patients with retinoblastoma and leukemia.[21]

MATRIX

The matrix of a solitary bone lesion refers to the acellular material produced by the mesenchymal cells composing the lesion. Three types include osteoid, chondroid, and fibrous. Although many bone lesions produce no matrix, its presence can indicate the predominant cell-type of the lesion, namely osteoblasts, chondroblasts, or fibroblasts, which further refine the differential diagnosis. It is important to note, however, that there is significant overlap between these categories because some tumors produce more than one matrix type. For

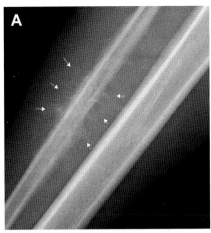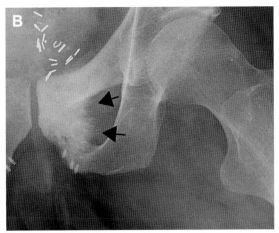

Fig. 18. Sunburst periosteal reaction in patients with (A) osteosarcoma (arrows) and (B) metastatic prostate cancer (arrows).

example, even if a minority of cells in a malignant tumor produce osteoid, it is histologically classified as osteosarcoma, which may then be further subdivided into osteoblastic, chondroblastic, or fibroblastic, depending on the prevailing cell-type.[7] Therefore, it is possible that an osteosarcoma would present radiographically with a chondroid matrix. Thus, matrix analysis of solitary bone lesions may serve as a guideline for establishing a diagnosis. However, this analysis must be placed in the context of other radiographic features. Furthermore, the matrix of a lesion may be difficult to detect on radiography. If there is clinical suspicion for a mineralized lesion, a CT scan is a more sensitive modality for the detection of subtle calcification.

An osseous, or osteoid, matrix is the result of abnormal osteoid production by tumor cells. It is often described as amorphous, fluffy, cloud-like, solid, cotton-like, or ivory-like on radiographs. It appears as homogeneously increased density within the bone and adjacent soft tissues. The prototype lesion with an osseous matrix is osteosarcoma (**Fig. 19**A). The location of the abnormal matrix aids in further classifying the lesion as intramedullary (conventional) or as a surface (parosteal or periosteal) lesion. Approximately 90% of osteosarcomas show some degree of osteoid matrix on radiographs.[7] In contrast, osteoblastomas, which are benign osteoblastic tumors, have a variable radiographic presentation from purely lytic to mixed lytic and sclerotic, despite the production

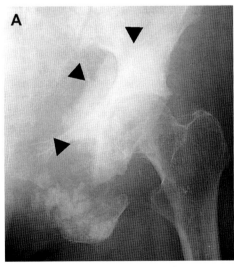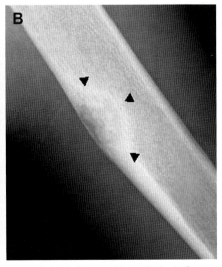

Fig. 19. Osseous matrix. (A) Osseous matrix from osteosarcoma of the ischium with pathologic fracture (arrowheads). (B) Osteoid osteoma with surrounding solid periosteal reaction and faintly mineralized matrix (arrowheads).

of osteoid. This is explained by histologic evidence that the osteoid produced by osteoblastomas is occasionally not mineralized by calcium hydroxyapatite and other inorganic salts, rendering it undetectable on radiographs.[22–24] Other osteoid-producing tumors include osteoid osteoma, the nidus of which shows variable degrees of mineralization often only appreciated on a CT scan (see **Fig. 19**B). Bone islands, or enostoses, are common hamartomas that are comprised of mature lamellar bone that appear radiographically as small foci of sclerosis.[22]

A cartilaginous or chondroid matrix is seen in lesions comprised of chondrocyte proliferation. The radiographic appearance can be described as ring-and-arc, punctate, curved, stippled, or coarser flocculent foci of calcification (**Fig. 20**A). The mineralization in cartilaginous lesions mimics that which occurs at the zone of provisional calcification during normal developmental enchondral bone formation.[24] Cartilage-containing tumors include benign lesions, such as osteochondromas, chondromas (including enchondromas and surface chondromas), and chondroblastomas, as well as malignant chondrosarcoma. The radiographic presence of chondroid matrix implies mature cartilage production; however, this may be seen in both benign and malignant lesions.

For instance, a benign enchondroma may be radiographically identical to a low-grade chondrosarcoma in the absence of aggressive features such as cortical destruction and soft tissue extension. Historically, clinical symptoms have been considered helpful in differentiating chondrosarcoma, which causes pain in 95% of cases, from benign enchondromas, which are typically painless.[25] Although this may be true for higher grade chondrosarcoma, one study showed no statistical difference in symptoms between patients with low-grade chondrosarcoma and enchondroma.[26] Furthermore, it is known that some chondrosarcomas develop from enchondromas, with the risk for malignant degeneration of solitary enchondromas estimated to be 2% to 3% for lesions 3 to 7 cm in diameter.[27] In general, chondrosarcomas will be larger lesions, with the risk of malignancy significantly increasing in lesions greater than 4 to 5 cm (see **Fig. 20**B).[9]

The location of the chondroid matrix within the bone and the age of the patient help narrow the differential diagnosis. A chondroid lesion in the epiphysis of a pediatric patient is almost certainly a chondroblastoma[8] (**Fig. 21**A), whereas the same lesion in a 30-year-old patient may represent a clear cell chondrosarcoma (see **Fig. 21**B).[27] An intramedullary lesion in the metaphysis of an adult

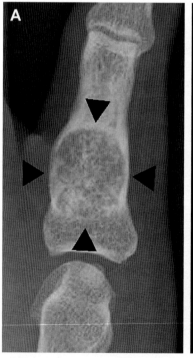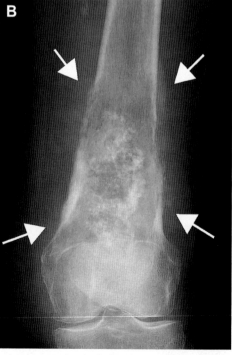

Fig. 20. Chondroid matrix. (*A*) Cartilaginous lesion in the proximal phalanx compatible with enchondroma (*arrowheads*). Most enchondromas in the hands and feet in fact show no matrix. (*B*) Aggressive-appearing lesion with chondroid matrix resulting in cortical erosion and periosteal reaction found to be high-grade chondrosarcoma (*arrows*).

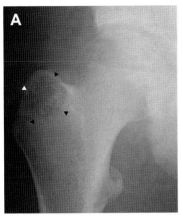
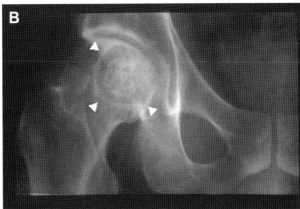

Fig. 21. Location of chondroid lesion. (A) Lesion in the greater trochanter, an epiphyseal equivalent, in a pediatric patient found to be chondroblastoma (*arrowheads*). (B) Lesion in proximal femoral epiphysis in a 30-year-old patient found to be clear cell chondrosarcoma (*arrowheads*).

patient may represent an enchondroma or chondrosarcoma. If chondroid matrix is seen along the surface of a bone, it may represent an osteochondroma, which can be differentiated from a periosteal chondroma by detecting contiguity with the underlying medullary space, as well as orientation away from the adjacent joint. Significant change in size or an aggressive appearance of an osteochondroma may indicate malignant degeneration to chondrosarcoma.

Occasionally, chondroid matrix may be occult on radiographs. A CT scan affords greater sensitivity for the detection of intralesional calcifications and may be helpful if a cartilaginous lesion is suspected on radiographs or MR imaging.

The final type of radiographically evident tumor matrix is the fibrous, or fibro-osseous, matrix. This matrix results from the conversion of fibroblasts to osteoblasts, resulting in mineralization of a fibrous lesion. The resultant bone is loosely organized as it intercalates with the randomly distributed collagen fibers composing the lesion. Radiographically, the matrix appears homogeneously hazy, described as ground glass, in reference to opaque glass used in privacy windows (**Fig. 22**). This appearance is virtually pathognomonic for fibrous dysplasia, although it can occasionally be seen in ossifying fibroma of the facial bones.[1,24,28]

Although not truly representing tumor matrix, a commonly encountered mineralized lesion on radiographs is focal osteonecrosis. Linear or patchy foci of calcification seen on radiographs correspond to the interface between necrotic and viable bone marrow that has undergone dystrophic mineralization.[24] These lesions may be radiographically indistinguishable from a cartilaginous lesion such as an enchondroma. However, if the calcifications take on a serpentine morphology, this is highly suggestive of infarction. Similar dystrophic calcification occurs within intraosseous lipomas at sites of fat necrosis, generally within the central portion of the lesion where the blood supply is most tenuous (see **Fig. 8A**).

Many lesions do not show a matrix and are excluded from the differential diagnosis of a lesion that shows one of the patterns described. Examples include unicameral and aneurysmal bone cysts, giant cell tumors, Ewing sarcoma, and lymphoma, to name just a few. Conversely, some lesions that produce a matrix never mineralize; hence, the matrix is undetectable by radiographs. Osteoblastomas, as mentioned previously, vary in their degree of mineralization depending on the location of the lesion, with 72% of vertebral lesions and 65% of long bone lesions showing a radiographically detectable matrix.[29] Similarly, only 25% of chondroblastomas show chondroid matrix on radiographs.[6]

SIZE

The size of a lesion can be helpful in assessing its aggressiveness, although size alone is not an adequate predictor of malignancy or benignity. As a rule, lesions larger than 6 cm are statistically more likely to be malignant, although other radiographic features such as rate of growth and cortical destruction must be taken into account.[6]

Several specific lesions have size criteria that are important in their radiographic analysis. For instance, periosteal chondroma and chondrosarcoma may appear similar on radiographs. Statistically, however, lesions less than 3 cm at gross pathology are overwhelmingly benign chondromas, whereas lesions greater than 5 cm are

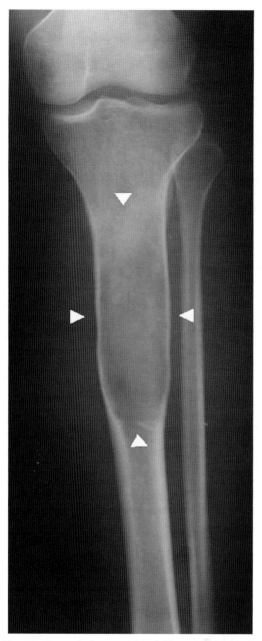

Fig. 22. Ground glass matrix of fibrous dysplasia in the proximal tibia (*arrowheads*).

malignant, whereas lesions less than 2 cm are more likely to be benign.[9,31]

Lesion size can also help differentiate osteoid osteoma from osteoblastoma. The lucent nidus of osteoid osteoma will rarely measure greater than 2 cm in diameter, with the majority of cases less than 1 cm at gross pathology.[4,32] Some investigators suggest using 1.5 cm as the cut-off, with lesions greater than 1.5 cm more likely to be osteoblastoma.[22] At gross pathology, one series measured osteoblastomas ranging in size from 1 to 11 cm, with an average of just greater than 3 cm.[4]

SOFT TISSUE EXTENSION

The presence of a radiographically evident soft tissue mass associated with a solitary bone lesion increases the likelihood the lesion is malignant. Exceptions include giant cell tumor, which demonstrates locally aggressive biologic behavior but is considered benign, and aneurysmal bone cyst, which may result in severe thinning of the adjacent cortex, rendering it invisible on radiographs.[17] Lesions commonly showing a soft tissue component include metastases and primary bone sarcomas, though soft tissue involvement is also usually seen with osteomyelitis. In addition to differing clinical presentations, cross-sectional imaging may help differentiate neoplasm from infection because infection would be expected to show associated inflammation that is generally more prominent than that seen with neoplasm.[17]

The lack of a radiographically evident soft tissue mass, however, does not suggest benignity, given the inherent low sensitivity of radiography for soft tissue disease. If there is radiographic evidence of an aggressive bone lesion or question of cortical disruption, cross-sectional imaging is generally warranted, with MR imaging being the preferred modality. MR imaging is useful for the detection and characterization of a suspected soft tissue component, as well as staging the lesion using the Enneking Staging System or the American Joint Committee on Cancer Staging System for primary malignant tumors of bone.[33,34]

It has been observed that some primary bone sarcomas do not generate matrix in their soft tissue components, even though the bone components were mineralized. This may render the soft tissue component undetectable by conventional radiography and cross-sectional imaging should be considered. Additionally, this observation has lead to speculation that percutaneous biopsy of the nonmineralized soft tissue component may yield unreliable results because it may not reflect the true biologic behavior of the parent lesion.[24]

usually malignant chondrosarcomas.[4] Furthermore, for lesions arising in osteochondromas, the size of the cartilage cap on MR imaging corresponds to the likelihood of malignant degeneration, with caps greater than 1.5 cm in adults considered suspicious for chondrosarcoma.[30]

Intramedullary chondroid lesions may also be characterized by size. Whereas there is significant overlap in size of benign enchondromas and chondrosarcomas, lesions greater than 5 to 6 cm on radiographs are statistically more likely to be

RADIOGRAPHIC ANALYSIS OF SOFT TISSUE MASSES

The term soft tissue is used to refer to various anatomic structures in medical literature and practice. The authors use the term to refer specifically to tissues derived from the mesenchyme, namely adipose, skeletal muscle, fibrous connective tissue, blood vessels, and nerves. Palpable soft tissue masses are a common reason for primary care clinic visits, although it is estimated that a primary care practitioner may only see two soft tissue sarcomas over the course of a career.[35]

Conventional radiography plays a limited, but important, role in the analysis of soft tissue masses. The American College of Radiology Appropriateness Criteria recommends radiographs of the area of interest, assigning them its highest rating of appropriateness. However, they recognize their limitations by commenting that, "radiographs may not preclude the need for advanced imaging."[36] Although MR imaging is broadly considered the test of choice for the evaluation of soft tissue tumors, studies have shown that MR imaging may lead to the correct histologic diagnosis in only 25% of cases.[37] Therefore, only the specific radiographic findings of soft tissue masses that may limit the differential diagnosis are reviewed, with special attention paid to features precluding further imaging evaluation. The MR imaging appearances of soft tissue masses are discussed later in this issue by Walker and colleagues and also Navarro.

Many soft tissue masses will be radiographically occult. Some will simply show soft tissue opacity, often referred to as "soft tissue swelling" in reports. The location of the opacity may be helpful, as in the case of periarticular opacity suggestive of a ganglion cyst. However, because these findings are not specific, they may warrant further evaluation with MR imaging or ultrasound.

Some soft tissue masses will show specific radiographic features (**Fig. 23**). For instance, radiographs may reveal the cause of a clinically evident mass to be an underlying bone lesion, such as an osteochondroma or deformity related

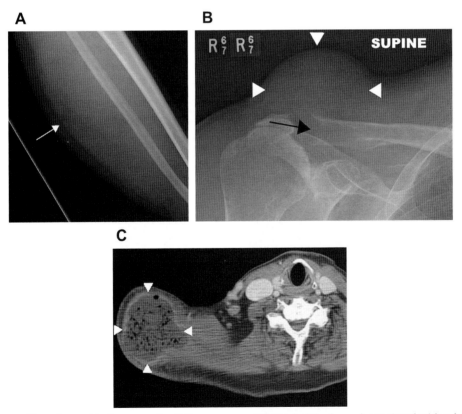

Fig. 23. Specific radiographic features of soft tissue masses. (*A*) Phleboliths (*arrow*) associated with a lobulated soft tissue mass on radiographs suggest the presence of a benign vascular lesion, confirmed on MR imaging (not shown). (*B*) Foci of gas density within a soft tissue mass superior to the acromioclavicular joint (*arrowheads*) and erosion of the distal clavicle (*arrow*) indicate an abscess with associated osteomyelitis on radiographs, confirmed by (*C*) contrast-enhanced CT scan (*arrowheads*).

to prior fracture, often precluding further imaging evaluation. Periarticular calcifications or ossifications may indicate intraarticular loose bodies and perhaps the presence of synovial osteochondromatosis. The presence of phleboliths within a soft tissue mass strongly suggests a benign vascular lesion.[38,39] Occasionally, foci of gas density are detected within a soft tissue mass, highly suggestive of an abscess.

Other soft tissue masses may show mineralization suggesting the presence of chondroid or osteoid matrix. A soft tissue mass showing peripheral ossification is highly suggestive of myositis ossificans,[37,40] a benign posttraumatic lesion that may require no further imaging evaluation if classic in appearance, and should be biopsied with caution because it may mistaken histologically for a sarcoma (**Fig. 24**). Other mineralized soft tissue masses are less specific in appearance, including rare lesions such as extraskeletal osteosarcoma, soft tissue chondroma, extraskeletal chondrosarcoma, and dedifferentiated liposarcoma, which may show disorganized or central mineralization warranting further evaluation with MR imaging.[40,41] In a young adult patient, a soft tissue mass containing scattered calcifications not characteristic of phleboliths should be considered a synovial sarcoma until proven otherwise, also warranting MR imaging.[37,40]

Additional benign processes may result in mineralized soft tissue masses recognizable on

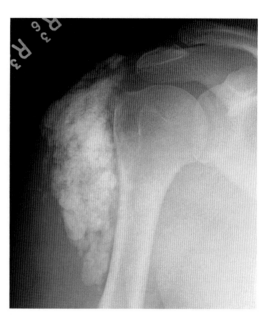

Fig. 25. Bulky amorphous calcification around the shoulder of a patient with primary tumoral calcinosis.

radiographs. Gouty tophi frequently mineralize and may be associated with classic-appearing bone erosions.[40] Discrete soft tissue calcifications in the expected location of tendons or bursae likely represent calcific tendinosis or bursitis, respectively. Approximately 25% of cases of melorheostosis show ossified soft tissue masses, usually adjacent to the typical bone findings.[42] Tumoral calcinosis is a rare disorder of phosphate metabolism characterized by large, painless, periarticular calcified masses (**Fig. 25**).[43]

In addition to characterizing the soft tissue mass itself, care should be taken to assess the adjacent bone. Frank bone invasion favors a malignant process in the absence of clinically evident soft tissue infection. Scalloping and periosteal reaction of the adjacent bone may indicate a slow-growing soft tissue tumor. However, they are not useful in predicting whether the lesion is benign or malignant.[37]

SUMMARY

Detailed radiographic analysis of solitary bone lesions and soft tissue masses is essential to the appropriate management of patients. The role of the radiograph varies from characterization, to excluding or making a diagnosis, to serving as a gateway to other modalities such as MR imaging. The radiologist plays an essential role in the detection and characterization of lesions, as well as the clinical management of the patient through recommending further imaging and providing biopsy services. Whereas the analysis

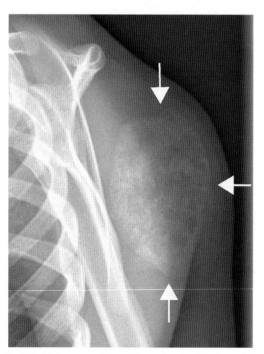

Fig. 24. Mature myositis ossificans (*arrows*) that was followed clinically and radiographically without biopsy.

is multifactorial, simple clinical and imaging features can aid the radiologist in formulating a sound differential diagnosis and properly managing the patient.

REFERENCES

1. Smith SE, Kransdorf MJ. Primary musculoskeletal tumors of fibrous origin. Semin Musculoskelet Radiol 2000;4(1):73–88.
2. Helms CA. Fundamentals of skeletal radiology. 3rd edition. Philadelphia (PA): WB Saunders; 2004.
3. Murphey MD, Nomikos GC, Flemming DJ, et al. Imaging of giant cell tumor and giant cell reparative granuloma of bone: radiologic-pathologic correlation. Radiographics 2001;21:1283–309.
4. Unni KK, Inwards CY. Dahlin's bone tumors. 6th edition. Philadelphia: Lippincott; 2010.
5. Reinus WR, Gilula LA. Radiology of Ewing's sarcoma: intergroup Ewing's Sarcoma Study (IESS). Radiographics 1984;4:929–44.
6. Kricun ME. Radiographic evaluation of solitary bone lesions. Orthop Clin North Am 1983;14(1):39–64.
7. Murphy MD, Robbin MR, McRae GA, et al. The many faces of osteosarcoma. Radiographics 1997; 17:1205–31.
8. Gardner DJ, Azouz EM. Solitary lucent epiphyseal lesions in children. Skeletal Radiol 1988;17:497–504.
9. Miller TT. Bone tumors and tumorlike conditions: analysis with conventional radiography. Radiology 2008;246(3):662–74.
10. Levine SM, Lambiase RE, Petchprapa CN. Cortical lesions of the tibia: characteristic appearances at conventional radiography. Radiographics 2003;23: 157–77.
11. Mulligan ME. Myeloma and lymphoma. Semin Musculoskelet Radiol 2000;4(1):127–35.
12. Robinson P, White LM, Sundaram M, et al. Periosteal chondroid tumors: radiologic evaluation with pathologic correlation. AJR Am J Roentgenol 2001;177: 1183–8.
13. Madewell JE, Ragsdale BD, Sweet DE. Radiologic and pathologic analysis of solitary bone lesions. Part I: internal margins. Radiol Clin North Am 1981;19(4): 715–48.
14. Lodwick GS. A probabilistic approach to the diagnosis of bone tumors. Radiol Clin North Am 1965; 3(3):487–97.
15. Hwang S, Panicek DM. The evolution of musculoskeletal tumor imaging. Radiol Clin North Am 2009; 47:435–53.
16. O'Donnell P. Evaluation of focal bone lesions: basic principles and clinical scenarios. Imaging 2003;15: 298–323.
17. Priolo F, Cerase A. The current role of radiography in the assessment of skeletal tumors and tumor-like conditions. Eur J Radiol 1998;27:S77–85.
18. Ragsdale BD, Madewell JE, Sweet DE. Radiologic and pathologic analysis of solitary bone lesions. Part II: periosteal reactions. Radiol Clin North Am 1981;19(4):749–83.
19. Edeiken J, Hodes PJ, Caplan LH. New bone production and periosteal reaction. AJR Am J Roentgenol 1966;97(3):708–18.
20. Yochum TR, Rowe LJ. Essentials of skeletal radiology. Philadelphia: Lippincott; 2005.
21. Lehrer HZ, Maxfield WS, Nice CM. The periosteal "sunburst" pattern in metastatic bone tumors. AJR Am J Roentgenol 1970;108(1):154–61.
22. White LM, Kandel R. Osteoid-producing tumors of bone. Semin Musculoskelet Radiol 2000;4(1):25–43.
23. Cerase A, Priolo F. Skeletal benign bone-forming lesions. Eur J Radiol 1998;27:S91–7.
24. Sweet DE, Madewell JE, Ragsdale BD. Radiologic and pathologic analysis of solitary bone lesions. part III: matrix patterns. Radiol Clin North Am 1981;19(4):785–814.
25. Murphey MD, Walker EA, Wilson AJ, et al. Imaging of primary chondrosarcoma: radiology-pathologic correlation. Radiographics 2003;23:1245–78.
26. Geirnaerdt MJ, Hermans J, Bloem JL, et al. Usefulness of radiography in differentiating enchondroma from central grade 1 chondrosarcoma. AJR Am J Roentgenol 1997;169:1097–104.
27. Brien EW, Mirra RJ, Kerr R. Benign and malignant cartilage tumors of bone and joint: their anatomic and theoretical basis with an emphasis on radiology, pathology, and clinical biology. Skeletal Radiol 1997; 26:324–53.
28. Kumar R, Madewell JE, Lindell MM, et al. Fibrous lesions of bone. Radiographics 1990;10:237–56.
29. Kroon HM, Schurmans J. Osteoblastoma: clinical and radiologic findings in 98 new cases. Radiology 1990;175:783–90.
30. Murphey MD, Choi JJ, Kransdorf MJ, et al. Imaging of osteochondroma: variants and complications with radiologic-pathologic correlation. Radiographics 2000;20:1407–34.
31. Murphey MD, Flemming DJ, Boyea SR, et al. Enchondroma versus chondrosarcoma in the appendicular skeleton: differentiating features. Radiographics 1998;18:1213–37.
32. Chai JW, Hong SH, Choi JY, et al. Radiologic diagnosis of osteoid osteoma: from simple to challenging findings. Radiographics 2010;30:737–49.
33. Stacy GS, Mahal RS, Peabody TD. Staging of bone tumors: a review with illustrative examples. AJR Am J Roentgenol 2006;186:967–76.
34. Morrison WB, Zoga AC, Daffner RH, et al. Primary bone tumors. In: ACR Appropriateness criteria. Reston (VA): American College of Radiology; 2009. p. 1–6.
35. Rosenthal TC, Kraybill W. Soft tissue sarcomas: integrating primary care recognition with tertiary care center treatment. Am Fam Physician 1999;60:567–72.

36. Morrison WB, Zoga AC, Daffner RJ, et al. Soft tissue masses. In: ACR Appropriateness criteria. Reston (VA): American College of Radiology; 2009. p. 1–7.

37. Kransdorf MJ, Murphey MD. Radiologic evaluation of soft-tissue masses: a current perpective. AJR Am J Roentgenol 2000;175:575–87.

38. Olsen KI, Stacy GS, Montag A. Soft-tissue cavernous hemangioma. Radiographics 2004;24:849–54.

39. Murphey MD, Fairbairn KJ, Parman LM, et al. Musculoskeletal angiomatous lesions: radiologic-pathologic correlation. Radiographics 1995;15: 893–917.

40. Kransdorf MJ, Meis JM. Extraskeletal osseous and cartilaginous tumors of the extremities. Radiographics 1993;13:853–84.

41. Yu L, Jung S, Hojnowski L, et al. Dedifferentiated liposarcoma of soft tissue with high-grade osteosarcomatous dedifferentiation. Radiographics 2005; 25:1082–6.

42. Murray R, McCreide J. Melorheostosis and the sclerotomes: a radiologic correlation. Skeletal Radiol 1979; 4:57–71.

43. Olsen KM, Chew FS. Tumoral calcinosis: pearls, polemics, and alternative possibilities. Radiographics 2006;26:871–85.

44. Garceau GJ, Gregory CF. Solitary unicameral bone cyst. J Bone Joint Surg Am 1954;36:267–80.

45. Tausend ME, Marcus M. Solitary unicameral bone cyst in a seven-week-old infant. N Engl J Med 1959; 260:129–31.

Benign Bone Tumors

Kambiz Motamedi, MD*, Leanne L. Seeger, MD

KEYWORDS

- Benign bone tumor • Radiography • Computed tomography
- Magnetic resonance imaging

The imaging characteristics of benign bone tumors reflect their histopathologic appearance. A solid knowledge of this underlying histopathology aids in differential diagnoses of these tumors. Important factors in diagnosis of a bone tumor include patient age and gender; the bone involved; the location of the tumor along, within, or on the bone; lesion margin; matrix proliferation; and periosteal reaction. This article provides a review of the origin of the tumor matrix and its influence on the imaging properties of these tumors.

TUMORS WITH AN OSTEOID MATRIX

These tumors contain a matrix derived from the bone and cartilage progenitor cells of the embryonal mesenchyme. They encompass only 3.6% of biopsied bone tumors.

Enostosis

These osteoblastic lesions, commonly known as "bone islands," are usually asymptomatic and considered incidental findings. There is no gender or age preference, yet bone ensotoses are unusual in children. They are usually less than 2 cm in diameter, although larger variants have been described as giant bone islands. Histologically, ensotoses consist of dense intramedullary lamellar bone with normal haversian canals, which blend in with the normal surrounding trabecular bone. They are most commonly found in the axial skeleton (spine, pelvis, and ribs). In the long bones they are usually located in the epiphysis or metaphysis (**Table 1**).[1]

An enostosis characteristically appears on radiography and computed tomography (CT) as an oval, densely sclerotic intramedullary focus with a spiculated or thorny margin.[2] This translates into a low signal focus on MR imaging on all pulse sequences with a normal surrounding marrow signal (**Fig. 1**). Enostosis is usually inactive on bone scintigraphy. Further work-up is rarely necessary and biopsy is generally not indicated. A bone island may slightly fluctuate in size because of intrinsic osteoblastic or osteoclastic activity, but a growth of more than 25% over 6 months is unusual and may warrant a biopsy. The differential diagnosis includes sclerotic metastasis, but a metastatic lesion often demonstrates increased activity on bone scintigraphy and displays a halo of surrounding bone marrow edema on MR imaging on fluid-sensitive sequences.[3]

Multiple bone islands may be associated with osteopoikilosis (osteopathia disseminata); striped osteopathy (Voorhoeve disease); or melorheostosis. Osteopoikilosis consists of numerous circular or ovoid bone islands, usually on both sides of joints, whereas striped osteopathy is characterized by bandlike sclerotic foci in the bones. Melorheostosis is characterized by long segments of thickened cortical bone.[2]

Osteoma

This benign slow-growing osteoid tumor is usually an incidental finding. At times it becomes symptomatic because of its location. There is no age or gender predilection for this tumor. Histologically, an osteoma is composed of both woven and dense bone and arises strictly from the cortex of the bone. It is most commonly found in the skull and occasionally in the long bones (see **Table 1**). In the sinuses it can cause headache, sinusitis, and other symptoms related to obstruction of the paranasal airspace.

On all imaging modalities an osteoma is a sharply defined bony surface lesion arising from the cortex.

The authors have nothing to disclose.

Musculoskeletal Imaging, UCLA Radiology, David Geffen School of Medicine, University of California, 200 Medical Plaza, Suite 160-59, Los Angeles, CA 90095, USA

* Corresponding author.

E-mail address: kmotamedi@mednet.ucla.edu

Radiol Clin N Am 49 (2011) 1115–1134

doi:10.1016/j.rcl.2011.07.002

Table 1
Location of benign bone tumors

Matrix	Bone Tumor	Location in Skeleton		Location Within the Bone	
		Most common	Other locations	Long axis	Short axis
Osteoid					
	Enostosis	Axial skeleton	Anywhere	Epiphysis and metaphysis	Medullary
	Osteoma	Sinuses, skull	Rarely in long bones	Anywhere	Cortical
	Ostoid osteoma	Femur and tibia	Other long bones > spine > hand and foot	Diaphysis	Cortex or adjacent
	Osteoblastoma	Spine, femur, and tibia	Skull > hands and feet > pelvis	Diaphysis or metaphysis	Central
Chondroid					
	Osteochondroma	Long bones	Ilium and scapula	Metaphysis	Surface
	Enchondroma	Long bones	Hand and feet	Metaphysis	Central
	Juxtacortical chondroma	Long bones	Humerus > femur > tibia > hands and feet	Metaphysis	Surface
	Chondroblastoma	Long bones	Femur > tibia > proximal humerus, hands and feet	Epiphysis	Eccentric
	Chondromyxoid fibroma	Tibia	Other long bones	Metaphysis	Eccentric in long bones, central in short bones
Fibrous					
	Fibroxanthoma	Long bones	Around the knee	Metaphysis	Eccentric
	Fibrous dysplasia	Long bones, skull	Femur > tibia > skull and facial bones > ribs	Diaphysis	Central
	Osteofibrous dysplasia	Tibia and fibula	Tibia > fibula	Diaphysis	Cortex
	Desmoplastic fibroma	Long bones	Femur > tibia > humerus > radius	Metadiaphysis	Central
Fat					
	Intraosseus lipoma	Calcaneus	Calcaneus > femur > tibia	Metaphysis	Central
Vascular					
	Osseous hemangioma	Vertebrae	Calvarium > calncaneus > long bones	Metaphysis	Central
Unknown origin					
	Giant cell tumor	Long bones	Femur > tibia > radius > humerus	Epiphysis and metaphysis	Eccentric
	Simple bone cyst	Long bones	Fumerus > femur > calcaneus	Metaphysis	Central
	Aneurysmal bone cyst	Long bones > spine	About knee > spine	80% metaphsys, 20% diaphysis	Eccentric

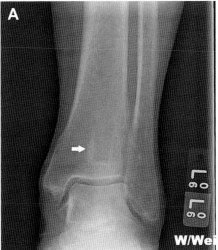
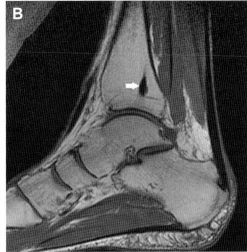

Fig. 1. A 58-year-old man with a bone island in the distal tibia (*arrow*). (*A*) Frontal radiograph of the ankle shows the elongated sclerotic focus in distal tibia. (*B*) Sagittal T1-weighted MR image shows the low signal bone island with surrounding normal marrow.

It demonstrates a density identical to cortex on radiography and CT (**Fig. 2**), and follows the low signal intensity characteristics of cortex on all MR imaging pulse sequences.[2] Multiple osteomas are associated with Gardner syndrome and tuberous sclerosis.

Osteoid Osteoma

Osteoid osteoma (OO) is a painful benign bony lesion of unknown cause. Although OO most commonly occurs in the long bones, it is the most common cause of painful scoliosis in a skeletally immature patient; the lesion is usually located along the concavity of the scoliosis. Pain, which can be worse at night, is usually relieved with nonsteroidal anti-inflammatory drugs through inhibition of prostaglandin 2. OO is more common in males (2–3:1) and mostly affects patients between 5 and 25 years of age. The "nidus," representing the actual lesion, is usually less than 1 cm in diameter, although the lesion diameter can vary between 0.1 and 2 cm. Histologically, the nidus is composed of osteoid and woven bone on a background of highly vascularized fibrous connective tissue. This nidus may be surrounded by a variable degree of sclerosis depending on the location within or along the bone. The cortical variant is the most common and is usually located in the shaft of the long bones. Less common locations are cancellous (subcortical), intra-articular, and subperiosteal.[2] The most common locations in the skeleton and within the bone are listed in **Table 1**.

The radiographic and CT imaging characteristics of OO depend on its location. The nidus appears as an osteolucent focus, which may or may not have

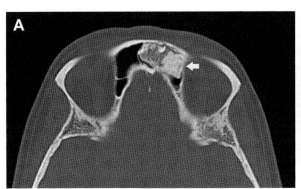
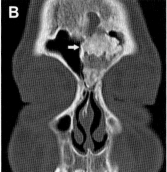

Fig. 2. A 45-year-old man with an osteoma in the left frontal sinus (*arrow*). (*A*) Axial head CT. (*B*) Head CT, coronal reformation. (*Courtesy of* Ali Sepahdari, MD, University of California, Los Angeles, CA.)

a dense central focus of mineralization. In long bones, surrounding extensive fusiform sclerosis is the hallmark of this lesion. Cancellous and intra-articular lesions may have no or only limited surrounding sclerosis. The rare subperiosteal lesion may have no adjacent sclerosis and may present as only subtle erosion.[2] On MR imaging the intense bone marrow edema adjacent to the nidus is paramount for detection and localization of the lesion (Fig. 3). The nidus itself may not be readily visible on MR imaging depending on its size and the degree of mineralization.[4] Adjacent soft tissue edema and periosteal reaction are often noted. An intra-articular lesion may be masked by reactive changes in the surrounding tissue; in a child with joint pain, and synovitis, joint effusion, and adjacent marrow edema on MR imaging, OO should be strongly considered. A CT examination, preferably with triplanar reformatted images, demonstrates the nidus.[2] The differential diagnosis for OO in the long bones includes stress fractures and osteomyelitis (Brodie abscess). Toxic and inflammatory synovitis can be considered in the differential diagnosis for the intra-articular lesions.

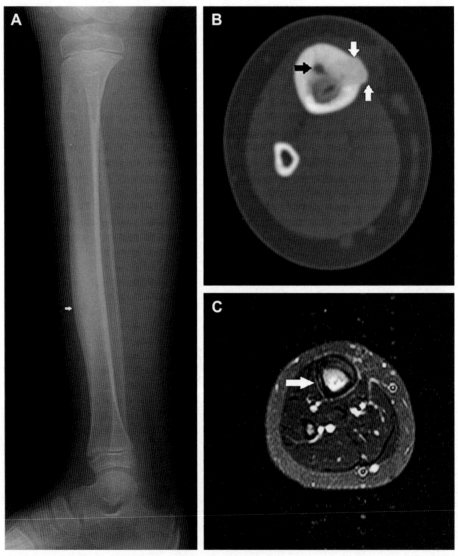

Fig. 3. An 8-year-old girl with an osteoid osteoma of mid-tibial shaft. (*A*) Lateral radiograph with anterior tibial cortical thickening (*arrow*). (*B*) Axial CT shows the nidus (*black arrow*). *White arrows* mark tracks of a previously attempted biopsy. (*C*) Axial fat-saturated T2-weighted MR image with marrow edema and cortical thickening (*arrow*).

Osteoblastoma

Osteoblastoma (OB) is a rare osteoid-producing tumor that on routine histologic analysis is essentially indistinguishable from OO. A tumor size of 2 cm or larger is the main histopathologic criterion to distinguish this lesion from an OO. OB exhibits different clinical behavior: it presents with a dull ache and possible swelling that may not be worse at night and usually does not respond to nonsteroidal anti-inflammatory drug intake. Scoliosis is common with spinal OB along with neurologic symptoms in up to 40% of cases in the spine. The patients are usually younger than 30 years of age and the lesion is more common in males (by ≃2:1). The common locations in the skeleton are the spine (particularly the posterior elements) and long bones. In most cases in long bones an eccentric location in the diaphysis or metaphysis is noted (see **Table 1**).[2,5]

OB may have three different presentations on radiographs. The first presentation is similar to OO, only larger; this is termed a "giant osteoid osteoma." Second, it may have an expansile appearance with a mineralized matrix and a narrow zone of transition. This is typical of the spinal OB. Finally, it may appear more aggressive with prominent bone expansion, partial cortical destruction, and soft tissue infiltration. This is more common in long bones. CT examination may better demonstrate the mineralization and the lesion margin. In complex bony structures, such as in the spine or pelvis, CT demonstrates the extent of the lesion and helps differentiate between bone and soft tissue components.[2,5] MR imaging may show reactive marrow edema of the surrounding bone, usually less than with OO, with a variable degree of increased T2 signal depending on matrix mineralization and cellularity of the lesion (**Fig. 4**). MR imaging helps to determine the extension of the spinal lesions into the neural foramina and spinal canal.[6]

Approximately 16% of OBs have components of aneurysmal bone cyst (ABC). Aggressive-appearing inflammatory variants have been described.[7] A malignant transformation into an osteosarcoma is rare.

TUMORS WITH A CHONDROID MATRIX

Cartilage-forming tumors have imaging characteristics that aid with their diagnosis. In particular, the chondroid "ring and arc" mineralization pattern is often a prominent imaging feature. Chondroid lesions encompass approximately 14% of biopsied primary bone tumors.

Osteochondroma

Osteochondroma (OC) is a relatively common surface lesion of the bone composed of lamellar bone covered by a cartilage cap.[8] Clinically, it presents most commonly as painless swelling and cosmetic deformity. Further clinical presentations may include neurovascular impingement, fracture, overlying bursal or pseudoaneurysm development, and malignant transformation. There is a male predominance, and 75% of patients are younger than 20 years of age. Its growth comes to a halt by the time the physis closes, and the cartilage cap usually involutes after skeletal maturity. This lesion is usually classified as a neoplasm, but it is generally believed that it occurs as a result of physeal cartilage displacement onto the bone surface. This displacement may be secondary to trauma or radiation. OC can arise from any bone undergoing enchondral maturation, but it is most common in tubular bones and in particular around the knee. The ilium and scapula are the two most commonly affected flat bones. In long bones it is located at the metaphysis and grows away from the joint (see **Table 1**).[8]

On imaging, OC is a surface lesion that demonstrates cortical and medullary continuity. It may be on a stalk (pedunculated) or broad based (sessile). Cross-sectional imaging with CT and MR imaging may demonstrate a cartilage cap (**Fig. 5**). After skeletal maturity the cartilage cap should not be thicker than 2 cm; if it is, then transformation to chondrosarcoma should be considered. Ultrasound or contrast-enhanced CT and MR imaging aid in distinguishing bursa formation over the cap from the actual cap. Cartilage cap growth after skeletal maturity and pain are worrisome for malignant transformation.[9,10] Associated entities include hereditary multiple exostoses and Trevor disease (dysplasia epiphysealis hemimelica, or epiphyseal OC).

Enchondroma

Enchondroma (EC) is a common incidental finding in long bones. EC comprises 3% to 5% of biopsied primary bone lesions. EC is encountered equally in men and women and has a peak incidence in the third decade. Histologically it is characterized by rests of hyaline cartilage within the medullary bone intermixed at times with a myxoid matrix. EC may have a variable degree of amorphous matrix mineralization. It is common in bones of the hand and feet and in long bones. EC occurs mostly as a central lesion in the metaphysis (see **Table 1**).[11]

On radiography EC presents as an expansile lucent lesion with a narrow zone of transition; varying degree of chondroid mineralization (rings and arcs); and often cortical thinning (endosteal scalloping). EC in long bones of the hands and

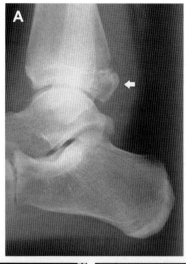

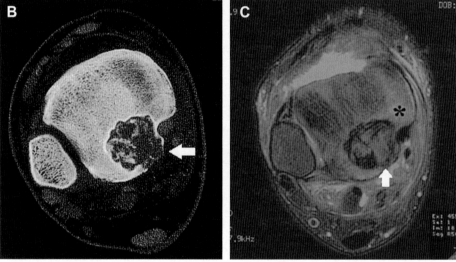

Fig. 4. A 13-year-old boy with an osteoblastoma of distal tibia. (*A*) Lateral radiograph demonstrates the expansile lesion of the distal tibia (*arrow*). (*B*) Axial CT shows mineralization within the lesion (*arrow*). (*C*) Axial fat-saturated T2-weighted MR image shows the lesion (*arrow*) and surrounding bone marrow edema (*asterisk*).

feet often lacks any degree of matrix mineralization. In other locations CT readily detects chondroid mineralization, even in those cases with only subtle or no radiographic evidence of matrix mineralization. MR imaging properties reflect the high water content of the hyaline cartilage (ie, high signal on fluid-sensitive sequences with scattered low signal foci of chondroid mineralization). A lobular margin can usually be identified in larger central ECs on all imaging modalities (**Fig. 6**). These lesions may undergo a chondrosarcomatous transformation, presenting with a more destructive lytic lesion with a soft tissue mass. However, the most sensitive indicator of sarcomatous transformation is pain. Ollier disease (multiple

enchondromatosis) and Maffucci syndrome (enchondromatosis and soft tissue hemangiomas) are associated entities. Both of these entities are associated with an increased rate of malignant transformation of ECs.[11]

Juxtacortical Chondroma

Juxtacortical or periosteal chondroma (JC) compromises less than 2% of primary bone lesions and presents as focal swelling. It is most common in men younger than the age of 30. Histologically, JC demonstrates a lobular cartilaginous growth limited to the cortex and beneath the periosteum without an extension into the medullary cavity. It

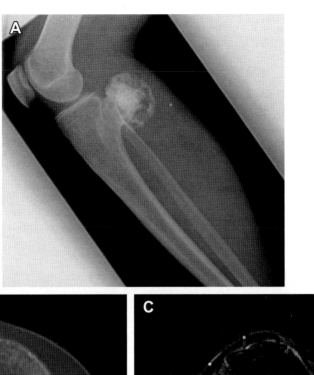

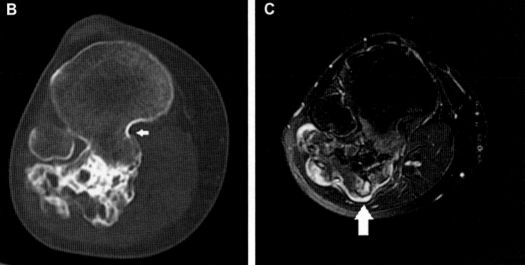

Fig. 5. A 35-year-old woman with a large osteochondroma arising from the posterior cortex of the proximal tibia. (A) Lateral radiograph. (B) Axial CT clearly demonstrates the continuity of cortex with underlying bone (arrow). (C) Fat-saturated T2-weighted MR image with a thin cartilage cap (arrow).

is most common in the proximal humerus followed by the femur, tibia, hands, and feet (see **Table 1**). Pelvis and ribs are uncommon sites.[9]

On radiography JC presents as a focus of cortical saucerization with a soft tissue mass that may contain a chondroid matrix. A well-defined sclerotic margin separates the lesion from the medullary cavity. Overhanging cortical edges may be present and may entirely cover the lesion. CT aids in demonstration of the matrix mineralization and MR imaging shows the high water content of the cartilage tissue. Both modalities confirm the lack of communication of this lesion with the medullary canal (**Fig. 7**). The main differential

diagnosis is a surface chondrosarcoma, which usually presents later in life; is larger (>3 cm); and on imaging demonstrates invasion of the medullary cavity. Other lesions that may arise from the surface of bone, such as a surface osteosarcoma, ABC, or chondromyxoid fibroma (CMF), also need to be excluded.[12]

Chondroblastoma

Chondroblastoma (CB) is an uncommon lesion compromising less than 2% of benign primary bone neoplasms. It occurs close to joints and may present with some loss of joint function. CB

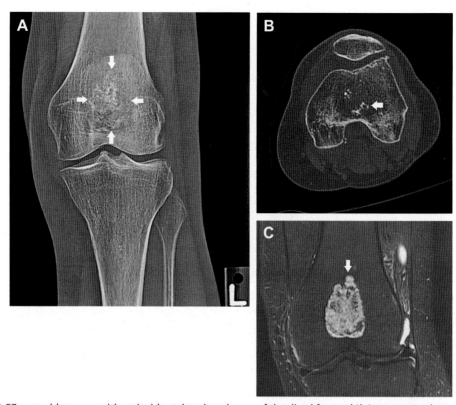

Fig. 6. A 57-year-old woman with an incidental enchondroma of the distal femur. (*A*) Anteroposterior radiograph of the knee shows a central mineralized lesion (*arrows*). (*B*) Axial CT shows the chondroid matrix with characteristic "ring-and-arc" mineralization (*arrow*). (*C*) Coronal fat-saturated proton density MR image demonstrates the high signal lesion (*arrow*) with lobulated superior margins.

is twice as common in males as females, and most cases occur between the ages of 5 and 25 years. Histologically, it presents as a sharply marginated and lobulated lesion containing chondroblasts, occasional giant cells, and abundant chondroid matrix. ABC components may be present in up to 15% of cases and matrix mineralization occurs in a lacelike pattern with a histologic appearance similar to chicken wire. CB occurs predominantly in the epiphyses or epiphysis equivalents (apophyses and sesamoids). It is most commonly seen in the proximal femur followed by the distal femur, proximal tibia, proximal humerus, and hands and feet (see **Table 1**).[9]

On radiographs CB presents as a lucent lesion of the epiphysis with a thin sclerotic rim. It may have a subtle chondroid matrix, which is better demonstrated on CT. CT also may characterize the adjacent periosteal reaction, which is usually an inflammatory response. CB may appear more expansile depending on the size of the ABC component. A more aggressive appearance may be encountered featuring cortex destruction and invasion of the surrounding soft tissues or the joint space. MR imaging readily demonstrates the surrounding marrow edema and the typical low-to-intermediate signal of the tumor on fluid-sensitive sequences (**Fig. 8**). This is a distinguishing feature of this cartilage lesion, which has been attributed to the high hemosiderin content or highly cellular matrix. The differential diagnosis for epiphyseal lesions includes giant cell tumor (GCT), subchondral cyst, infection, Langerhans cell histiocytosis, OB, and clear cell chondrosarcoma.[9,13]

Chondromyxoid Fibroma

CMF is rare (<1% of primary bone tumors). It is composed of varying degrees of cartilaginous, fibrous, and myxoid components. It presents with swelling and may occasionally be painful. CMF has a slight male predilection and affects a wide range of age between 3 and 70 years; however, most cases occur younger than age 30. Histologically, CMF presents as a sharply demarcated lesion containing the aforementioned components with small foci of calcification and common multinucleated giant cells, usually at the periphery of

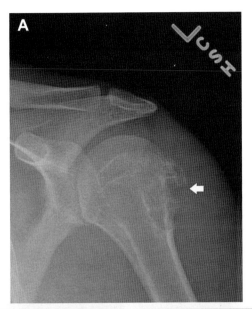

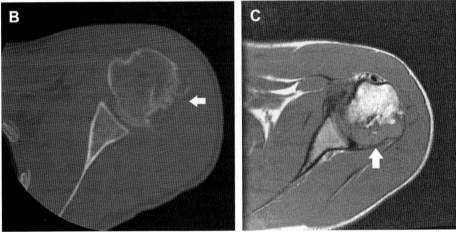

Fig. 7. A 21-year-old man with a JC arising from the proximal humerus (*arrow*). (*A*) Frontal shoulder radiograph in internal rotation shows a surface lesion of the humeral head and neck. (*B*) Axial CT shows mineralization of the lesion. (*C*) Axial T1-weighted MR image shows a low-to-intermediate signal surface lesion of the proximal humerus.

the cartilaginous lobules. It arises most often around the knee with the proximal tibia as the single most common location. The foot and pelvic bones also are common sites. CMF is usually located in the metaphysis of the long bones as an eccentric lesion, and it is often cortical (see Table 1).[9]

On radiography CMF presents as an eccentric, expansile metaphyseal lesion of the long bones with an inner narrow zone of transition with the adjacent normal bone and a thinned or absent outer margin simulating a more aggressive lesion. In the foot and flat bones it presents as a central expansile lesion. CT may reveal trabeculation and a mineralized matrix. CT and MR imaging

may demonstrate a lobulated margin. MR imaging also demonstrates the characteristic high signal water-laden cartilage matrix (**Fig. 9**).[9]

TUMORS FORMING OR ARISING FROM FIBROUS TISSUE

The common feature of these often eccentric benign tumors is a fibrous matrix with adjacent bone sclerosis.

Fibroxanthoma

The histopathologic term "fibroxanthoma" (FX) covers both the larger nonossifying fibroma and the smaller fibrous cortical defect. FX encompasses

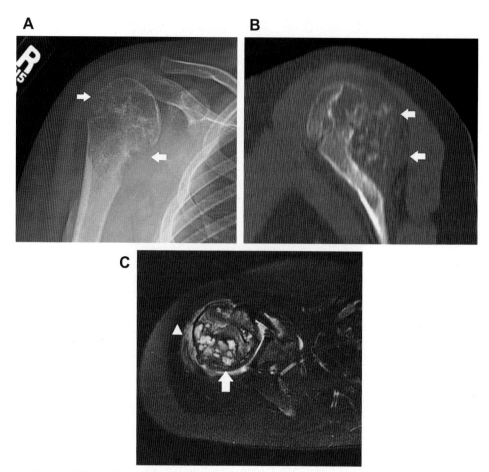

Fig. 8. An 11-year-old boy with a chondroblastoma of the proximal humerus. (*A*) Frontal shoulder radiograph in internal rotation shows a lucent lesion (*arrows*) involving the humeral head and neck. (*B*) Sagittal reformatted CT images demonstrates epiphyseal location of the lesion with extension into the metaphysis (*arrows*) and matrix mineralization suggesting a chondroid lesion. (*C*) Axial fat-saturated T2-weighted MR image shows the chondroblastoma (*arrow*) with surrounding soft tissue edema (*arrowhead*).

about 2% of biopsied primary bone tumors. This lesion is usually asymptomatic and demonstrates a tendency for spontaneous healing. The larger nonossifying fibroma may present with a painful pathologic fracture. FX is more common in males with a peak incidence in the first two decades of life. Histologically, it presents with bundles of fibrous tissue with a few multicentric giant cells along with foam or xanthoma histiocytes. Occasional foci of necrosis and hemorrhage (hemosiderin) may be visible.[14] FX is a metaphyseal lesion that can migrate into the diaphysis with growth. It affects in up to 90% of cases the long tubular bones. FX is eccentric ("cortically based") and up to 55% of cases arise about the knee (femur, tibia, and fibula). It is uncommon in the upper extremity (see **Table 1**).[15]

Radiographically, the main differentiation between nonossifying fibroma and fibrous cortical

defect is the size of the lesion. An exact size criterion may be unnecessary because histologically they have a similar pattern. The fibrous cortical defect is smaller, cortically based, and well marginated. The nonossifying fibroma tends to be lobulated and expansile with trabeculation and a longitudinal growth pattern. A rim of sclerosis and thinned or absent cortices may be encountered on radiographs, CT, and MR imaging. Because of the high fibrous content FX is often of predominantly low signal on all MR pulse sequences (**Fig. 10**). The involuted lesion may appear as normal bone with mild expansion or contain a sclerotic matrix. This lesion has a typical appearance in long bones and a differential diagnosis is often unnecessary. The most well-known associated entity is the Jaffe-Campanacci syndrome with multiple FXs, skin changes, and mental retardation.[14,15]

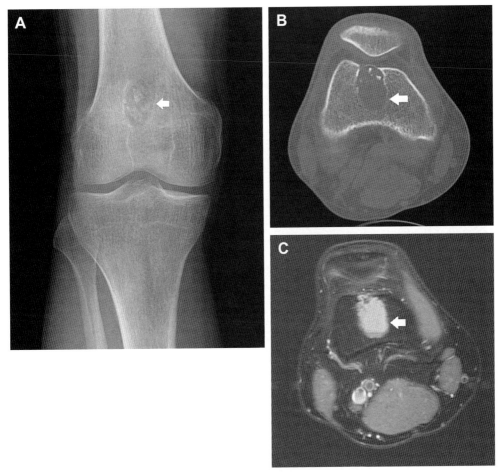

Fig. 9. A 33-year-old man with a distal femoral chondromyxoid fibroma (*arrow*). (*A*) Frontal radiograph of the knee shows a lucent metaphyseal lesion with small foci of mineralization. (*B*) Axial CT scan shows the thin anterior margin of lesion with foci of calcification. (*C*) Axial fat-saturated T2-weighted MR image demonstrates the partially lobulated margins of the intermediate-to-high signal lesion.

Fibrous Dysplasia

Fibrous dysplasia (FD) is usually a noninherited developmental anomaly of bone formation in which the normal bone marrow and cancellous bone is replaced by immature bone and fibrous tissue. It compromises up to 7% of benign bone tumors and less than 1% of biopsied bone tumors. FD is usually an incidental finding unless complicated by a pathologic fracture or rare malignant transformation. Males and females are equally affected, and although the lesion can be detected at any age, there is a peak incidence between 2 and 30 years. Histologically, it presents as a fibro-osseous metaplasia with islands of pure woven bone creating a typical "alphabet soup" pattern. ABC components also may be present. Most cases are monostotic (70%–80%), but up to 30% may be polyostotic. FD is most commonly found in the femur followed by tibia, skull and facial bones, and ribs. It is uncommon in the hand and foot, spine, and clavicle. In the long bones it presents as a medullary diaphyseal lesion (see **Table 1**).[16]

The radiographic features include a usually well-defined lucent expansile lesion with a sclerotic rim. FD may be multiloculated and the woven bone creates a "ground glass" appearance. Because of growth disturbance or underlying fracture, it may create a bowing deformity of the bone. CT can aid in detailing these radiographic features. On MR imaging FD is of low signal on T1-weighted images with a variable appearance on T2-weighted images ranging from intermediate to high signal intensity (**Fig. 11**). The differential diagnosis may include a simple bone cyst (SBC), Paget disease, and in the skull meningioma. The risk of a pathologic fracture depends on the location of the lesion and may

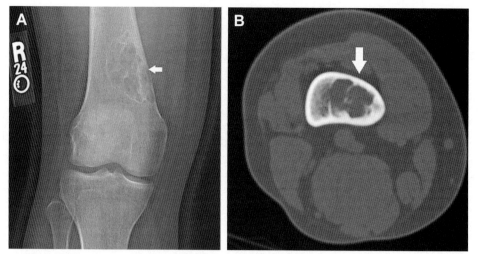

Fig. 10. A 17-year-old boy with a distal femur nonossifying fibroma (*arrow*). (*A*) Frontal radiograph shows an eccentric lesion with sclerotic lobulated margins. (*B*) Axial CT scan confirming the eccentricity of the lesion and lack of a mineralized matrix.

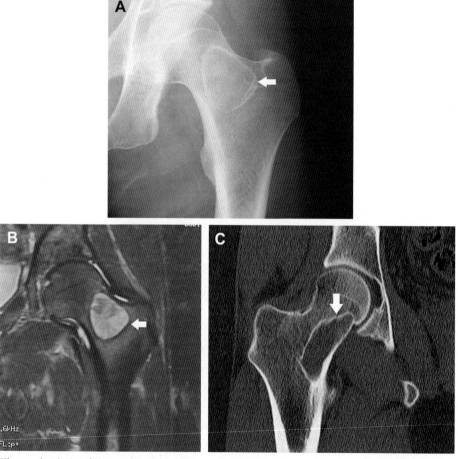

Fig. 11. Fibrous dysplasia of the proximal femur (*arrow*). (*A, B*) A 46-year-old man. Frontal radiograph (*A*) shows a lesion with a "ground glass" appearance and sclerotic margins in the femoral neck. Fat-saturated proton density weighted MR image (*B*) shows a hyperintense lesion with low signal intensity margins. (*C*) A 37-year-old man. CT (coronal reformation) shows the sclerotic rim (*arrow*) and foci of ground glass density along the lesion margin.

be related to the size of the ABC component. Malignant transformation into a sarcoma occurs in only 1% of cases and presents with pain and swelling; radiologically, cortical destruction and a soft tissue mass are prominent features. Syndromes associated with the polyostotic variant include McCune-Albright (precocious puberty and skin pigmentation in girls) and Mazabraud (rare combination with soft tissue myxomas).[16]

Osteofibrous Dysplasia

Osteofibrous dysplasia (OFD) is an unusual lesion compromising less than 0.2% of biopsied benign bone tumors. It presents with focal swelling and is painless unless complicated by a fracture. The patients are usually younger than 10 years and rarely older than 16. There is no gender predilection. Histologically, OFD presents with a vascularized fibrous stroma similar to FD without the alphabet soup woven bone pattern. Up to 80% of cases are found in the tibia, the remainder occurring in the fibula only or in combination with a fibular lesion. Radius and ulna lesions are extremely rare. OFD is usually based in the anterior cortex of the tibia (see **Table 1**).[17]

On radiographs and CT, OFD presents as an expansile lytic lesion of the anterior tibial cortex with a mixed lytic and sclerotic matrix. On MR imaging, OFD is usually of intermediate signal on T1- and high on T2-weighted images (**Fig. 12**). In many cases, patients with OFD can simply be observed closely after biopsy confirms the diagnosis; however, the most crucial entity in the differential diagnosis is the adamantinoma, a low-grade malignant tumor. OFD and adamantinoma components may both be present in a lesion and needle biopsy may not be conclusive. Imaging features suggesting adamantinoma, such as a more locally aggressive appearance with multiple lytic lesions, invasion of the medullary canal, and a soft tissue mass, may aid in the differential diagnosis; however, in these cases the entire lesion should undergo curettage and histologic investigation.[17]

Desmoplastic Fibroma

Desmoplastic fibroma (DF) is a rare lesion accounting for only 0.1% of benign bone tumors. It is considered the bony counterpart of the more common soft tissue desmoid. The clinical presentation is nonspecific and may include pain and swelling. There are controversial reports about gender distribution, but one review mentions a 1.5:1 male to female ratio.[18] DF is mostly found in the third and fourth decades of life. On histologic analysis it reveals a similar appearance to its soft tissue counterpart with a white-to-gray mass containing fibroblasts producing well-formed collagen. DF is mostly located centrally in the metadiaphysis of tubular bones around the knee (femur and tibia) followed by the humerus and radius (see **Table 1**).[19]

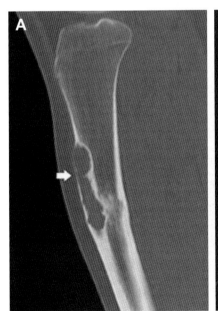
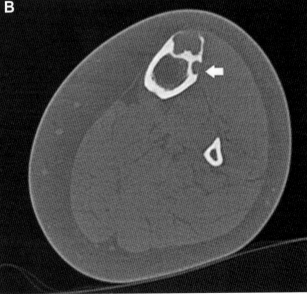

Fig. 12. A 15 year old with anterior tibial osteofibrous dysplasia. (*A*) CT, sagittal reformation shows readily the location of the lesion in the anterior cortex of the bone (*arrow*). (*B*) CT, axial image shows the location of the lesion within the anterior cortex and an additional lucent focus in the lateral cortex of the tibia (*arrow*).

On radiography DF frequently has an aggressive appearance presenting as a lytic expansile lesion. The lesion may have internal trabeculation and a sclerotic margin. CT confirms lack of a mineralized matrix and may demonstrate cortical breaching and a soft tissue component. The hallmark of DF on MR imaging is intermediate-to-low signal intensity on fluid-sensitive sequences because of the high collagen content of its fibrous component (**Fig. 13**).[18] The differential diagnosis includes a low-grade central osteosarcoma and FD. Rare association with FD has been described.[19]

HISTIOCYTIC OR FIBROHISTIOCYTIC TUMORS

The main benign representative of this group is the Langerhans cell histiocytosis, which is discussed elsewhere in this issue.

TUMORS WITH A FATTY MATRIX
Intraosseous Lipoma

Intraosseous lipoma (IL) is the main benign variant of this group. It is usually an incidental finding and only presents with pain if there is an associated

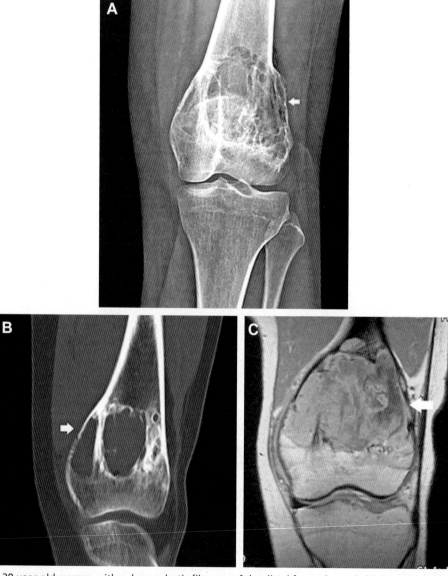

Fig. 13. A 28-year-old woman with a desmoplastic fibroma of the distal femur (*arrow*). (*A*) Anteroposterior radiograph of the knee shows a large lucent lesion of the metaphysis with expansile remodeling and trabeculation. (*B*) CT, coronal reformation shows a sclerotic margin and lack of matrix mineralization. (*C*) Coronal proton density weighted MR image confirms presence of low-to-intermediate signal components within the lesion.

fracture. IL has been considered to be a very rare bone tumor, although a general increase in use of cross-sectional imaging has resulted in more frequent reporting. The absolute etiology of this tumor is not well known and speculation includes its possible association with focal stress, osteoporosis, or involution of an underlying primary bone tumor. There is an equal gender distribution with a possible slight male predominance. There is a wide age range (from 4–85 years) with a mean of 40 years. Histologically, IL demonstrates a mature fatty matrix devoid of medullary trabeculation. Areas of fat necrosis with associated foamy histiocytes or cyst formation are encountered. It is most commonly found in the calcaneus followed by the metaphysis of the long bones, such as femur, tibia, and fibula. It is usually centrally located within the bone (see **Table 1**).[20]

On radiography IL presents as a well-defined lucent lesion with a narrow zone of transition without remodeling of the bone. A central calcification or ossification may be present. The mature fatty matrix can be confirmed by Hounsfield measurement on CT and fat-saturation on MR imaging (**Fig. 14**). On CT and MR imaging a central ossification is readily visible and cystic components are encountered commonly. The differential diagnosis includes a metastatic or myeloma lesion on radiography; however, demonstration of a fatty matrix on cross-sectional imaging secures the correct diagnosis, with no further work-up necessary.[20]

TUMORS WITH A VASCULAR MATRIX

The main representatives of this tumor type in the bone are osseous hemangioma (OH) and the glomus tumor (GT). Solitary or multiple osseous lymphangiomas may have an appearance similar to bony hemangiomas, but are not as common.

Osseous Hemangioma

The predominant matrix of an OH is vascular. The capillary subtype is most common; however, mixed tumors with other vascular subtypes may be present. OH is usually an incidental finding and asymptomatic. It is twice as common in males as females, and affects individuals in the fourth or fifth decade of life. Histologically, OH demonstrates vascular replacement of the marrow with possible calcified or cystic foci and a reactive sclerotic margin. One article reports that up to 75% of OH occur in the vertebrae, but they also occur in the calvarium, calcaneus, and the long bones.[21] Hemangiomas in the vertebrae may partially or completely replace the vertebral body. OH commonly presents in the long bones as a central metaphyseal lesion (see **Table 1**).[22]

Vertebral hemangiomas demonstrate a typical striated appearance on radiography similar to corduroy. This translates into a polka dot appearance on axial CT.[23] In other bones OH presents as a lytic lesion with a honeycomb pattern and cortical erosion. Advanced imaging with CT and MR imaging may show a soft tissue component with

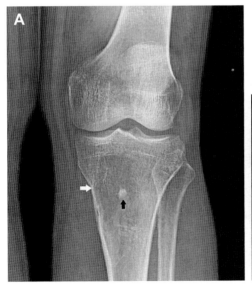
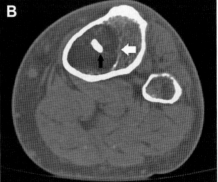

Fig. 14. A 78-year-old man with an incidental intraosseous lipoma of the proximal tibia (*white arrow*) with a central ossification (*black arrow*). (*A*) Anteroposterior radiograph of the knee. (*B*) CT, axial image. Note attenuation of the lesion similar to that of subcutaneous fat.

phleboliths. On MR imaging the fatty component interspersed between the vascular channels may exhibit high T1 signal; the predominant T2 signal is usually high (**Fig. 15**).[6,22] The differential diagnosis of extraspinal OH on plain radiography may include infection and metastatic disease, although cross-sectional imaging usually confirms the presence of a hemangioma. OH may be encountered as the smaller component of extensive diffuse soft tissue hemangiomatosis.

Glomus Tumor

GT is a rare benign lesion that almost exclusively occurs in the subungual region of the terminal phalanx. It is technically a soft tissue tumor that arises from the specialized arteriovenous anastomosis responsible for thermoregulation of the fingertips. GT commonly erodes into the tuft of the distal phalanx, thus simulating a bony tumor.[24] GT is described in further detail elsewhere in this issue.

TUMORS OF MISCELLANEOUS OR UNKNOWN ORIGIN

This group consists of bony lesions of unknown etiology. The more common representatives are discussed next. Other entities commonly grouped in this category but not discussed here include epidermoid inclusion cyst, subchondral cyst, intraosseous ganglion, and posttraumatic cyst.

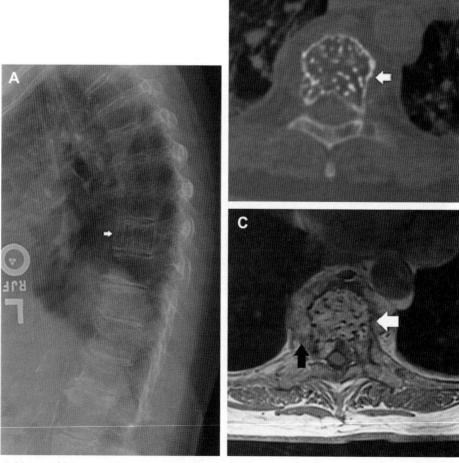

Fig. 15. A 86-year-old woman with a hemangioma of T8 (*white arrow*). (*A*) Lateral radiograph of the thoracic spine shows the "corduroy" appearance of the hemangioma. (*B*) CT, axial image demonstrates the characteristic polka dot appearance. (*C*) Axial T1-weighted MR image shows the replacement of the vertebral body with a soft tissue mass with low signal striation and extraosseous soft tissue component (*black arrow*).

Giant Cell Tumor

GCT of the bone is a relatively common bone tumor comprising up to 10% of primary bone tumors. It may present with pain, swelling, and at times a pathologic fracture. GCT may grow with pregnancy or intake of oral contraceptives. It is slightly more common in females and affects individuals after skeletal maturity with a peak incidence in the third decade of life. Histologically, GCT presents with an abundance of multinucleated giant cells on a background of mononuclear cells. The stroma is usually vascular with numerous capillaries, thus microscopic foci of internal hemorrhage and ABC-like components are possible. GCT is usually located at the ends of the tubular bones extending to the subchondral bone and typically is eccentric in location (see Table 1).[25]

Radiography reveals a characteristic expansile lytic lesion at the end of the bone with a narrow zone of transition. CT may reveal a partially sclerotic rim and confirms the lack of matrix mineralization. CT and MR imaging may demonstrate a soft tissue component. On MR imaging a low-to-intermediate signal intensity prevails on T1-weighted and the fluid-sensitive sequences (Fig. 16). The lower T2 signal compared with other subarticular lesions may be caused by hemosiderin deposition or increased cellularity. GCT has a high recurrence rate (up to 25%) after curettage or resection. It is the most common lesion associated with secondary ABC. The term "benign metastasizing GCT" is reserved for a histologically benign tumor with aggressive growth and distant metastatic deposits.[25]

Simple Bone Cyst

A SBC is a true cystic lesion of the bone. Other terms used, such as a "unicameral," "solitary," or "juvenile" bone cyst are misleading because the lesion may be multiloculated, rarely multiple, and occasionally seen in adults. SBC comprises about 3% of all biopsied primary bone tumors. SBC frequently presents with pain after a pathologic fracture; however, incidental asymptomatic occurrence is not uncommon. There is a predilection for males with a male to female ratio of 2.5:1. SBC mostly occurs in the first two decades of life with

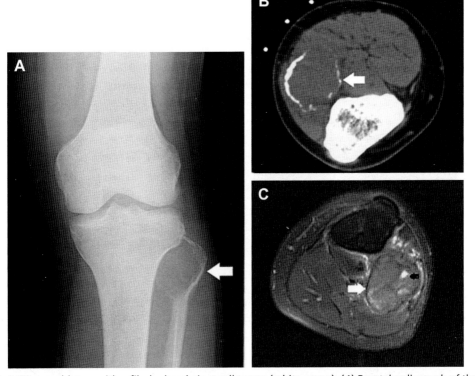

Fig. 16. A 27-year-old man with a fibular head giant cell tumor (*white arrow*). (*A*) Frontal radiograph of the knee shows the extension of the metaphyseal lesion into the epiphysis and subcortical bone. (*B*) CT, axial image, confirms lack of a mineralized matrix and thinning of the cortex. (*C*) Axial fat-saturated T2 image shows the predominantly intermediate signal lesion with a cystic focus (*black arrow*).

less than 15% occurring after 20 years of age. Histologically, the uncomplicated SBC demonstrates a thin cyst wall composed of a single layer of mesothelial cells. The serous fluid content is usually under pressure. SBC complicated by a fracture contains serosanguinous fluid and fibro-osseous repair tissue. In the pediatric population up to 60% of cases occur in the proximal humerus followed by 30% in the proximal femur. In the adult population there is a preference of location in the calcaneus and iliac bones adjacent to the sacroiliac joints. SBC is usually located centrally in the metaphysis of the bone (see **Table 1**).[26,27]

In a child SBC presents radiographically as a mildly expansile lucent lesion of the metaphysis invariably abutting the open growth plate. With skeletal growth the lesion migrates into the diaphysis, which has been termed the "latent" form. The appearance may be more complex with an underlying fracture. A "fallen fragment" sign has been described as a pathognomic finding with the fracture fragment in the dependent portion of the lesion confirming the "simple" fluid content of the lesion. This has been reported in up to 5% of lesions. The "rising bubbles" sign is based on similar priniciples.[28] MR imaging, and in particular CT, may better demonstrate the details of an underlying pathologic fracture. In an uncomplicated SBC, CT and MR imaging exhibit characteristic features of a lesion with simple fluid content (ie, a Hounsfield unit equal to simple fluid on CT and high T2 signal on MR imaging) (**Fig. 17**).[26]

Aneurysmal Bone Cyst

ABC is a benign bone lesion that is neither a cyst nor a neoplasm.[29] Several theories have been postulated regarding its origin. The most entertained is a reactive vascular process of native bone caused by antecedent trauma or a precursor tumor. ABC is rare (<2% of biopsied benign bone lesions) and usually presents with pain and swelling. A juxta-articular ABC may be the source of limited range of motion and the spinal variants may cause nerve and cord impingement. Pathologic fractures occur in up to 20% of patients. ABC is slightly more common in females and is seen in patients younger than age 20. The gross pathologic appearance has been described as that of a blood-filled sponge. On histology, cavernous blood-filled spaces lined by fibrous walls and osteoclast-rich giant cells prevail. A primary ABC has no associated underling lesion. A secondary ABC refers to those associated with an underlying bone tumor, most commonly GCT, followed by CB, OB, and FD. Over half of ABC cases occur in long bones and about 20% are encountered in the spine (predominantly the posterior elements). Pelvic bones are the most common flat bones affected. In long bones an eccentric metaphyseal location is seen in 80% of cases. A diaphyseal location, usually cortical or subperiosteal, is seen in approximately 20% of cases (see **Table 1**).[26,27]

ABC is the only bone lesion named for its radiographic appearance. Three phases have been

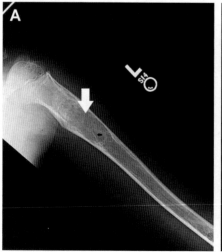
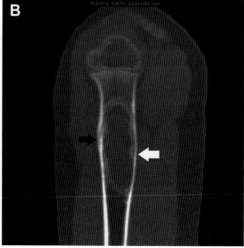

Fig. 17. A 10-year-old boy with a simple bone cyst of the proximal humerus (*white arrow*). (*A*) Lateral radiograph of the humerus with a "fallen fragment" (*black arrow*). (*B*) CT, coronal reformation image with a cortical fracture (*black arrow*).

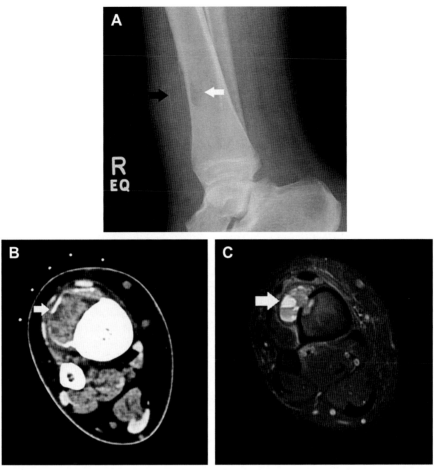

Fig. 18. A 15-year-old boy with a subperiosteal distal tibia aneurysmal bone cyst (*white arrow*). (*A*) Lateral radiograph of the ankle. *Black arrow* points to the extraosseous component. (*B*) CT, axial image, demonstrates a thin sclerotic rim. (*C*) Axial fat-saturated T2-weighted MR image shows the fluid–fluid levels in the lesion.

described. Initially, a focal area of osteolysis may be seen mimicking other benign bone tumors, such as FD or SBC. This is followed by an active or growth phase characterized by locally aggressive enlargement, bone destruction, and marked expansile remodeling. The outer border demonstrates extreme thinning, whereas the inner margin appears usually less aggressive. Periosteal reaction may occur suggesting a malignant tumor, although bone expansion with an intact rim of cortex usually supports the presence of a benign lesion. The stabilization phase is characterized by progressive calcification and ossification of the rim. CT imaging aids in excluding a mineralized matrix and reveals in up to 35% of cases one or multiple fluid–fluid levels. MR imaging is more sensitive in revealing the fluid–fluid levels, which may have a variable T1 and T2 appearance depending on the stage of blood products (Fig. 18). With secondary ABC, MR imaging also more readily demonstrates the solid underlying primary tumor. The differential diagnosis includes teleangiectatic osteosarcoma, GCT, OB, and CB, all of which may also contain fluid–fluid levels in the absence of a secondary ABC.[26,27]

SUMMARY

At first glance the benign bone tumors may appear confusing. However, thorough knowledge of radiologic characteristics of these benign lesions aids in a succinct differential diagnosis. The radiologic appearance of this group of bone tumors plays a major role in appropriate clinical management, preventing unnecessary patient anxiety, medical intervention, and ultimately added healthcare cost.

REFERENCES

1. Greenspan A. Bone island (enostosis): current concept: a review. Skeletal Radiol 1995;24:111–5.
2. Cerase A, Priolo F. Skeletal benign bone forming lesions. Eur J Radiol 1998;27:91–7.
3. Schweitzer ME, Levine C, Mitchell DG, et al. Bull's eyes and halos: useful MR discriminators of osseous metastases. Radiology 1993;188:249–52.
4. Davies M, Cassar-Pullicino VN, Davies MA, et al. The diagnostic accuracy of MR imaging in osteoid osteoma. Skeletal Radiol 2002;31:559–69.
5. Kroon HM, Schurmans J. Osteoblastoma: clinical and radiographic findings in 98 new cases. Radiology 1990;175(3):783–90.
6. Motamedi K, Ilaslan H, Seeger LL. Imaging of the lumbar spine neoplasms. Semin Ultrasound CT MR 2004;25:474–89.
7. Crim JR, Mirra JM, Eckardt JJ, et al. Widespread inflammatory response to osteoblastoma; the flare phenomenon. Radiology 1990;177(3):835–6.
8. Jaffe HL. Hereditary multiple exostosis. Arch Pathol 1943;36:335–57.
9. Robbin MR, Murphey MD. Benign chondroid neoplasms of the bone. Semin Musculoskelet Radiol 2000;4(1):45–58.
10. Murphey MD, Choi JJ, Kransdorf MJ, et al. Imaging of osteochondroma: variants and complications with radiographic-pathologic correlation. Radiographics 2000;20(5):1407–34.
11. Murphey MD, Flemming DJ, Boyea SR, et al. Enchondroma versus chondrosarcoma in the appendicular skeleton: differentiating features. Radiographics 1998; 18(5):1213–37.
12. Robinson P, White LM, Sundaram M, et al. Periosteal chondroid tumors: radiologic evaluation with pathologic correlation. AJR Am J Roentgenol 2001; 177(5):1183–8.
13. Nomikos GC, Murphey MD, Jelinek JS, et al. Advanced imaging of chondroblastoma. Radiology 2001;221(P):232.
14. Mankin HJ, Trahan CA, Fondren G, et al. Non-ossifying fibroma, fibrous cortical defect and Jaffe-Campanacci syndrome: a biologic and clinical review. Musculoskelet Surg 2009;93:1–7.
15. Jee WH, Choe BY, Kang HS, et al. Non-ossifying fibroma: characteristics at MR imaging with pathologic correlation. Radiology 1998;209(1):197–202.
16. Fitzpatrick KA, Taljanovic MS, Speer DP, et al. Imaging findings of fibrous dysplasia with histopathologic and intraoperative correlation. AJR Am J Roentgenol 2004;182(6):1389–98.
17. Khanna M, Delancy D, Tirabosco R, et al. Osteofibrous dysplasia, osteofibrous dysplasia-like adamantinoma and adamantinoma: correlation of radiological imaging features with surgical histology and assessment of the use of radiology in contributing to needle biopsy diagnosis. Skeletal Radiol 2008;37:1077–84.
18. Frick MA, Sundaram M, Unni KK, et al. Imaging findings in desmoplastic fibroma of bone: distinctive T2 characteristics. AJR Am J Roentgenol 2005;184: 1762–7.
19. Robbin MR, Murphey MD, Temple HD, et al. Imaging of musculoskeletal fibromatosis. Radiographics 2001; 21:585–600.
20. Campbell RS, Grainger AJ, Mangham DC, et al. Intraosseous lipoma: report of 35 new cases and a review of the literature. Skeletal Radiol 2003;32: 209–22.
21. Llauger J, Palmer J, Amores S, et al. Primary tumors of the sacrum: diagnostic imaging. AJR Am J Roentgenol 2000;174:417–24.
22. Baudrez V, Galant C, Vande Berg BC. Benign vertebral hemangiomas: MR-histological correlation. Skeletal Radiol 2001;30:442–6.
23. Persaud T. The polka dot sign. Radiology 2008;246: 980–1.
24. Baek HJ, Lee SJ, Cho KH, et al. Subungual tumors: clinicopathologic correlation with US and MR imaging findings. Radiographics 2010;30:1621–36.
25. Murphey MD, Nomikos GC, Flemming DJ, et al. From the archives of AFIP. Imaging of giant cell tumor and giant cell reparative granuloma of bone: radiologic-pathologic correlation. Radiographics 2001;21(5): 1283–309.
26. Parman LM, Murphey MD. Alphabet soup: cystic lesions of bone. Semin Musculoskelet Radiol 2000; 4(1):89–101.
27. Sim F, Esther R, Wenger DE. Tumor-like lesions of bone. In: Szendroi M, Sim FH, editors. Color atlas of clinical orthopedics. Berlin Heidelberg: Springer-Verlag; 2009. p. 209–29.
28. Jordanov MI. The "rising bubble" sign: a new aid in the diagnosis of unicameral bone cyst. Skeletal Radiol 2009;38:597–600.
29. Mirra JM. Aneurysmal bone cyst. In: Mirra JM, Picci P, Gold RH, editors. Bone tumors: clinical, radiologic, and pathologic correlation. Philadelphia: Lea & Febiger; 1989. p. 1267–311.

Imaging of Primary Malignant Bone Tumors (Nonhematological)

Prabhakar Rajiah, MBBS, MD, FRCR*, Hakan Ilaslan, MD,
Murali Sundaram, MD, FRCR

KEYWORDS

• Tumors • CT • MR imaging • Radiograph • Bone

Primary malignant bone tumors are uncommon, accounting for only 0.2% of all primary malignancies and 5.0% of all pediatric malignancies.[1,2] Metastatic tumors, benign tumors, and tumor mimics (eg, bone cysts, nonossifying fibroma, inflammatory lesions, fibrous dysplasia, Paget disease) are more common than primary bone malignancies. The estimated prevalence of primary malignant bone tumors in the United States is 8 per 1,000,000, with 2500 new cases diagnosed each year. Although primary bone malignancies can occur at any age, there is a peak at age 10 to 20 years, with a second peak after age 40.[1,3]

CLASSIFICATION

Primary malignant bone tumors are classified based on their cell of origin. The current World Health Organization (WHO) system of classification for bone tumors, both benign and malignant, is shown in **Box 1**.[4] The relative frequencies of the more common primary bone malignancies are shown in **Table 1**.[1] Osteosarcoma, chondrosarcoma, and Ewing sarcoma account for 75% of primary bone malignancies.[3] Although the histologic grade for some malignancies is implied when the diagnosis is made (eg, dedifferentiated chondrosarcoma is a high-grade lesion, whereas chordoma is a low-grade to intermediate-grade tumor), for most of these tumors, the grade is determined pathologically. Some tumors, such as small-cell malignancies (eg, Ewing sarcoma), do not readily lend themselves to histologic grading.[4]

PREDISPOSING LESIONS AND ASSOCIATED SYNDROMES

Some benign lesions have a predisposition to develop bone malignancies; radiation of preexisting lesions and radiation of healthy bone can also lead to malignancy. Radiation has been shown to induce various tumors. Osteochondroma is seen in 10% to 29% of children younger than 5 years who receive 1500 to 5000 cGy of radiation, with a latent period of 3 to 18 years. Sarcoma is seen in 0.2% of patients who receive more than 3000 cGy of radiation over 3 weeks, with a latent period ranging from 4 to 55 years (mean, 11–14 years). Ninety percent of these tumors are osteosarcomas or spindle-cell sarcomas.[5] Two-thirds of these cases originate after general radiation, and one-third arise after irradiation of preexisting bone lesions. These tumors develop in the periphery of the radiation field, where cell mutation occurs without cell death. The presence of cortical destruction and soft tissue mass in a known radiation field should therefore suggest a sarcoma. The differential diagnosis for this condition includes radiation osteonecrosis or insufficiency fracture. Radiation osteonecrosis is generally indicated by a lack of bone destruction, soft tissue mass, contrast enhancement, and change over serial

The authors have nothing to disclose.
Division of Musculoskeletal Radiology, Imaging Institute, Cleveland Clinic Foundation, 9500 Euclid Avenue, A21, Cleveland, OH 44195, USA
* Corresponding author.
E-mail address: radprabhakar@gmail.com

Radiol Clin N Am 49 (2011) 1135–1161
doi:10.1016/j.rcl.2011.07.003

Box 1
WHO classification of primary bone tumors

Cartilage tumors
Osteochondroma
Chondroma
    Enchondroma
    Periosteal chondroma
    Multiple chondromatosis
Chondroblastoma
Chondromyxoid fibroma
Chondrosarcoma
    Central, primary, and secondary
    Peripheral
    Dedifferentiated
    Mesenchymal
    Clear cell

Fibrogenic tumors
Desmoplastic fibroma
Fibrosarcoma

Fibrohistiocytic tumors
Benign fibrous histiocytoma
Malignant fibrous histiocytoma

Giant-cell tumor
Giant-cell tumor
Malignancy in giant-cell tumor

Hematopoietic tumors
Plasma cell myeloma
Malignant lymphoma

Joint lesions
Synovial chondromatosis

Lipogenic tumors
Lipoma
Liposarcoma

Miscellaneous lesions
Aneurysmal bone cyst
Simple bone cyst
Fibrous dysplasia
Osteofibrous dysplasia
Langerhans cell histiocytosis
Erdheim-Chester disease
Chest wall hamartoma

Miscellaneous tumors
Adamantinoma

Metastatic malignancy

Neural tumors
Neurilemmoma

Notochordal tumors
Chordoma

Osteogenic tumors
Osteoid osteoma
Osteoblastoma
Osteosarcoma
    Conventional
        Chondroblastic
        Fibroblastic
        Osteoblastic
    Telengiectatic
    Small cell
    Low-grade central
    Secondary
    Paraosteal
    Periosteal
    High-grade surface

Primitive neuroectodermal tumor
Ewing sarcoma

Smooth muscle tumors
Leiomyoma
Leiomyosarcoma

Vascular tumors
Hemangioma
Angiosarcoma

Data from Fletcher CD, Unni KK, Mertens F, editors. World Health Organization classification of tumors. Pathology and genetics of tumours of soft tissue and bone (IARC WHO Classification of Tumours). Lyon (France): IARC Press; 2002.

radiographs, whereas a recurrent tumor or radiation-associated sarcoma is indicated by pain, soft tissue mass, increased osteolysis, and contrast enhancement. Tumor recurrence generally occurs within 5 years.[6]

Paget disease may undergo malignant transformation in 5% of patients. This transformation occurs more commonly in men, particularly in the sixth and seventh decades of life.[7] Osteosarcoma is the most common sarcoma followed by spindle-cell sarcoma and chondrosarcoma, and these tumors occur most commonly in the femur, pelvis, and

Table 1
Relative frequencies of common primary malignant bone tumors

Tumor	Frequency, %
Osteosarcoma	35.1
Chondrosarcoma	25.8
Ewing sarcoma	16.0
Chordoma	8.4
Malignant fibrous histiocytoma	5.7
Angiosarcoma	1.4
Unspecified	1.2
Others	6.4

Data from Dorman HD, Czerniak B. Bone cancers. Cancer 1995;75(Suppl 1):203–10.

humerus. Cortical destruction and large soft tissue mass are features of sarcoma, although the absence of these signs does not necessarily rule out malignancy: subtle periosteal effacement or osteolysis may be the initial signs and may be indistinguishable from osteolytic exacerbation of established Paget disease. On bone scan, a photopenic area develops within the high uptake of Pagetic bone. Giant-cell tumor (GCT) and enchondroma have also been reported in Pagetic bone.[8] Metastasis, lymphoma, and leukemia can also arise in bone with Paget disease. Magnetic resonance (MR) imaging shows fat signal in uncomplicated Paget disease; the loss of this fat signal indicates development of either tumor or fracture.[9] A pseudosarcomatous appearance can be produced by cortical destruction and soft tissue mass, but with this condition, the fat signal is preserved. Postimmobilization lysis and bisphosphonate-induced bone disease can also mimic a tumor when marked osteolysis is the dominant radiographic appearance. However, fatty T1 marrow signal is preserved in these cases.[9] Both Paget disease and tumor show dynamic MR imaging contrast enhancement.[7]

Bone infarction may also predispose patients to the development of sarcoma, with malignant fibrous histiocytoma (MFH) being the most common secondary bone malignancy. A recent study demonstrated that secondary MFH is more common in patients with bone infarct than in those who were exposed to radiation.[10] Fibrous dysplasia itself is not considered to be a premalignant lesion, but malignancies may arise sporadically in patients with this condition. Malignant transformation has been reported in 0.4% to 1.0% of patients with fibrous dysplasia, with most of these malignancies

identified as osteosarcoma, followed by fibrosarcoma. Recent studies have shown that most cases of malignancy from fibrous dysplasia rarely occur de novo and are instead secondary to radiation.[11] Additionally, malignancies occur rarely at sites of chronic osteomyelitis and orthopedic implants. Rare cases of bone malignancies arising in association with aneurismal bone cyst, GCT, and neurofibromatosis-1 have been reported.

Several syndromes, both inherited and sporadic, are associated with an increased risk of bone tumor development. These syndromes are listed in **Table 2**.[4]

PRIMARY MALIGNANT BONE TUMORS

The characteristics of the various primary malignant bone tumors are summarized in **Table 3**.

Osteosarcoma

Osteosarcoma is a malignant tumor that is characterized by production of osteoid matrix (immature bone). Osteosarcoma is the most common primary nonhematologic bone malignancy and is the most common primary bone malignancy in children. There are various subtypes of osteosarcoma, each with distinct clinical and imaging characteristics. Osteosarcomas can be classified as intramedullary (high grade, telangiectatic, low grade, small cell, osteosarcomatosis, gnathic), juxtacortical (parosteal, periosteal, intracortical, high-grade surface), or secondary lesions.[12]

Conventional osteosarcoma
Conventional intramedullary osteosarcoma is the most common subtype of osteosarcoma, accounting for 75% of all cases. Conventional osteosarcoma is a high-grade neoplasm that is pathologically characterized by the production of tumor osteoid that originates centrally within the bone and involves the entire width of the bone. Conventional osteosarcoma is often pleomorphic and can produce variable amounts of cartilage, fibrous tissue, or other components. Depending on the dominant cell type, it can be classified as osteoblastic (50%–80%), fibroblastic-fibrohistiocytic (7%–25%), chondroblastic (5%–25%), telangiectatic (2.5%–12%), or small cell (1%). Giant cells and osteoblastomalike cells can also be seen. This malignancy is more common in the second and third decades of life, peaking when patients are aged 10 to 15 years. Conventional osteosarcoma is uncommon in patients younger than 6 years or older than 60 years and is more common in white patients and men. This condition usually occurs sporadically but may be familial. Conventional osteosarcoma is seen in the long bones (70%–80%),

Table 2
Syndromes associated with bone tumors

Syndrome	Inheritance	Manifestations
Osteochondromatosis	Autosomal dominant	Multiple osteochondromas; secondary chondrosarcoma or osteosarcoma (less likely)
Ollier disease	Sporadic	Multiple enchondromas
Maffucci syndrome	Sporadic	Multiple enchondromas; chondrosarcoma; hemangioma/venous malformation; spindle-cell hemangioma; angiosarcoma
McCune-Albright syndrome	Sporadic	Polyostotic fibrous dysplasia; hyperpigmentation; endocrine disorder; osteosarcoma
Mazabraud syndrome	Sporadic	Polyostotic fibrous dysplasia; intramuscular myxoma; osteosarcoma
Familial Paget disease	Autosomal dominant	Osteosarcoma
Retinoblastoma	Autosomal dominant	Osteosarcoma; soft tissue sarcomas
Familial expansile osteolysis	Autosomal dominant	Osteosarcoma
Li-Fraumeni syndrome	Autosomal dominant	Early onset of malignancies, including osteosarcoma; soft tissue sarcomas
Werner syndrome	Autosomal recessive	Premature aging; increased risk of bone and soft tissue sarcomas
Bloom syndrome	Autosomal recessive	Growth deficiency; immunodeficiency; early development of cancers including osteosarcoma
Rothmund-Thomson syndrome	Autosomal recessive	Poikiloderma; sparse hair; small stature; skeletal abnormalities; increased risk of cancers including osteosarcoma
Langer-Giedion syndrome	Sporadic	Combination of tricho-rhino-phalangeal syndrome II and multiple osteochondromas; chondrosarcoma

Data from Fletcher CD, Unni KK, Mertens F, editors. World Health Organization classification of tumors. Pathology and genetics of tumours of soft tissue and bone (IARC WHO Classification of Tumours). Lyon (France): IARC Press; 2002.

most commonly near the knee, in the femur, tibia, and humerus. This lesion originates in the metaphysis, with extension to the epiphysis (seen in up to 80% of MR imaging studies). Primary involvement of the diaphysis or epiphysis is uncommon. Patients with conventional osteosarcoma may present with pathologic fractures. Skip lesions occur in about 5% of patients with this condition. The lungs are the most common site for metastatic osteosarcoma; lung metastasis often shows ossification and may be associated with spontaneous pneumothorax. Hemorrhage and necrosis may also be observed. The intraosseous and extraosseous extent of tumor should be measured and documented. Joint involvement is seen in 19% to 24% of cases and is diagnosed when hyaline cartilage is penetrated. Synovial involvement is rare.

Radiographic findings for conventional osteosarcoma are characteristic, showing a large aggressive lesion with osteoid matrix (90%) with a pattern of fluffy opacities that destroy the cortex, with aggressive periosteal reaction (laminated, hair-on-end, sunburst, or Codman triangle) and with a soft tissue mass (Fig. 1A, B). Although the most common pattern is mixed lytic and sclerotic, purely lytic (fibroblastic) or sclerotic (osteoblastic) types may also be seen. MR imaging is the examination of choice for local staging and for planning biopsies or surgery. The entire bone should be scanned to evaluate for skip metastases. The lytic areas show low signal on T1-weighted images and high signal on T2-weighted images, whereas the mineralized matrix shows low signal on both T1-weighted and T2-weighted images (see Fig. 1C, D).

Treatment includes chemotherapy followed by wide surgical resection and limb salvage or amputation. The 5-year survival rate for conventional osteosarcoma is 60% to 80%; higher long-term survival is seen if there is greater than 90% tumor necrosis after chemotherapy. Local recurrence is

Table 3
Characteristic features of various malignant bone tumors

Tumor	Age	Sex	Bones	Location	Pattern	Margins	Cortical Destruction	Cortical Thickening	Periosteal Reaction	Soft Tissue Invasion
Conventional osteosarcoma	10–30	M>F	Distal femur, proximal tibia	Metaphysis; may extend to epiphysis	Mixed lytic and sclerotic; osteoid matrix	Ill defined	+	–	+	+
Telangiectatic osteosarcoma	10–30	M>F	Femur, tibia, humerus	Metaphysis	Geographic, lytic, expansile	Ill defined	+	–	+	+
Small-cell osteosarcoma	10–30	M = F	Distal femur, proximal tibia	Metaphysis; extension to epiphysis; may be isolated to diaphysis	Permeative with osteoid matrix; may be purely lytic	Ill defined	+	–	+	+
Low-grade central osteosarcoma	20–40	M = F	Distal femur, proximal tibia	Metaphysis; may extend to epiphysis	Lytic; may be expansile; diffuse sclerosis may be seen	Well defined, sclerotic rim; ill defined may be seen	May be subtle	–	May be subtle	May be subtle
Parosteal osteosarcoma	20–50	F>M	Distal femur (posterior), proximal humerus	Metaphysis	Juxtacortical ossific mass	Well defined	Rarely seen	+	–	+ in high grade
Periosteal osteosarcoma	10–30	M>F	Femur, tibia	Diaphysis or metadiaphysis	Juxtacortical mass; involves 50% of circumference	Well defined	–	+	+	Juxtacortical
High-grade surface osteosarcoma	10–40	M>F	Distal femur, shoulder	Diaphysis or metaphysis	Juxtacortical mass; involves entire circumference	Well defined	–	+	+	Juxtacortical
Intracortical osteosarcoma	10–20	M>F	Tibia, femur	Diaphysis	Intracortical, geographic with osteoid	Smooth	–	+	–	–
Central chondrosarcoma	50–80	M>F	Pelvis, femur, proximal humerus, ribs	Metaphysis or metadiaphysis	Geographic lytic; chondroid or amorphous calcification	Depends on grade	Scalloping or penetration	+	Mild	+ in high grade

(continued on next page)

Table 3
(continued)

Tumor	Age	Sex	Bones	Location	Pattern	Margins	Cortical Destruction	Cortical Thickening	Periosteal Reaction	Soft Tissue Invasion
Clear-cell chondrosarcoma	25–60	M>F	Proximal femur, humerus	Epiphysis	Lytic with chondrogenic calcification; can be expansile	Well defined with thin sclerotic rim	–	Thinning	–	–
Mesenchymal chondrosarcoma	10–40	M = F	Jaws, ribs, pelvis, spine	Metaphysis or metadiaphysis	Geographic lytic; chondroid or amorphous calcification	Depends on grade	Scalloping or penetration	+	Mild	+ in high grade
Dedifferentiated chondrosarcoma	50–70	M>F	Pelvis, femur, humerus	Metaphysis	Bimorphic appearance; cartilaginous and noncartilaginous appearances	Ill defined	+	–	–	+
Juxtacortical chondrosarcoma	17–65	F>M	Femur	Metaphysis	Lytic with striated calcification	Ill defined	Scalloping on periosteal side	–	Thick radial	+ Surface lesion
Secondary chondrosarcoma	20–60	M>F	Pelvis, hip, shoulder	Metaphysis	Geographic lytic; chondroid or amorphous calcification	Depends on grade	Scalloping or penetration	+	Mild	+ in osteochondroma
Ewing sarcoma	5–30	M>F	Pelvis, long bones of upper and lower extremities	Diaphysis or metadiaphysis	Permeative	Ill defined	+	–	Laminated, onion peel, Codman triangle	+
Chordoma	30–80	M>F	Sacrococcygeal, skull base, vertebrae	Midline	Lytic	Ill defined or may be well defined owing to slow growth	+	May be seen	–	+

Malignant fibrous histiocytoma	40–70 M>F	Appendicular > flat bones; distal femur, proximal tibia	Diametaphysis	Permeative	Ill defined	+	Rarely seen	–	+
Fibrosarcoma	20–50 M = F	Femur, tibia	Metaphysis, may extend to epiphysis	Lytic, moth eaten	Ill defined	+	–	Uncommon	+
Hemangioendothelioma	10–60 M>F	Femur, tibia	Diaphysis, may be seen in metaphysis, metaepiphysis	Lytic; mixed and sclerotic may be seen; multifocal	Well defined	Uncommon	Expansion and thinning	Uncommon	Uncommon
Epithelioid hemangioendothelioma	10–30 M>F	Calvarium, spine, femur, tibia, feet	Metaphysis or epiphysis	Lytic, multifocal	Ill defined	Uncommon	Expansion uncommon	Rare	+
Angiosarcoma	20–50 M>F	Spine, pelvis, hip, shoulder	Metaphysis or diaphysis	Lytic, mixed	Ill defined	+	–	Uncommon	+
Adamantinoma	10–30 M>F	Tibia	Diaphysis	Intracortical, eccentric, mixed lytic	Variable	–	Soap bubble	May be seen	May be seen
Malignant giant-cell tumor	20–60 F>M	Knee, pelvis, shoulder	Epiphysis	Lytic, expansile	Ill defined	+	–	+	+
Leiomyosarcoma	30–70 M = F	Long bones, around major joints	Metaphysis; extension to epiphysis or diaphysis	Lytic	Ill defined	+	–	+	+

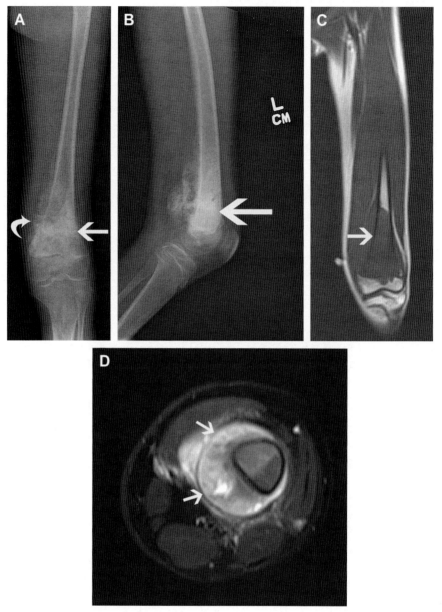

Fig. 1. Conventional high-grade osteosarcoma. Anteroposterior (AP) (*A*) and lateral (*B*) radiographs show a mixed sclerotic and lytic lesion (*straight arrow*) in the distal femur, with spiculated periosteal reaction (*curved arrow*) and a Codman triangle. (*C*) Coronal T1-weighted image shows a large, low-signal mass in the distal femur (*arrow*) with extension into the epiphysis. (*D*) Axial T2-weighted image shows a high-signal mass (*arrows*), which is circumferentially surrounding the distal femur.

high if there has been a pathologic fracture. A large tumor and advanced stage indicate a poor prognosis.[13]

Telangiectatic osteosarcoma

Telangiectatic osteosarcoma is pathologically characterized by dilated cavities filled with blood and septa and a rim that contains high-grade osteosarcomatous cells.[14] This type of lesion accounts for 2.5% to 12% of osteosarcomas. Age, sex distribution, and lesion location are similar to those seen with conventional osteosarcoma. Telangiectatic osteosarcomas are located in the metaphysis of long bones and show a geographic pattern of bone destruction, with ill-defined margins, expansive remodeling, cortical destruction, periosteal reaction, and soft tissue mass (**Fig. 2**A). More aggressive osteolysis or parallel striations attributable to hypertrophied veins have also been reported.

Bone scans of these lesions show heterogeneous uptake with central photopenia. The central region has low attenuation on computed tomography (CT), low signal on T1-weighted MR imaging, and high signal on T2-weighted MR imaging. Fluid-fluid levels are seen in up to 90% of these lesions (see **Fig. 2**B). The imaging and pathologic features of these lesions may be confused with those of aneurysmal bone cysts, but telangiectatic osteosarcomas are distinguished by the presence of solid and viable tumor, osteoid matrix, and aggressive growth pattern. The presence of thick, nodular, solid tissue within or around the cystic spaces, best seen on contrast-enhanced MR imaging, is also helpful in making the diagnosis. Matrix mineralization in these lesions may be subtle on radiographs, as viable tumor cells constitute only 10% of the tumor, and these cells are better seen on CT. Imaging can be used to guide biopsy of the viable tumor cells. Treatment is similar to that for conventional osteosarcoma; prognosis is also similar, with a 5-year survival rate of 68%.[15]

Small-cell osteosarcoma

Small-cell osteosarcoma is a rare subtype, accounting for only 1% to 4% of osteosarcomas. These lesions contain small, round, blue cells along with tumor osteoid. The age distribution of affected patients and location of the lesions are similar to those seen with conventional osteosarcoma, but an equal number of men and women have small-cell osteosarcoma. These lesions are most commonly seen in the metaphysis, with occasional extension to the epiphysis, but they are isolated to the diaphysis in 15% of cases. Small-cell osteosarcoma is an intramedullary, permeative lytic lesion with ill-defined margins that is associated with cortical destruction, aggressive periosteal reaction, and soft tissue mass. Although osteoid matrix is typically seen, purely lytic lesions may occur in up to 40% of cases. The prognosis is worse than that of conventional osteosarcoma.[15]

Gnathic osteosarcoma

Osteosarcoma of the jawbones is considered a distinct entity, accounting for 6% of all osteosarcomas. The mean age of affected patients is 34 to 36 years. The imaging appearance of gnathic osteosarcoma is similar to that of conventional osteosarcoma, including osteoid matrix, aggressive periosteal reaction, soft tissue mass, and opacification of maxillary sinuses. Treatment is difficult, and although distant metastasis is uncommon, the local recurrence rate is high (50%–80%).[15]

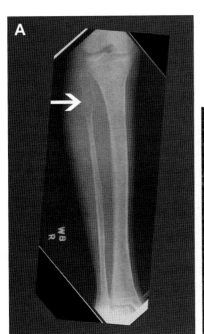
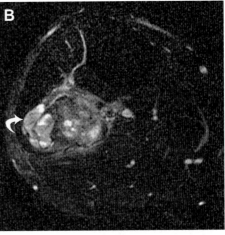

Fig. 2. Telangiectatic osteosarcoma. (*A*) AP radiograph shows an expansile lytic lesion in the proximal fibula (*arrow*). (*B*) T2-weighted axial MR image shows the expansile mass within the proximal fibula, extending into the surrounding soft tissue and showing multiple focal fluid-fluid levels suggestive of intralesional hemorrhage (*curved arrow*).

Low-grade central osteosarcoma

Low-grade central osteosarcoma (well differenti- ated, sclerosing) accounts for 1% to 2% of all osteosarcomas. This condition occurs in a slightly older age group (third decade) than the conven- tional type and is seen equally in men and women. Low-grade central osteosarcoma affects the same bones as conventional osteosarcoma. The radio- logic and pathologic findings mimic those of fibrous dysplasia, often resulting in erroneous radiographic and microscopic diagnosis (**Fig. 3**). Any bone tumor with the appearance of fibrous dysplasia that also shows cortical effacement or destruction or a soft tissue mass should be con- sidered a low-grade osteosarcoma.[16] Even if the biopsy results suggest fibrous dysplasia, the samples should be reanalyzed based on imaging findings.[17] Wide excision typically leads to an excellent outcome and prognosis. Curettage can result in recurrences, with 15% transforming into high-grade osteosarcoma.

Juxtacortical osteosarcoma

Juxtacortical osteosarcoma accounts for 4% to 10% of all osteosarcomas. These lesions are further divided into parosteal, periosteal, high- grade surface, and intracortical osteosarcomas.

Parosteal osteosarcoma originates from the outer layer of the periosteum and accounts for 65% of juxtacortical osteosarcomas. This condi- tion is typically seen in the third and fourth decades and is more common in women. Paro- steal osteosarcoma is most commonly seen in the metaphysis of long bones, typically in the posterior distal femur and occasionally in the proximal humerus, tibia, and fibula. Pathologically, osteoid matrix and fibrous stroma with occasional cartilage foci are seen.[18] Radiographs show a large, cauliflowerlike, ossific juxtacortical mass, which in its early stages is separated by a radiolu- cent cleavage plane from the remaining cortical bone; in the later stages of growth, this plane may be obliterated (**Fig. 4**A, B). Cortical thickening without aggressive periosteal reaction may also be seen. Most parosteal osteosarcomas are low grade, but high-grade foci can be seen in 22% to 64% of cases; these foci may appear on CT or MR imaging as nonmineralized soft tissue components measuring larger than 1 cm^3 (see **Fig. 4**C). Extension into the medullary cavity may be seen in 8% to 59% of cases, and although this occurrence does not alter the prognosis of these patients, knowledge of this extension is important before the performance of complete surgical resection.[19] Prognosis in patients with pa- rosteal osteosarcoma is excellent, with a 10-year survival rate of 80%. High-grade foci warrant adjuvant chemotherapy. The main differential diagnosis for this condition includes myositis ossi- ficans, which has denser peripheral ossification and is not attached to the cortex.[20]

Periosteal osteosarcoma, which accounts for 25% of juxtacortical osteosarcomas, is an inter- mediate-grade tumor that originates from the deep periosteal layer. Pathologically, periosteal osteosarcoma is highly chondroblastic with small areas of osteoid. This condition is commonly seen in the second and third decades and has a slight male preponderance. Periosteal osteosarcoma most commonly occurs in the diaphysis or meta- diaphysis and involves 50% of the osseous circumference. This condition most commonly affects the tibia and femur, followed by the ulna and humerus. A broad-based soft tissue mass with perpendicular periosteal reaction is seen on the surface of the bone, with cortical scalloping, cortical thickening, and Codman triangle occur- ring at the upper or lower margins (**Fig. 5**A). Because these lesions are pathologically chon- droblastic, matrix ossification is not distinctly seen. The cartilaginous areas appear as low attenuation on CT, low signal on T1-weighted

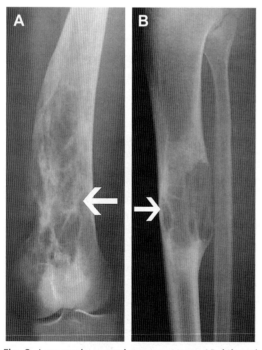

Fig. 3. Low-grade central osteosarcoma. AP (A) and lateral (B) radiographs show a coarsely trabeculated lesion in the distal femur with expansile remodeling and cortical destruction on its medial aspect (*arrow*). This is the most common pattern of low-grade central osteosarcoma, mimicking fibrous dysplasia.

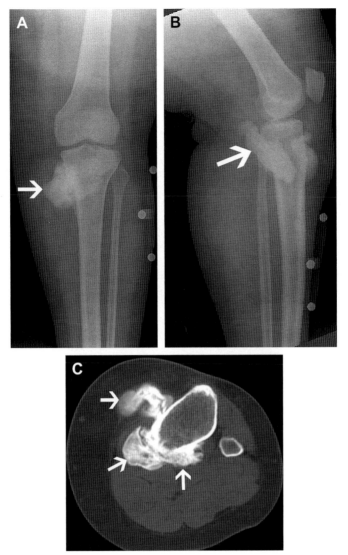

Fig. 4. Parosteal osteosarcoma. AP (*A*) and lateral (*B*) radiographs show dense ossification (*arrow*) surrounding the proximal tibial metaphysis. (*C*) Axial CT image shows dense tumor ossification defining the extent of tumor (*arrows*) and a cleavage plane partially evident at the proximal tibial metaphysis.

images, and high signal on T2-weighted images. Perpendicular periosteal reaction is seen as rays of low signal intensity on all MR imaging sequences (see **Fig.** 5B, C). Invasion of the marrow is rare; when seen, it is contiguous with the surface mass. However, reactive changes in the marrow occur in more than 50% of cases, appearing as low signal on T1-weighted images and high signal on T2-weighted images adjacent to but not contiguous with the mass.[21] Prognosis of patients with this condition is worse than the prognosis seen with parosteal osteosarcoma but better than that seen with conventional osteosarcoma. Treatment consists of wide local excision with limb salvage.

High-grade surface osteosarcoma accounts for 10% of juxtacortical osteosarcomas and is pathologically similar to conventional intramedullary osteosarcoma. This condition is less frequently encountered than parosteal and periosteal osteosarcoma. It is more common in the second and third decades and has a male predominance. High-grade surface osteosarcoma affects the diaphysis of long bones, such as the femur, humerus, and fibula. Radiologically, it appears similar to periosteal osteosarcoma but involves the entire circumference of the bone and may invade the medullary cavity.[15]

Intracortical osteosarcoma is a rare type of osteosarcoma that arises from the cortex. Pathologically,

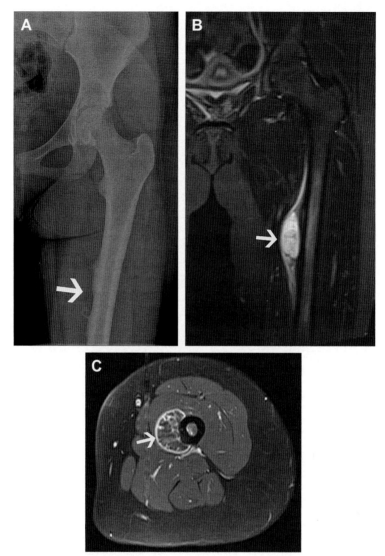

Fig. 5. Periosteal osteosarcoma. (*A*) AP radiograph shows a juxtacortical lesion in the medial aspect of proximal femur with an aggressive perpendicularly spiculated pattern of periosteal reaction (*arrow*). (*B*) Coronal T2-weighted MR image shows an aggressive periosteal mass with high T2 signal (*arrow*). (*C*) Axial T1-weighted MR image shows heterogeneous contrast enhancement, particularly of the septa (*arrow*).

intracortical osteosarcoma is a sclerosing osteosarcoma with foci of chondrosarcoma or fibrosarcoma. This condition is most common in the second decade and in men. These lesions are usually seen in the diaphysis of the tibia or femur and have a geographic pattern with variable amounts of mineralized osteoid. The lesions may also have smooth margins and cortical thickening. Medullary invasion is rare. High signal may be seen in and around the lesion on MR imaging. The common differential diagnosis for this condition includes osteoid osteoma or osteoblastoma. Metastasis and rickets have been reported in patients with intracortical osteosarcoma.[22]

Secondary osteosarcoma

Secondary osteosarcoma, which accounts for 5% to 7% of all osteosarcoma cases, is an osteosarcoma that originates from benign lesions, such as Paget disease (67%–90%), or that is secondary to radiation (6%–22%). Malignant transformation occurs in 5% of patients with Paget disease, with most malignancies manifesting as osteosarcoma (73%–84%), fibrosarcoma (9%–16%), chondrosarcoma (14%), or MFH (5%). Lytic or mixed lytic and blastic lesions with a soft tissue mass are seen, but periosteal reaction is not a dominant feature. The prognosis for these patients is poor. Among cases of malignancy that are secondary to radiation exposure, osteosarcoma is the most common lesion (50%–60%), followed by MFH (20%). This type of malignancy accounts for 3% to 5% of all osteosarcomas, with a latent period ranging from 4 to 30 years after exposure to radiation of 10,000 cGy or more.

Osteosarcomatosis (multifocal osteosarcoma) is a condition characterized by multiple intraosseous osteosarcomas that was earlier thought to represent multicentric osteosarcomas but is now believed to represent rapidly progressive multicentric metastatic disease. Most of these patients have a radiographically dominant lesion and pulmonary metastatic disease. Osteosarcomatosis accounts for 3% to 4% of all osteosarcomas and is bilaterally symmetric in skeletally immature patients but asymmetric in skeletally mature older patients. The dominant lesion is large, asymmetric, and contains osteoid, or the lesion may be purely lytic with metastatic foci that are smaller, sclerotic, well defined, and lacking periosteal reaction and cortical destruction. Mean survival for these patients is only 12 months.[15]

Chondrosarcoma

Chondrosarcoma is a malignant tumor of chondroid origin that accounts for 25% of malignant bone tumors. It is the third most common malignant bone tumor after myeloma and osteosarcoma. Chondrosarcoma can be classified based on location (central vs peripheral), histology (clear cell, dedifferentiated, or mesenchymal), origin (primary vs secondary), or grade (low, myxoid, high, or dedifferentiated). Secondary chondrosarcomas typically originate from an osteochondroma; enchondroma may dedifferentiate, showing areas of high-grade malignancy.[23]

Central chondrosarcoma
Primary central chondrosarcoma (conventional, intramedullary) is the most common type of chondrosarcoma, accounting for 90% of chondrosarcomas and 20% of all malignant bone tumors. Central chondrosarcoma is most commonly seen in the sixth decade, is more common in men (1.5:1.0), and typically occurs in or close to the trunk, particularly in the pelvis, proximal femur, proximal humerus, distal femur, and ribs. In the long bones, central chondrosarcoma is located in the metaphysis or metadiaphysis. Microscopically, most central chondrosarcomas are low grade. The imaging appearance of central chondrosarcoma depends on the grade of the lesion and ranges from a well-defined lucent lesion with chondroid matrix indistinguishable from an enchondroma to an aggressive, moth-eaten tumor with ill-defined margins, cortical destruction,

aggressive periosteal reaction, and soft tissue mass. Central chondrosarcoma most commonly appears as a large geographic type of lytic destruction, with cortical scalloping, cortical penetration, expansive growth, cortical thickening, mild periosteal reaction, and chondrogenic or amorphous calcification, with or without a pathologic fracture (**Fig. 6**A). On CT, central chondrosarcoma appears as chondrogenic calcification and cortical destruction (see **Fig. 6**B). On MR imaging, central chondrosarcoma has a lobular pattern with low T1 signal and high T2 signal because of the high water content of cartilage (see **Fig. 6**C). Central chondrosarcoma also demonstrates a "rings-and-arcs" pattern of enhancement of fibrovascular septae (tumors with this pattern are usually Grade II in histology). The differential diagnosis for lesions with chondrogenic calcification includes enchondroma; and for lesions without calcification, the differential diagnosis includes metastatis, lytic secondary osteosarcoma, MFH, and fibrosarcoma.[24]

Distinguishing a chondroma from a low-grade chondrosarcoma can be challenging, as chondromas have malignant potential and the borderline between enchondroma and low-grade chondrosarcoma is not well defined. Because of sampling errors, histology alone cannot help in this differentiation; therefore, radiology plays an important role in determining the growth pattern and biologic behavior of the lesion. The presence of atypical features is suggestive of a chondrosarcoma. These can include lesion-related pain, atypical location (enchondromas are rare in the axial skeleton, talus, and calcaneum, whereas chondrosarcomas are rare in the short tubular bones), progressive radiographic changes in the mature skeleton, large size (>5 cm), different calcification patterns within the lesion, deep cortical scalloping (>two-thirds of the cortical thickness), cortical penetration, periosteal reaction or cortical remodeling, soft tissue extension, and high uptake on bone scan (typically more than that of anterior iliac crest).[23,25] Cortical scalloping of eccentrically located cartilaginous lesions as a sign of chondrosarcoma is often misleading because there is no evidence that cortical scalloping associated with eccentrically located chondroid lesions in long tubular bones is a sign of malignancy.[26] These lesions, which abut the endosteal cortex, have been termed endosteal chondromas, distinguishing them from central chondromas, intra-aortic chondromas, and periosteal chondromas.[26] Chondroid lesions are largely named for their location.

Clear-cell chondrosarcoma
Clear-cell chondrosarcoma is a low-grade, slow-growing variant of chondrosarcoma that accounts for 1% to 2% of this lesion type. Clear-cell

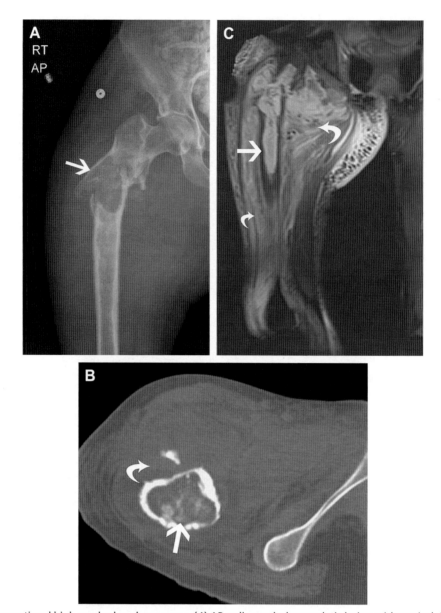

Fig. 6. Conventional high-grade chondrosarcoma. (*A*) AP radiograph shows a lytic lesion with cortical destruction and pathologic fracture in the proximal femur (*arrow*). (*B*) Axial CT image shows multiple areas of chondroid matrix within the lesion (*straight arrow*). There is also cortical destruction and soft tissue extension with calcification (*curved arrow*). (*C*) Coronal T2-weighted MR image shows extensive lesion in the proximal and mid femur (*straight arrow*), which is extending into the surrounding soft tissue (*curved arrows*).

chondrosarcoma is usually encountered in the third and fourth decades and is 3 times more common in men than in women. Lesions are seen in long bones, such as the femur and humerus, mainly in the epiphyseal equivalent area, and less commonly in the ribs, skull, spine, hands, and feet. Radiographically, these lesions may show well-defined margins, with a thin sclerotic rim, or may appear expansive with cortical thinning. Chondrogenic calcifications are seen in one-third of cases; periosteal reaction is rare (**Fig. 7**). The differential diagnosis for clear-cell chondrosarcoma includes chondroblastoma, intraosseous ganglion, metastasis, and avascular necrosis. Chondroblastoma occurs in younger patients with an open growth plate. Ganglion cyst does not have chondrogenic calcification, but may have a sclerotic rim; and metastasis

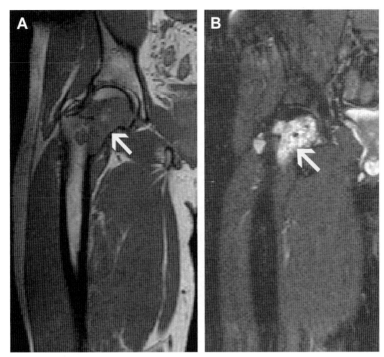

Fig. 7. Clear-cell chondrosarcoma. (*A*) T1-weighted MR image shows a low-signal lesion in the proximal femur that is extending outside the cortex, highlighting its aggressive nature (*arrow*). (*B*) T2-weighted MR image of the same patient shows high T2 signal of the lesion.

may appear more aggressive than clear-cell chondrosarcoma and does not show chondrogenic calcification.[23]

Mesenchymal chondrosarcoma

Mesenchymal chondrosarcoma is a rare type of chondrosarcoma that consists of highly differentiated cartilage cells and undifferentiated small round cells. The incidence of this condition peaks in the second and third decades and is equally seen in men and women. One-third of mesenchymal chondrosarcoma cases may originate in soft tissues. Osseous lesions are common in the craniofacial bones, ribs, ilium, and vertebrae. The imaging findings associated with this condition are similar to those seen with conventional chondrosarcoma. Most cases (75%) show chondrogenic calcification.[27]

Dedifferentiated chondrosarcoma

Dedifferentiated chondrosarcoma, which accounts for 10% of chondrosarcomas, is characterized by a bimorphic pattern of a well-differentiated chondrogenic lesion (low-grade chondrosarcoma, enchondroma, or osteochondroma) and a high-grade noncartilaginous lesion (MFH, fibrosarcoma, or osteosarcoma). This condition most commonly occurs in the fifth to ninth decades, has a slight

male predominance, and is typically seen in the pelvis, femur, and humerus. Imaging of dedifferentiated chondrosarcoma shows an intramedullary tumor with bimorphic appearance (on one-third of radiographs and one-half of CT scans), including a cartilaginous component showing chondrogenic calcification (50%) and a highly aggressive, noncartilaginous osteolytic component with ill-defined margins, cortical penetration, and soft tissue mass (**Fig. 8**). Biopsy should be performed on the suspected dedifferentiated component. Pathologic fractures may be seen in patients with this condition.[28,29]

Juxtacortical chondrosarcoma

Juxtacortical (periosteal) chondrosarcoma is a rare type of chondrosarcoma that originates on the surface of long bones. It is seen in patients aged 17 to 65 years and is more common in women. Juxtacortical chondrosarcoma occurs most commonly in the femur, usually in the distal posterior femoral metaphysis. The imaging appearance of this lesion resembles the appearance of a juxtacortical chondroma with a surface mass scalloping the cortex from the periosteal side; the lesion may have matrix calcifications. Compared with a chondroma, a juxtacortical chondrosarcoma is larger, has

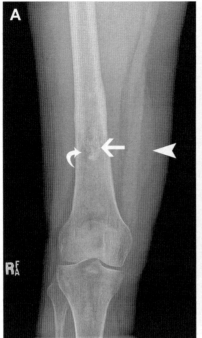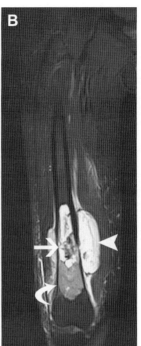

Fig. 8. Dedifferentiated chondrosarcoma. (*A*) AP radiograph shows a lobulated lesion with chondroid calcification (*straight arrow*) amidst areas of osteolysis (*curved arrow*) in the distal femur. There is also a soft tissue mass in the medial thigh (*arrowhead*). (*B*) T2-weighted coronal MR imaging shows a chondroid lesion in the distal femur (*straight arrow*) with an additional intramedullary noncartilaginous component associated with it (*curved arrow*), as well as extension of the tumor into the soft tissue of the thigh (*arrowhead*).

striated calcifications, and does not show an endosteal border of sclerosis. Reactive marrow involvement may be seen on MR imaging; a thick radial periosteal reaction may also be seen in some patients. The differential diagnosis for this condition includes periosteal osteosarcoma, which is a more aggressive tumor and may demonstrate a sunburst periosteal reaction and osteoid matrix.[30]

Secondary chondrosarcoma

Secondary chondrosarcoma originates from pre-existing benign cartilaginous lesions, such as enchondroma or osteochondroma (**Fig. 9**). The rate of conversion is higher when multiple lesions are present, such as in patients with osteochondromatosis (5%–25%), enchondromatosis (10%–25%), or Maffucci syndrome. It is more common in men (2:1) and has a younger age distribution than conventional chondrosarcomas (mean age, 34 years). This is typically a low-grade to intermediate-grade conventional chondrosarcoma, unlike a dedifferentiated chondrosarcoma, which has a high-grade tumor of different histology. In an osteochondroma, secondary chondrosarcoma is diagnosed when the cartilage cap is large (>2 cm) or irregular with inhomogeneous mineralization in

addition to new onset of pain and sudden growth of the lesion. This can be distinguished from bursae by the pattern of contrast enhancement, which is only peripheral in bursae. Distant metastasis is uncommon and prognosis is good with 5-year survival of 90%. Local recurrence is seen in 10% to 20%, particularly in the pelvis.[31]

Ewing Sarcoma/Primitive Neuroectodermal Tumors

Tumors with a common neuroectodermal origin, including Ewing sarcoma, primitive neuroectodermal tumor, adult neuroblastoma, malignant small-cell tumor of chest wall (Askin tumor), paravertebral small-cell tumor, and atypical Ewing sarcoma, have a common histogenesis and are therefore now referred to collectively as Ewing/primitive neuroectodermal tumors (PNET). Pathologically, these tumors contain monotonous small, round cells arranged in a sheetlike configuration. Reciprocal translocation between chromosomes 11 and 22 is seen in many of these cases. The Ewing/PNET family accounts for 5% of primary bone malignancies and is the second most common primary bone tumor in children. Approximately 75% of these tumors occur in

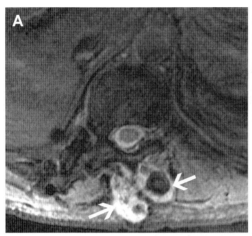
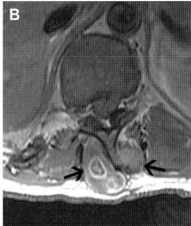

Fig. 9. Secondary chondrosarcoma. (A) Axial T2-weighted MR image of the spine obtained 2 years after resection of a thoracic spine osteochondroma shows a high-signal mass abutting the spinous process of the T11 vertebra (*arrows*). (B) Axial postcontrast T1-weighted image shows peripheral contrast enhancement (*arrows*). There is no destruction of the bone or extension into the spinal canal.

patients younger than 20 years; most affected patients are 5 to 25 years, with a peak in incidence between 10 and 20 years of age. These tumors are more common in men (2:1) and are rare in Afro-Caribbean patients. The lesions commonly affect the distal appendicular skeleton (27% femur and tibia), pelvic bones (21%), and ribs (6%–8%), and usually occur in the medullary cavity of the metadiaphysis or diaphysis.

Radiographs of patients with this condition show a permeative pattern of lytic bone destruction with a wide zone of transition, variably sclerotic matrix, laminated periosteal reaction (typically incompletely laminar with Codman triangle, but occasionally the classic multilamellated onion peel appearance, reflecting periodic activity of the tumor, or hair-on-end type), and a soft tissue mass that is often larger than the medullary component (**Fig. 10**A). Uncommon findings include cortical thickening, cystic component (unless necrotic), and bone expansion. Soft tissue calcification, honeycombing, sharp margins, and vertebra plana occur only rarely. Mixed sclerotic or lytic lesions occur in the flat bones or the spine. MR imaging is used for local staging, and bone scan is used to search for metastatic lesions (see **Fig. 10**B).

The differential diagnosis for this condition includes osteomyelitis, lytic osteosarcoma, neuroblastoma metastasis, Langerhans histiocytosis (LH), lymphoma, and leukemia. Osteomyelitis has similar imaging features, and the distinction is further confounded because purulent material may be aspirated from necrotic inflamed Ewing sarcoma. Osteosarcoma favors the metaphysis and shows evidence of osteoid formation. Metastatic neuroblastoma is usually seen in patients younger than 5 years; additionally, lesions are multiple, urinary metabolites are elevated, and a retroperitoneal/mediastinal mass is present in addition to a skeletal metastatic mass. Destructive LH occurs in a younger age group than does Ewing sarcoma and usually presents without a large soft tissue mass. Extraosseous disease in LH is attributed to reactive edema.

The prognosis of patients with Ewing/PNET depends partly on patient age: those who are younger than 10 have a better prognosis. Patients with an axial tumor site, large tumor, chromosome 22 translocation, or metastatic disease have a worse prognosis.[32]

Chordoma

Chordoma is a rare low-grade to intermediate-grade malignant tumor that originates from notochordal remnants. Chordoma accounts for 2% to 4% of all primary malignant bone tumors and is most common in the fifth and sixth decades and in men (2/3:1). This disease is rare in Afro-Caribbean individuals. Chordoma typically occurs as a solitary lesion and is exclusively seen in the axial skeleton, characteristically in the midline of the sacrococcygeal region (50%), spheno-occipital region (40%), or vertebra (5%). Chordoma accounts for 40% of all sacral tumors and is more commonly seen below the S3 level. Spheno-occipital tumors occur in younger patients and are generally smaller than sacrococcygeal

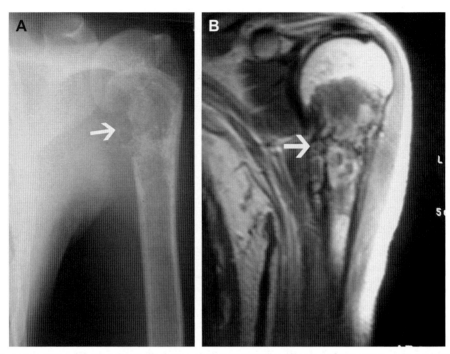

Fig. 10. Ewing sarcoma. (*A*) AP radiograph shows a lytic lesion with wide zone of transition and no matrix mineralization in the proximal humerus, with destruction of the medial cortex (*arrow*). (*B*) Coronal postcontrast T1-weighted image shows a contrast-enhancing lesion in the proximal humerus with soft tissue extension (*arrow*).

chordoma. Vertebral chordoma has equal sex distribution, can affect children, and is more common in the cervical region. Pathologically, these tumors display fluid and mucoid matrix, hemorrhage, necrosis, and sequestered bony fragments without a pseudocapsule. They have a lobular pattern with cohesive vacuolated (physaliferous) and nonvacuolated cells with atypia and infiltration of neighboring trabecular and cortical bone.[33]

Radiologically, these lesions appear advanced, as clinical presentation is delayed because of the slow-growing nature of these tumors and their occurrence in regions that are easily overlooked. Radiographs show a destructive lytic lesion with a soft tissue mass that may have nonspecific, amorphous calcification. A sclerotic margin and narrow transition zone may be present because of slow growth, particularly in spinal lesions (**Fig. 11**A).[34] CT scans show a destructive expansive lesion and a large lobulated soft tissue mass containing calcification. In sacral lesions, an anterior soft tissue mass is seen in 100% of patients and a posterior soft tissue mass is seen in 77% of patients. Calcification, along with residual bone fragments, is seen in 90% of sacral and 15% of vertebral lesions.[33] Because of the gelatinous matrix, the soft tissue mass has low

attenuation on CT and low T1 and high T2 signals on MR imaging (see **Fig. 11**B, C). Hemorrhage, when present, appears as a high T1 signal. Contrast enhancement is variable, appearing minimal in myxoid-containing lobules and moderate in vascular septa, which produces a criss-cross pattern.[35] A 99mTc–methylene diphosphate bone scan may produce negative or photopenic results because of poor reactive bone response. Sacral nerve root involvement is best seen on coronal MR images. Extension to sacroiliac joints, spinal nerves, and plexus should also be assessed. The differential diagnosis for this condition includes chondrosarcoma, plasmacytoma, metastasis, and lymphoma.

Vertebral chordoma lesions begin in the center of the body and extend to the posterior elements, with soft tissue masses seen anterior, posterior, and lateral to the bodies. When the epidural space is involved with breach of the posterior longitudinal ligament, the soft tissue mass may extend to involve multiple craniocaudal contiguous levels. Discal involvement is seen very late in the disease. Because chordoma and discs display the same MR imaging signal, disc involvement is not diagnosed based on MR imaging signal, but on the loss of end-plate integrity. The differential diagnosis for vertebral chordoma includes tuberculosis,

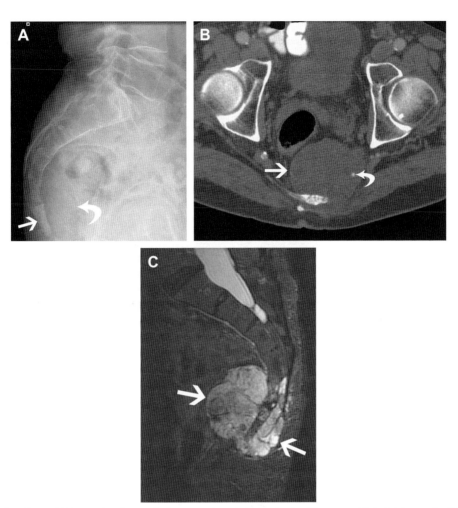

Fig. 11. Chordoma. (*A*) Lateral radiograph shows a sclerotic lesion in the S5 segment (*straight arrow*) with a large presacral soft tissue mass (*curved arrow*). (*B*) Axial CT scan shows destruction of S5 and a large soft tissue mass (*straight arrow*) extending anteriorly and posteriorly. Calcification is seen within the mass (*curved arrow*). (*C*) Sagittal T2-weighted MR image shows a heterogeneous hyperintense mass of the sacrum extending into the soft tissue (*arrows*).

chondrosarcoma, and metastasis from renal adenocarcinoma.[34,36]

Treatment for chordoma includes wide resection and surgical debulking; rectal involvement necessitates a colostomy. The mean survival in patients with chordoma is 5.7 years after the appearance of symptoms. The prognosis is better in younger patients and in those with lesions that are small or sacrococcygeal. Metastasis occurs late in the disease in 10% of patients with sacrococcygeal lesions and in 30% to 40% of patients with spinal lesions. Although metastasis is relatively uncommon, it is locally aggressive, often resulting in severe neurologic symptoms. There is a high rate of local recurrence (as high as 20%), particularly in the surgical bed, which is treated

with radiation. The 5-year survival for patients with chordoma is 50%.

The chondroid variant of chordoma contains cartilaginous areas. This variant accounts for 15% of chordomas, most occurring in the skull base. Imaging features for this condition resemble those of chondrosarcoma. CT and MR imaging show a lobulated tumor, with low attenuation areas and calcification and with low T1 and high T2 signal. Contrast enhancement is not lobular, but there is only mild septal enhancement compared with the lobular, nodular, or diffuse enhancement of chondrosarcomas. Occasionally, a rings-and-arcs pattern of enhancement may be seen. Chordomas (chondroid and nonchondroid) stain for cytokeratins, epithelial membrane antigen (EMA), and carcinoembryonic antigen (CEA), but these antigens are not expressed by chondrosarcomas.[37] Immunochemical studies demonstrate brachyury.[38] Dedifferentiated chordomas account for 6% to 9% of chordomas and can occur in either primary or recurrent chordoma. Dedifferentiated chordoma is more common in the sacrococcygeal region, particularly after radiation. Extra-axial chordomas have also been reported; patients with these lesions tend to have a better prognosis because the tumors are not near vital structures in the midline. CT and MR imaging show destructive lesions with internal hemorrhage and cyst formation.

It should be emphasized that the mere presence of chordoid tissue on biopsy does not confirm the presence of a chordoma; this finding must be correlated with imaging results to differentiate the lesion from a benign notochordal tumor (BNCT), which is typically intracompartmental and does not contain an extraosseous mass.[33]

Malignant Fibrous Histiocytoma

MFH (high-grade pleomorphic sarcoma) of the bone accounts for 2% to 5% of primary bone malignancies. Although most of these lesions arise de novo, 22% to 43% arise secondary to preexisting osseous lesions caused by previous irradiation, bone infarct, Paget disease, chronic osteomyelitis, fibrous dysplasia, aneurysmal bone cyst, GCT, neurofibromatosis-1, or orthopedic implants. Histologically, the MFH is composed of spindle-shaped cells that are arranged in a storiform pattern with varying atypical multinucleated giant cells, foamy cells, and chronic inflammatory cells. MFH is most commonly seen in the fifth to seventh decades of life, with peak incidence in the fifth decade, and is more common in men (3:2). Secondary MFH occurs in an older age group. These lesions are commonly seen at the end of long tubular bones, particularly in the distal diametaphysis of the femur and the proximal metaphysis of the tibia.[10]

Radiographs show an aggressive lytic lesion with permeative pattern of bone destruction. Soft tissue invasion is seen in 88% of cases. Rarely, well-defined margins and even a sclerotic rim have been described.[39] Periosteal reaction is rarely seen (**Fig. 12**). The appearance of these lesions on MR imaging is variable, ranging from isointense to slightly hyperintense relative to muscle on T1-weighted images and intermediate to slightly hyperintense relative to muscle on short TI inversion recovery and T2-weighted images, with nodular and inhomogeneous enhancement. This appearance makes MFH one of the few lytic malignant lesions without a very high T2 signal, similar to lymphoma and leiomyosarcoma,

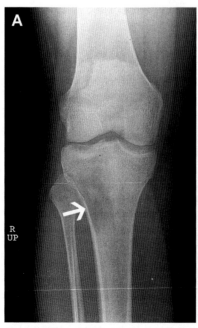
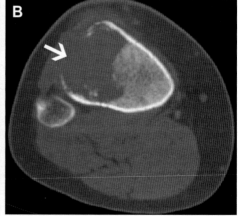

Fig. 12. Malignant fibrous histiocytoma. (*A*) AP radiograph reveals a large lytic lesion in the proximal tibial metaphysis laterally extending into the epiphysis (*arrow*). (*B*) Axial CT scan shows a large lytic lesion that is eccentrically located in the proximal tibial metaphysis and epiphysis with a narrow transition zone and no mineralization with disruption of the anterolateral cortex (*arrow*).

perhaps because of the histologic fibrous tissue matrix and variable cellularity in these lesions.[10] Other investigators have reported predominantly hypointense T1 and hyperintense T2 signals in patients with MFH, however.[40] In secondary MFH, the underlying bone lesion is seen along with MFH. Extraosseous disease is seen in almost all patients with MFH.

MFH has a high rate of local recurrence (80%) and metastasis (46%), particularly to lungs (32%–53%), bones (7%–15%), brain, kidneys, and heart. The 5-year survival rate is 34% to 53%.[10]

Fibrosarcoma

Fibrosarcoma is a malignant tumor composed of fibrous tissue. Like MFH, it can originate de novo or secondary to Paget disease, dedifferentiated chondrosarcoma, bone infarction, radiation, or chronic osteomyelitis. Fibrosarcoma is commonly seen in patients aged 20 to 50 years and occurs equally in men and women. This condition is more common in the long bones, with 50% of lesions arising in the lower limb around the knee joint. The femur is involved in 40% of cases, and the tibia in 15%. Lesions may also occur in the pelvis, humerus, and jaw. Lesions are typically seen in the metaphysis but may extend to the epiphysis. Pure diaphyseal lesions are rare, reported in only 7% of cases. Fibrosarcoma usually occurs as a lytic lesion with a moth-eaten pattern of bone destruction and a wide zone of transition. Patients with fibrosarcoma may have a pathologic fracture. Periosteal reaction is uncommon, but a small soft tissue mass may be seen. Calcification, if present, is typically punctate.[41]

Malignant Vascular Lesions

Malignant vascular lesions are uncommon in the bone and often present with nonspecific clinical and radiologic features. Tumors in this group include hemangioendothelioma, epithelioid hemangioendothelioma, and angiosarcoma. The presence of multifocal lesions within bones, particularly distal to the elbow or knee joints, in young to middle-aged patients warrants consideration of a vascular tumor of bone.

Hemangioendothelioma

Hemangioendothelioma, which includes tumors that were previously called low-grade hemangioendothelioma, hemangioendothelial sarcoma, or angiosarcoma, is a low-grade endothelial neoplasm that can occur at any age between 10 and 60, more commonly in males.[42] It is more common in the lower limb (femur, tibia), followed by vertebrae, upper limb, and flat bones. It is

common in the diaphysis, but also found in the metaphysis or meta-epiphysis.[42] Approximately 25% of affected patients have multicentric disease. The presence of multiple lesions in a solitary bone or extremity or multifocal lesions in various bones is a clue to the diagnosis of this condition. Pathologically, the tumor is vasoformative, with plump endothelial cells lining vascular spaces, which can show poor to high differentiation. Typically, the lesion is purely lytic, although mixed lytic-sclerotic and purely sclerotic lesions may also be seen. Cortical and/or medullary bone is involved in patients with hemangioendothelioma. Osseous expansion, cortical thinning, and endosteal erosion have been reported; periosteal reaction, cortical destruction, and soft tissue masses are uncommon. The differential diagnosis for a multifocal lesion in children includes LH, fibrous dysplasia, brown tumor, and metastasis; the differential diagnosis in adults includes metastasis, myeloma, and lymphoma, and brown tumors and fibrous dysplasia may also present in adults. A solitary lesion can be confused with fibrous dysplasia, fibrous cortical defect, solitary bone cyst, osteosarcoma, fibrosarcoma, or Ewing sarcoma.

Prognosis for these patients is variable and depends on the histologic grade, level of differentiation, and unifocal or multifocal nature of the tumor. Unifocal tumors are treated with surgery and adjuvant therapy, whereas multifocal tumors require radiation therapy.[43] A few cases have been cured with radiofrequency ablation.[44]

Epithelioid hemangioendothelioma is a rare malignant vascular neoplasm that involves multiple skeletal sites and has nonspecific imaging features. This condition can occur across a wide age range, mostly in the second and third decades, and is more common in men. It typically occurs in the calvarium, spine, femur, tibia, and feet. In the long bones, it is seen in the metaphysis or epiphysis. Pathologically, epithelioid hemangioendothelioma is composed of hyalinized stroma and cords or plump cells with abundant eosinophilic cytoplasm. Radiographs show lytic lesions, 40% of which are multifocal and mostly involve a single anatomic site or extremity (Fig. 13). Cortical destruction and expansion are common, whereas periosteal reaction and matrix mineralization are rare. A soft tissue mass is seen in 40% of cases. It is uncertain if patients with multifocal disease have a better prognosis than those with unifocal lesions.[43]

Angiosarcoma

Angiosarcoma is a high-grade malignant vascular tumor that includes such pathologic entities as high-grade angiosarcoma, high-grade hemangioendothelioma, and hemangioendothelial sarcoma.

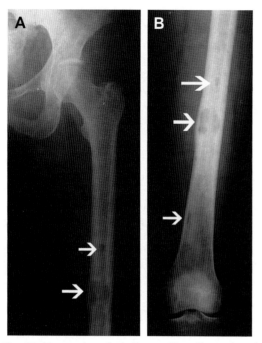

Fig. 13. Hemangioendothelioma. AP radiographs of the left femur (*A, B*) show multiple lytic lesions in the left femur (*arrows*).

Pathologically, these tumors are vasoformative, although less so than hemangioendothelioma or hemangioma, with variable atypical cells and vascular channels. This condition can present at any age, although peak incidence occurs in the third and fourth decades; it is more common in men. The lesions can be unifocal or multifocal, involving 1 or more anatomic regions.[43] Radiologic findings for this condition are nonspecific. Radiographs show a lytic lesion with ill-defined margins, although mixed lytic and sclerotic lesions have also been described. Purely sclerotic lesions are very rare. Endosteal erosion, cortical destruction, and extraosseous extension are common, but periosteal reaction and pathologic fracture are uncommon. The differential diagnosis for this condition includes other primary sarcomas and metastasis. Prognosis for these patients is poor. Management of the disease depends on age; size, number, and location of the tumor; and the amount of intraosseous and extraosseous extension. Treatment options include amputation, limb salvage, radical local resection, and radiation therapy.[43]

Adamantinoma

Adamantinoma is a low-grade epithelioid malignant lesion that is characterized by squamous, alveolar, and vascular tissues of unknown origin.[45] Adamantinoma is commonly seen in the second and third decades and is more common in men. The tibia is the bone most commonly affected (83%), followed by the fibula, humerus, and femur. The classic location is the anterior tibial diaphysis in its mid or proximal portions. Radiographs show an eccentric, intracortical, expansile mixed lytic lesion, which can extend longitudinally in the cortex or destroy the cortex and extend into the medulla (**Fig. 14**). The margins are variable. Multilocularity with thin walls produces a soap bubble appearance. Periosteal reaction and soft tissue mass may be seen. Adamantinoma can be multifocal in the same bone or can involve multiple bones. The differential diagnosis for this condition includes fibrous dysplasia and osteofibrous dysplasia, both of which are based in the cortex. However, fibrous dysplasia arises at a younger age and has ground glass opacity (with or without intralesional opacifications) and anterior tibial bowing without periosteal reaction or moth-eaten

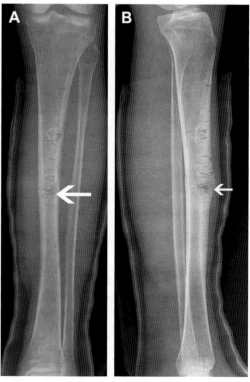

Fig. 14. Adamantinoma. AP (*A*) and lateral (*B*) radiographs of the leg show an osteolytic lesion with peripheral sclerosis involving the anterior cortex of the tibia (*arrow*). Biopsy revealed adamantioma. Additional multiple transverse linear lucencies within the cortex are of uncertain etiology, perhaps representing stress fractures related to underlying weakened bone.

destruction. Unlike adamantinoma, osteofibrous dysplasia occurs in patients younger than 10 years and is typically intracortical without medullary extension. Age is a helpful discriminator when imaging findings overlap.[46] A variant of adamantinoma is differentiated adamantinoma (osteofibrous dysplasialike adamantinoma), a diagnosis that is based on histology. It has a prolonged course similar to osteofibrous dysplasia and is treated less aggressively.[47] Although adamantinoma is locally nonaggressive and can be indolent for many years, metastasis, particularly to the lung, bones, and lymph nodes, is seen in 20% of patients. Adamantinoma is treated with wide local excision, but recurrence is common. The 10-year survival rate is higher than 80%.[46]

Malignant Giant-Cell Tumor

Malignant GCT is a term loosely applied to a heterogeneous group of tumors containing giant cells that have aggressive local behavior and systemic metastasis. The malignant GCT classification can be divided into categories of malignancy in GCT, giant-cell–containing sarcoma, secondary malignant GCT, and benign metastasizing GCT.[48,49] Malignancy in GCT and secondary malignant GCT account for 6% of all GCTs. Malignancy in GCT (13%) contains sarcomatous areas juxtaposed with typical benign GCT in patients with no history of radiation, resection, or curettage (**Fig. 15**); when a sarcoma develops in patients with a history of radiation, resection, or curettage of conventional GCT, the lesion is labeled secondary malignant GCT (87%). A history of radiation is present in 76% of these secondary GCT cases, with a latent period of 10 years or longer. Secondary malignant GCT in the absence of radiation is an exceptional event, with fewer than 6 well-documented cases.[50] Malignancy in GCT is said to occur in an older population than conventional GCTs. In our opinion, however, because these cases are so few, no firm conclusion can be drawn about age distribution. Giant-cell–containing sarcoma is an anaplastic variant of the typical benign GCT, but without evidence of tumor osteoid, bone, or cartilage. It is often associated with Paget disease and should be differentiated pathologically from giant-cell–rich sarcoma variants, such as osteosarcoma, fibrosarcoma, and MFH. Benign metastasizing GCT is a term used for skeletal GCT with pulmonary metastasis that is histologically identical to GCT. It is seen in 1.8% to 5% of GCTs. Local recurrence is seen in 48% of these patients. The prognosis for these patients is good. Metastasectomy is recommended when feasible.[49,51]

Leiomyosarcoma

Primary bone leiomyosarcoma is a rare malignant spindle-cell tumor with smooth muscle differentiation, believed to arise from smooth muscle cells of blood vessels or mesenchymal myofibroblasts. Only 120 cases have been reported in the literature to date.[52] Leiomyosarcoma is most commonly seen in the fourth through seventh decades, with equal sex distribution. The lesions typically occur in the medullary cavity of long tubular bones, centered in the metaphysis with extension to the epiphysis or diaphysis. The radiographic features of this condition are nonspecific and show an osteolytic lesion with aggressive features and ill-defined tumor margins. Periosteal reaction, Codman triangle, pathologic fracture, and soft tissue extension are commonly seen. A remarkable feature of this condition is the length of the lesion (up to 11 cm), which is unlike a metastasis but similar to lymphoma (**Fig. 16**A). CT of these lesions shows contrast enhancement in hypervascular areas. The tumor is isointense to hypointense relative to skeletal muscle on T1-weighted images (see **Fig. 16**B) and isointense to hypointense relative to fat on nonfat-suppressed T2-weighted images. This low T2 signal is an unusual feature for a lytic lesion and is caused by the smooth muscle component. A similar appearance is seen on scans of lymphoma. Leiomyosarcoma appears hyperintense on T2-weighted images with fat saturation. High uptake is seen on bone scans. Metastatic disease from the uterus or gastrointestinal tract should be excluded before a lesion is diagnosed as a primary leiomyosarcoma of bone. The mean survival of patients with this condition is 33 months; the tumor often metastasizes to the lung, lumbar spine, skin, and liver.[52]

Liposarcoma

Primary intraosseous liposarcoma is extremely rare. A sarcoma arising from a fat-containing bone infarct is more common than primary intraosseous liposarcoma, and the diagnosis of primary liposarcoma of bone is made only after exclusion of other tumor elements and metastatic spread from a soft tissue liposarcoma. Primary intraosseous liposarcoma affects all ages, is more common in those 24 to 45 years old, and is more common in men than in women. These lesions occur in the long bones, particularly the femur and tibia, and can be seen in epiphysis, metaphysis, or diaphysis. Radiographic appearances of these lesions are nonspecific, showing a lytic lesion associated with cortical destruction. Fluid-fluid levels may also be seen. Although fat-containing lesions are generally considered

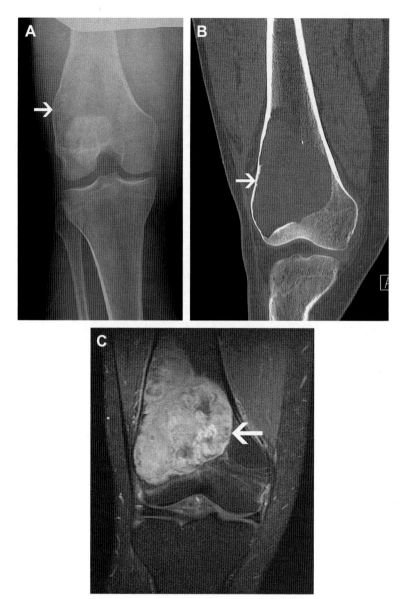

Fig. 15. Malignancy in a giant-cell tumor. (*A*) AP radiograph shows a well-defined expansile lesion in the distal femur (*arrow*) extending to its subarticular end with no periosteal reaction or cortical destruction. (*B*) Coronal CT image demonstrates the expansile lesion of the distal femur (*arrow*). (*C*) Coronal postcontrast T1-weighted MR image shows heterogeneous enhancement with areas of necrosis (*arrow*). The imaging appearances are suggestive of a benign giant cell tumor; however, biopsy of this lesion revealed a tumor with giant cells and malignant osteoid, not thought to be sufficient to histologically label it as giant-cell–rich osteosarcoma.

benign, the presence of cortical destruction and soft tissue mass is suggestive of malignancy and warrants a biopsy.[53]

Anaplastic Sarcoma

Anaplastic sarcoma is a highly malignant bone tumor composed of immature cells; the cell of origin for these tumors cannot be determined. The imaging appearances are nonspecific and typically include a lytic locally aggressive lesion.

SUMMARY

Primary malignant bone tumors are uncommon. Diagnosis of these conditions is typically based

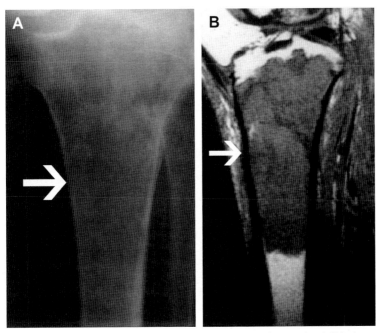

Fig. 16. Leiomyosarcoma. (*A*) AP radiograph shows a large lytic lesion in the proximal tibia (*arrow*) without significant matrix, the most common appearance for leiomyosarcoma. (*B*) Sagittal T1-weighted MR image shows homogeneous hypointense tumor involving the proximal tibial metaphysis and diaphysis (*arrow*). Often, MR imaging reveals a lesion longer than suggested by radiographs, a feature that leiomyosarcoma shares with lymphoma.

on the radiographic features combined with clinical and demographic features. CT and MR imaging scans are useful in further staging the tumors by determining intraosseous and extraosseous spread.

ACKNOWLEDGMENTS

The authors thank Megan Griffiths, scientific writer for the Imaging Institute, Cleveland Clinic, for her help in the preparation of this article.

REFERENCES

1. Dorman HD, Czerniak B. Bone cancers. Cancer 1995;75(Suppl 1):203–10.
2. Unni KK, Inwards CY, Bridge JA, et al. Tumors of the bones and joints. 4th series ed. AFIP Atlas of tumor pathology, series 4. Washington, DC: American Registry of Pathology; 2005.
3. Kindblom LG. Bone tumors: epidemiology, classification, pathology. In: Davies AM, Sundaram M, James SJ, editors. Imaging of bone tumors and tumor-like lesions. Berlin: Springer; 2009. p. 1–15.
4. Fletcher CD, Unni KK, Mertens F, editors. World Health Organization classification of tumors. Pathology and genetics of tumours of soft tissue and bone (IARC WHO Classification of Tumours). Lyon (France): IARC Press; 2002.
5. Sheppard DG, Libshitz HI. Post-radiation sarcomas: a review of the clinical and imaging features in 63 cases. Clin Radiol 2001;56(1):22–9.
6. Davies AM, James SL. Radiation-induced tumors. In: Davies AM, Sundaram M, James SJ, editors. Imaging of bone tumors and tumor-like lesions. Berlin: Springer; 2009. p. 503–13.
7. Davies AM, Pluot E, James SL. Tumor and tumor-like conditions associated with Paget's disease of bone. In: Davies AM, Sundaram M, James SJ, editors. Imaging of bone tumors and tumor-like lesions. Berlin: Springer; 2009. p. 515–28.
8. Smith SE, Murphey MD, Motamedi K, et al. From the archives of the AFIP. Radiologic spectrum of Paget disease of bone and its complications with pathologic correlation. Radiographics 2002;22(5):1191–216.
9. Sundaram M, Khanna G, El-Khoury GY. T1-weighted MR imaging for distinguishing large osteolysis of Paget's disease from sarcomatous degeneration. Skeletal Radiol 2001;30(7):378–83.
10. Koplas MC, Lefkowitz RA, Bauer TW, et al. Imaging findings, prevalence and outcome of de novo and secondary malignant fibrous histiocytoma of bone. Skeletal Radiol 2010;39(8):791–8.
11. Ruggieri P, Sim FH, Bond JR, et al. Malignancies in fibrous dysplasia. Cancer 1994;73(5):1411–24.

12. White LM, Kandel R. Osteoid-producing tumours of bone. Semin Musculoskelet Radiol 2000;4(1):25–43.

13. Bielack SS, Kempf-Bielack B, Delling G, et al. Prognostic factors in high-grade osteosarcoma of the extremities or trunk: an analysis of 1,702 patients treated on neoadjuvant cooperative osteosarcoma study group protocols. J Clin Oncol 2002;20(3):776–90.

14. Murphey MD, wan Jaovisidha S, Temple HT, et al. Telangiectatic osteosarcoma: radiologic-pathologic comparison. Radiology 2003;229(2):545–53.

15. Kransdorf MJ, Murphey MD. Osseous tumors. In: Davies AM, Sundaram M, James SJ, editors. Imaging of bone tumors and tumor-like lesions. Berlin: Springer; 2009. p. 251–306.

16. Andresen KJ, Sundaram M, Unni KK, et al. Imaging features of low-grade central osteosarcoma of the long bones and pelvis. Skeletal Radiol 2004;33(7):373–9.

17. Sundaram M. Imaging of Paget's disease and fibrous dysplasia of bone. J Bone Miner Res 2006;21(Suppl 2):P28–30.

18. Okada K, Frassica FJ, Sim FH, et al. Parosteal osteosarcoma. A clinicopathologic study. J Bone Joint Surg Am 1994;76(3):366–78.

19. Jelinek JS, Murphey MD, Kransdorf MJ, et al. Parosteal osteosarcoma: value of MR imaging and CT in the prediction of histologic grade. Radiology 1996;201(3):837–42.

20. Nuovo MA, Norman A, Chumas J, et al. Myositis ossificans with atypical clinical, radiographic, or pathologic findings: a review of 23 cases. Skeletal Radiol 1992;21(2):87–101.

21. Murphey MD, Jelinek JS, Temple HT, et al. Imaging of periosteal osteosarcoma: radiologic-pathologic comparison. Radiology 2004;233(1):129–38.

22. Griffith JF, Kumta SM, Chow LT, et al. Intracortical osteosarcoma. Skeletal Radiol 1998;27(4):228–32.

23. Ludwig K. Cartilage tumors. In: Davies AM, Sundaram M, James SJ, editors. Imaging of bone tumors and tumor-like lesions. Berlin: Springer; 2009. p. 225–50.

24. Murphey MD, Walker EA, Wilson AJ, et al. From the archives of the AFIP: imaging of primary chondrosarcoma: radiologic-pathologic correlation. Radiographics 2003;23(5):1245–78.

25. Flemming DJ, Murphey MD. Enchondroma and chondrosarcoma. Semin Musculoskelet Radiol 2000;4(1):59–71.

26. Bui KL, Ilaslan H, Bauer TW, et al. Cortical scalloping and cortical penetration by small eccentric chondroid lesions in the long tubular bones; not a sign of malignancy? Skeletal Radiol 2009;38(8):791–6.

27. Nakashima Y, Unni KK, Shives TC, et al. Mesenchymal chondrosarcoma of bone and soft tissue. A review of 111 cases. Cancer 1986;57(12):2444–53.

28. MacSweeney F, Darby A, Saifuddin A. Differentiated chondrosarcoma of the appendicular skeleton: MRI-pathological correlation. Skeletal Radiol 2003;32(12):671–8.

29. Littrell LA, Wenger DE, Wold LE, et al. Radiographic, CT, and MR imaging features of dedifferentiated chondrosarcomas: a retrospective review of 174 de novo cases. Radiographics 2004;24(5):1397–409.

30. Vanel D, De Paolis M, Monti C, et al. Radiological features of 24 periosteal chondrosarcomas. Skeletal Radiol 2001;30(4):208–12.

31. Lin PP, Moussallem CD, Deavers MT. Secondary chondrosarcoma. J Am Acad Orthop Surg 2010;18:608–15.

32. Vanhoenacker FM, Kerkhove FV, Peersman B, et al. Ewing's sarcoma/PNET tumors. In: Davies AM, Sundaram M, James SJ, editors. Imaging of bone tumors and tumor-like lesions. Berlin: Springer; 2009. p. 337–50.

33. Cassar-Pullicino VN, Mangham DC. Notochordal tumors. In: Davies AM, Sundaram M, James SJ, editors. Imaging of bone tumors and tumor-like lesions. Berlin: Springer; 2009. p. 375–92.

34. deBruine FT, Kroon HM. Spinal chordoma: radiologic features in 14 cases. AJR Am J Roentgenol 1988;150(4):861–3.

35. Sung MS, Lee GK, Kang HS, et al. Sacrococcygeal chordoma: MR imaging in 30 patients. Skeletal Radiol 2005;34(2):87–94.

36. Papagelopoulos PJ, Mavrogenis AF, Galanis EC, et al. Chordoma of the spine: clinicopathological features, diagnosis, and treatment. Orthopedics 2004;27(12):1256–63.

37. Rosenberg AE, Brown GA, Bhan AK, et al. Chondroid chordoma—a variant of chordoma. A morphologic and immunohistochemical study. Am J Clin Pathol 1994;101:36–41.

38. Vujovic S, Henderson S, Presneau N, et al. Brachyury, a crucial regulator of notochordal development, is a novel biomarker for chordomas. J Pathol 2006;209(2):157–65.

39. Yokoyama R, Tsuneyoshi M, Enjoji M, et al. Prognostic factors of malignant fibrous histiocytoma of bone. A clinical and histopathologic analysis of 34 cases. Cancer 1993;72(6):1902–8.

40. Link TM, Haeussler MD, Poppek S, et al. Malignant fibrous histiocytoma of bone: conventional x-ray and MR imaging features. Skeletal Radiol 1998;27(10):552–8.

41. Papagelopoulos PJ, Galanis EC, Trantafyllidis P, et al. Clinicopathologic features, diagnosis, and treatment of fibrosarcoma of bone. Am J Orthop 2002;31(5):253–7.

42. Campanacci M, Boriani S, Giunti A. Hemangioendothelioma of bone. Cancer 1980;46:804–14.

43. Wenger DE, Wold LE. Malignant vascular lesions of bone: radiologic and pathologic features. Skeletal Radiol 2000;29(11):619–31.

44. Rosenthal DI, Treat ME, Mankin HJ, et al. Treatment of epithelioid hemangioendothelioma of bone using a novel combined approach. Skeletal Radiol 2001; 30(4):219–22.

45. Van der Woude HJ, Hazelbag HM, Bloem JL, et al. MRI of adamantinoma of long bones in correlation with histopathology. Am J Roentgenol 2004;183(6):1737–44.

46. Mannava S, Sundaram M. Fibrous dysplasia, osteofibrous dysplasia, and adamantinoma. In: Davies AM, Sundaram M, James SJ, editors. Imaging of bone tumors and tumor-like lesions. Berlin: Springer; 2009. p. 411–24.

47. Kahn LB. Adamantinoma, osteofibrous dysplasia and differentiated adamantinoma. Skeletal Radiol 2003;32(5):245–58.

48. Kransdorf MJ, Murphey MD. Giant cell tumor. In: Davies AM, Sundaram M, James SJ, editors. Imaging of bone tumors and tumor-like lesions. Berlin: Springer; 2009. p. 321–36.

49. Mirra JM. Giant cell tumor. In: Mirra JM, Picci P, Gold RH, editors. Bone tumors: clinical, radiologic, and pathologic correlations. 2nd edition. Philadelphia: Lea and Febiger; 1989. p. 941–1020.

50. Schajowicz F, Granato DB, McDonald DJ, et al. Clinical and radiological features of atypical giant cell tumors of bone. Br J Radiol 1991;64(766):877–89.

51. Viswanathan S, Jambhekar NA. Metastatic giant cell tumor of bone: are there associated factors and best treatment modalities? Clin Orthop Relat Res 2010; 468(3):827–33.

52. Simpfendorfer C, Sundaram M. Smooth muscle tumors. In: Davies AM, Sundaram M, James SJ, editors. Imaging of bone tumors and tumor-like lesions. Berlin: Springer; 2009. p. 393–400.

53. Campbell RS. Lipogenic tumors of the bone. In: Davies AM, Sundaram M, James SJ, editors. Imaging of bone tumors and tumor-like lesions. Berlin: Springer; 2009. p. 401–10.

Hematopoietic Tumors and Metastases Involving Bone

Sung H. Kim, MD[a], Stacy E. Smith, MD[b],
Michael E. Mulligan, MD[a],*

KEYWORDS

- Metastases • Myeloma • Lymphoma • Leukemia
- Langerhans cell histiocytosis

Diseases involving marrow replacement are commonly encountered pathologic processes that often present with vague nonspecific symptoms. Imaging findings of marrow replacement are frequently subtle on screening radiographs and often require a high level of suspicion on the part of the radiologist. Whether focal or diffuse in nature, an appreciation of the underlying pathophysiologic basis for each process helps radiologists to not only better understand the related imaging features but also facilitate accurate staging, aid in subsequent imaging follow-up, and be better aware of the types and appearances of potential complications. This review explores in depth the most common malignant process involving the bone, namely metastatic disease, as well as some of the more common proliferative forms of hematopoietic disease of bone marrow.

METASTATIC DISEASE

Metastatic disease to bone is the most common malignant process in the skeleton. It is 25 to 35 times more common than any primary bone tumor and accounts for approximately 140,000 new cases in the United States annually.[1] More than 80% of adult cases arise from prostate, breast, lung, thyroid, and renal carcinomas. Neuroblastoma accounts for most cases in children.

Bone metastases often present with pain and may be complicated by fracture, spinal cord and/or nerve root compression (**Fig. 1**), hypercalcemia, and infection from bone marrow suppression. Statistically, osseous metastatic involvement is most common, followed by lung and liver metastases.[2] Bone marrow vascular permeability allows hematopoietic precursors ready access to the circulation as well as reverse transport of metastatic cells to the nutrient-rich environment the marrow provides. As a result, metastatic spread through the venous system is more common than lymphatic or arterial spread. The lung and liver act as effective venous filters and trap malignant cells, thus explaining the high incidence of metastatic disease in these organs. Despite the high prevalence of gastrointestinal cancers, metastatic bone involvement from these tumors is low.

Osseous metastases can occur without disease in the liver or the lung. This is in large part due to the existence of Batson plexus.[3] This extensive network of valveless paraspinal veins was shown by Batson to communicate directly with the deep pelvic veins and caval venous system. Batson plexus now has been shown to form extensive communications with the azygous, intercostal, posterior bronchial, parietal, and pleural venous systems as well as the upper-extremity and lower-extremity veins and occasionally renal veins

The authors have nothing to disclose.

[a] Department of Radiology, University of Maryland Medical Center, 22 South Greene Street, Baltimore, MD 21201, USA

[b] Musculoskeletal Radiology, Department of Radiology, Brigham and Women's Hospital, 75 Francis Street, Boston, MA 02115, USA

* Corresponding author. Department of Radiology, UMMS, 22 South Greene Street, Baltimore, MD 21201.
E-mail address: mmulligan@umm.edu

Radiol Clin N Am 49 (2011) 1163–1183
doi:10.1016/j.rcl.2011.07.004
0033-8389/11/$ – see front matter © 2011 Elsevier Inc. All rights reserved.

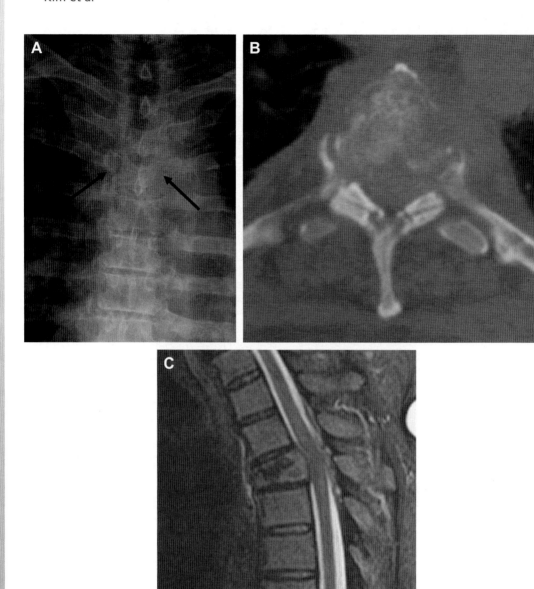

Fig. 1. A 50-year-old man with metastatic hepatocellular carcinoma presents with back pain. (*A*) Frontal view of the thoracic spine shows absence of T4 vertebral body pedicles (*arrows*). (*B*) CT through the T4 level shows pathologic compression fracture with metastatic deposit involving the vertebral body and both pedicles. (*C*) T2 STIR MR imaging shows the pathologic compression fracture with characteristic convexity into the spinal canal. Resulting spinal cord compression and contusion is demonstrated with increased signal change in the central cord.

in addition to pelvic viscera. Clinically, this results in the majority of bone metastases occurring in the axial skeleton and the proximal long bones.

Because arterial spread metastatic disease typically occurs secondary to bronchogenic carcinoma invading a pulmonary vein, distant metastases (below the elbow joint or knee joint) are most commonly due to lung cancer, although they have been reported secondary to many other primary malignancies. Although direct local invasion occurs less commonly, it nevertheless comprises a significant route of disease spread. Two important examples are (1) Pancoast tumor (**Fig. 2**), which spreads to adjacent ribs and vertebra, and (2) malignant paraspinal lymph node invasion of adjacent vertebra.

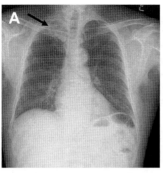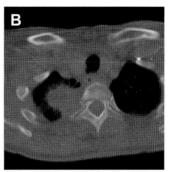

Fig. 2. A 60-year-old man with Pancoast tumor who presented with right shoulder pain. (*A*) Posteroanterior chest radiograph shows a right apical opacity (*arrow*). (*B*) CT scan shows a right apical tumor with direct extension through the pleura, destroying the adjacent posterior third rib medially.

IMAGING APPEARANCE

Most metastatic foci are lytic (**Fig. 3**) largely due to activation of osteoclasts and synthesis of collagenase by osteoclasts. Osteoclast-stimulating factors, which act to stimulate the osteoclastic bone resorption, have been isolated from primary bone tumors (myeloma and lymphoma) and in certain cases of metastases.[4] Also, parathyroid hormone–related protein, in addition to being responsible for hypercalcemia, leads to unchecked osteoclastic activity. Coupled with the hypervascularity of metastatic lesions, increased osteoclastic destruction often results in myriad complications not limited to pathologic fractures. Alternatively, blastic metastatic lesions (**Fig. 4**), such as those seen in prostate cancer, result when there is unchecked osteoblastic stimulation. New bone formation has been shown to result from stimulation with endothelin-1.

Due to its tremendous frequency, any new bone lesion in a patient older than 40 years of age is considered metastatic until proved otherwise. Imaging work-up must depend on clinical history, physical examination, and appropriate laboratory studies and must be directed with the goal of establishing a diagnosis of primary tumor or metastatic involvement as well as determining the extent of disease. In some cases, a primary tumor may not be located. In one study, 60% of the primary tumors could not be found despite extensive work-up, including laparotomy.[5]

The ideal imaging technique for initial staging and monitoring would quickly and accurately identify all active sites of disease. No single imaging modality satisfies all the criteria in all different situations. Current whole-body imaging techniques include positron emission tomography (PET), PET/CT, MR imaging, CT, and nuclear scintigraphy (**Fig. 5**) using various agents. Any of these may be the "right" study for an individual patient. The work-up should, therefore, be tailored for individual circumstances depending on various clinical factors.

Metastases can and do have a varied radiographic appearance, ranging from purely lytic to purely blastic with mixed lytic/blastic types and lytic blowout patterns in between. Lytic metastases are most common and range in appearance

Fig. 3. A 73-year-old man with metastatic lung cancer. A large lytic lesion is present in the humeral head with a pathologic fracture through the surgical humeral neck.

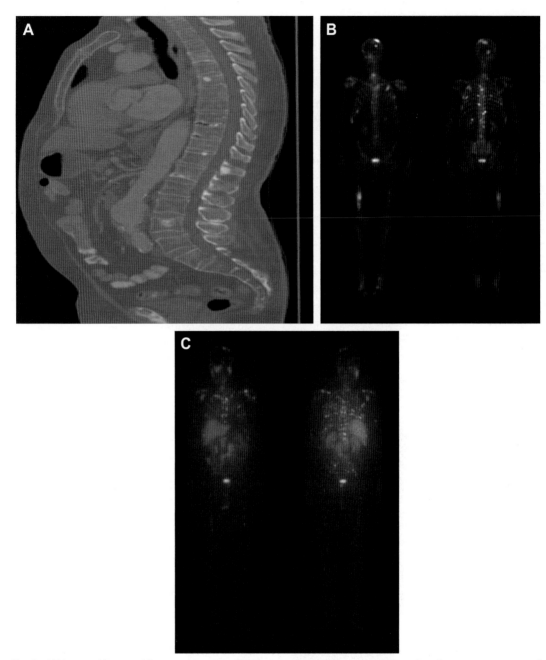

Fig. 4. A 74-year-old man with prostate cancer. (*A*) Reconstructed sagittal CT of the spine shows numerous purely blastic metastatic foci involving vertebral bodies and posterior spinal elements. (*B*) Whole-body technetium Tc99m MDP bone scan allows quick overall assessment of the entire skeleton. (*C*) Indium In 111 capromab pendetide (ProstaScint) scintigraphy is a whole-body imaging technique specific for evaluating prostate cancer.

from geographic to permeative (**Fig. 6**). Breast and lung are the most common primary sites. If a breast cancer patient presents solely with bone metastasis, the patient has a better prognosis than those with additional visceral metastatic disease.[6] Lytic blowout patterns are seen typically with renal cell (**Fig. 7**) and thyroid carcinomas but can be seen with breast and lung carcinomas as well. A mixed lytic/blastic pattern is sometimes seen, particularly with breast, lung, and gastrointestinal tract tumors. Purely blastic metastases are most often seen with prostate cancer (see **Fig. 4**A) with lesser

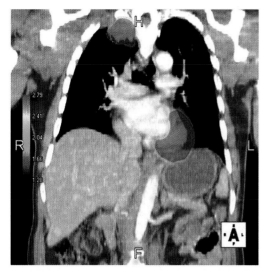

Fig. 5. Whole-body imaging techniques. MR imaging, PET, CT, and MDP bone scan are some current available options. PET/CT image of the Pancoast tumor (seen in **Fig. 2**) shows hypermetabolic activity in the apical mass but no other focus of abnormal metabolic activity.

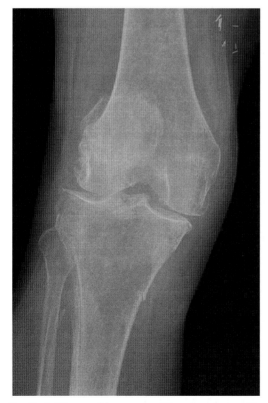

Fig. 6. A 78-year-old woman with colon cancer. The metastatic focus to the proximal right tibia shows a purely lytic geographic pattern on radiograph.

percentages reported from carcinoid, medulloblastoma, breast (**Fig. 8**), and small cell lung carcinomas.

The increased availability of multislice helical CT scanners allows high-quality routine coronal and sagittal plane reformatted images to be obtained easily. This technique is especially valuable in the pelvis and in the peripheral skeleton, especially in patients who cannot undergo MR imaging.

The basic MR imaging sequences for evaluating metastatic disease include T1-weighted and fat-saturated T2-weighted or inversion recovery sequences in multiple planes. Inversion recovery sequences are often superior especially for large fields of view, with metal artifacts, and other instances of field inhomogeneity. Intravenous gadolinium contrast is not routinely needed when evaluating osseous metastasis. The decision to use gadolinium should be made on an individual basis, such as in those patients requiring concurrent evaluation of visceral organs or in those patients with a lesion that is difficult to characterize. Diffusion-weighted imaging and in-and-out-of-phase imaging can also be used in certain circumstances. With regard to in-phase and out-of-phase imaging, a signal drop of at least 20% on out-of-phase imaging relative to in-phase imaging reliably rules out a metastatic lesion with 95% specificity and sensitivity.[7]

Bone scintigraphy with technetium Tc 99m methylene diphosphonate (MDP) is an invaluable modality that provides a quick overall survey of the entire skeleton (see **Fig. 4**B). Up to 64% of all solitary axial skeletal lesions have been shown to be metastatic, with the caveat that if the lesion is rib based, only 10% to 17% represent a metastatic focus.[8,9] Multiplicity of lesions increases the probability of metastatic disease, although other polyostotic processes are listed in **Box 1**.

Fluorodeoxyglucose F 18 (FDG)-PET/CT has established itself as the modality of choice in initial staging and subsequent follow-up of many primary carcinomas. Its reliability was demonstrated recently by a study that indicates that even solitary lesions have a 98% positive predictive value for metastatic disease when FDG-PET and CT findings are concordant.[10] Lytic lesions tend to exhibit higher uptake than sclerotic lesions and thus are more conspicuous (see **Fig. 5**; **Fig. 9**). Carbon C11 choline–PET has been shown, however, to be more sensitive and specific than FDG-PET/CT and technetium Tc 99m skeletal scintigraphy for evaluation of prostate cancer metastasis.[11] Usefulness for evaluating multiple myeloma also has been demonstrated recently.[12]

Due to its pathophysiologic features, including its rich blood supply and active red marrow, the

A   **B**

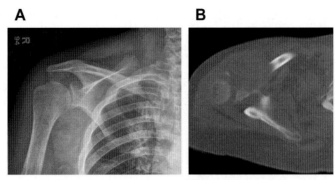

Fig. 7. A 51-year-old woman with metastatic renal cell carcinoma. The coracoid process is absent on the conventional radiograph (*A*) due to a large lytic blowout metastatic lesion better seen on CT (*B*).

vertebral body is the most common site of metastatic deposit. Thoracic and lumbar vertebrae are more frequently affected than cervical vertebrae. Clinical presentation can range from asymptomatic to back and/or radicular pain, weakness, sensory deficits, bowel/bladder dysfunction, pathologic fracture, cord compression and paralysis.

Vertebral body lesions may not be detectable on radiographs until 50% to 75% of the vertebral body has been destroyed.[13] Vertebral collapse is a common manifestation of metastasis but up to 30% of patients may have a nonmalignant cause of compression in the setting of known stage IV cancer.[14] A few features can help guide differentiation between benign and malignant causes. Intravertebral gas is usually specific for a benign vertebral fracture or avascular necrosis and usually rules out a malignant fracture. Benign

compression fractures of cervical and upper thoracic vertebra (above T6 level) are rare. Bony destruction and acute angular endplate deformities are features rarely seen with osteoporotic fractures and bring forth the possibility of metastatic involvement.[15] Pedicle involvement is typical of metastasis but it is a late finding (see **Fig. 1**).[16]

For evaluation of vertebral bone marrow, MR imaging is currently the modality of choice. Neoplastic involvement typically shows focal marrow replacement with tumoral tissue, which shows lower T1 signal than adjacent skeletal muscle and accompanying high T2 signal (see **Fig. 1C**). If the lesion is sclerotic, it may demonstrate low signal on both T1-weighted and

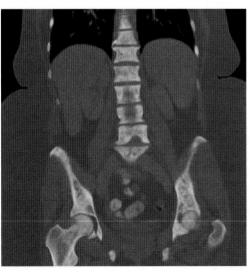

Fig. 8. A 58-year-old woman with metastatic breast cancer showing diffuse blastic metastasis throughout the lumbar spine.

Box 1
Osseous metastatic disease mimics

- Multiple myeloma
- Multifocal infection/inflammation
  - Chronic recurrent multifocal osteomyelitis
  - Synovitis, acne, pustulosis, hyperostosis, and osteitis syndrome
- Polyostotic fibrous dysplasia
- Sarcoidosis
- Brown tumors
- Primary lymphoma of bone (PLB) (multifocal type)
- Angiomatosis
  - Bacillary
  - Systemic
- Tuberous sclerosis
- Langerhans cell histiocytosis
- Myofibromatosis

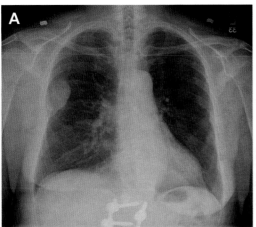
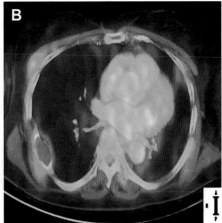

Fig. 9. A 72-year-old woman with breast cancer. Large expansile right sixth rib lesion seen on chest radiograph (*A*) led to survey with nuclear scintigraphy. (*B*) The left sixth rib lesion also demonstrates hypermetabolic activity on FDG-PET scan on fused PET/CT image.

T2-weighted sequences. Red marrow involvement, especially in children, is better appreciated on T2-weighted or short tau inversion recovery (STIR) imaging. The lesions may be focal or may involve the entire vertebra.

Several features on MR imaging can help distinguish benign and malignant causes of vertebral collapse. A benign osteoporotic fracture is suggested when a retropulsed fragment is present, when T1 fat signal is preserved without increased T2 signal, and when a horizontal fracture plane is seen. The fracture plane may be better demonstrated after contrast administration. A malignant cause of fracture is suggested when the posterior cortex is convex toward the spinal canal (see **Fig. 1**C), when an epidural mass is present, when the pedicles are involved, and when high or heterogeneous signal is seen on T2 sequences or with contrast administration.[17]

MR imaging also can be used for problem solving when the radiologist is confronted with difficult lesions. Dynamic contrast imaging studies have shown a 100% positive predictive value of metastatic involvement when there is rapid wash in and early washout.[14] For a focal lesion, a high–signal intensity T2 rim has been termed, the *halo sign*, and is associated with malignancy. Chemical shift may allow differentiation of fracture-related edema from tumor marrow replacement by nulling out fluid signal in a local fat rich environment, such as that present with benign compression fractures. Diffusion-weighted imaging is another technique by which benign compression and malignant fractures can be distinguished. High signal intensity on diffusion-weighted images seen with pathologic fractures may be explained by decreased water

mobility resulting from dense packing of tumorous tissue and decreased extracellular free water.[18]

CT can be used for detecting metastatic bony lesions, albeit with less sensitivity than with MR imaging. Nevertheless, it plays an important role, especially in patients who for various reasons are not able to be evaluated with MR imaging. Many morphologic findings discussed in regard to radiographs and MR imaging apply to this modality.

PET and nuclear scintigraphy often demonstrate scattered foci of increased uptake, which are typically not in a linear orientation (see **Fig. 4**B). Localization of activity at the vertebral endplates or at the facets suggests a benign entity rather than metastatic disease.

Findings of an ivory vertebral body (**Fig. 10**) merit special mention. The term, *ivory vertebral body*, refers to a homogeneously dense vertebral body and has been associated with metastatic disease in approximately 50% of cases.[19] Hodgkin disease accounts for approximately 30% of all cases of ivory vertebra. Slightly less frequent are metastases from all other sources. The other 50% of ivory vertebrae are usually due to Paget disease. Rare entities, such as osteomyelitis or chordoma, also have been described as occasionally having an ivory vertebral body appearance.

Hypertrophic osteoarthropathy is seen in 3% to 10% of patients with bronchogenic carcinoma.[20] Mesothelioma has higher association but is much less common than primary lung cancer. The etiology of hypertrophic osteoarthropathy is still unclear and it has been associated with many conditions (**Fig. 11**). Clinically, patients present with clubbing and/or articular pain and swelling. Periostitis is most pronounced along

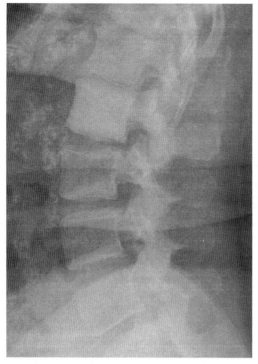

Fig. 10. A 31-year-old woman with ivory vertebra. The patient presented after trauma and was, unfortunately, lost to follow-up.

uncommon, focal proliferative periosteal reaction can be seen with metastatic disease. Underlying sclerotic lesions with florid focal periosteal reaction are seen most commonly with prostate cancer and can mimic primary osteosarcoma. Neuroblastoma, bronchogenic carcinoma, and gastrointestinal tumors also have been shown to have focal proliferative periosteal reaction pattern.

Less-common manifestations of metastatic disease include cortical, soft tissue, and synovial involvement. The cookie bite (Fig. 12) appearance of cortical metastasis is most often seen with lung cancer although other primary cancers also may be causative.[21] Soft tissue metastases are frequently small and subcutaneous in location. Larger deeper lesions can represent foci of bronchogenic carcinoma soft tissue metastasis. In such circumstances, however, a primary soft tissue tumor should strongly be considered in the differential diagnosis. Synovial metastatic involvement is rare. It may occur as direct extension from adjacent bone. The knee is the most commonly affected joint with breast and lung cancers accounting for most of the known cases. Findings are nonspecific with thickening of the synovium. Rare calcifications may be seen. Joint aspiration

the paired long bones of the radius/ulna and tibia/fibula, typically along the metadiaphysis sparing the epiphysis. Frequently, thick, solid, smooth, and undulating periostitis is noted on radiographs. Nuclear scintigraphy is more sensitive and its findings consist of increased uptake in a parallel manner along the long bones. Although

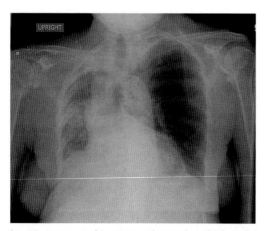

Fig. 11. Hypertrophic osteoarthropathy. Thick, solid, undulating periosteal reaction is seen along the metadiaphysis of both humeri.

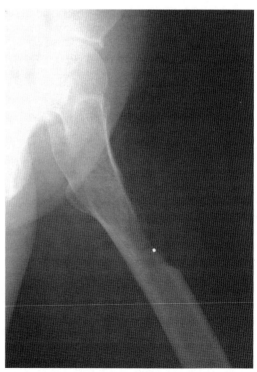

Fig. 12. A 50-year-old woman with breast cancer shows a cortical metastasis to the proximal femur.

can be performed for cytologic diagnosis whereas synovial biopsy frequently provides the definitive diagnosis.

PATHOLOGIC FRACTURE

The incidence of pathologic fracture ranges between 7% and 27%.[22] It is more common in the lower extremity. Breast cancer patients have the highest rate of pathologic fracture, occurring in approximately 39%.[22] Melanoma rarely results in pathologic fractures. Nontraumatic fractures, transverse fractures (see **Fig. 3**), and nontraumatic avulsion of the lesser trochanter are some specific patterns associated with pathologic fractures.

Histologically, reparative and/or resorptive changes often mimic malignancy, especially in the setting of previous irradiation. The ability to differentiate between a pathologic fracture and insufficiency fracture by imaging alone is important to avoid unnecessary biopsy. The linear or band-like nature of insufficiency fractures exhibited in the sacrum (described as the Honda sign) and also in the pubic rami on scintigraphic studies can be used for discernment. These changes are also evident on CT as well as MR imaging.

Identifying impending pathologic fracture is another important radiologic contribution to patient management. This not only serves to avoid pain and decreased function but also may potentially decrease metastatic spread because pathologic fractures may be associated with increased risk of developing pulmonary metastasis.[23] Two criteria for prophylactic fixation of an impending long bone pathologic fracture include (1) a well-defined cortical lesion involving greater than 3 cm of the cortex in length and (2) 50% or greater total cortical destruction on anteroposterior (AP)

and lateral radiographs.[24,25] These criteria are somewhat limited by their definitions and overlook blastic disease. Other scoring systems have been developed; one of these, developed by Mirels,[26] assesses location, size, appearance, and associated pain, with each factor graded from 1 to 3. Lesions with scores greater than 8 are typically treated surgically. The Harrington classification (**Fig. 13**) is used for lytic acetabular lesions. Class I lesions are small with intact lateral cortices and intact superior and medial acetabular walls. Class II lesions have some deficiency of the medial wall, and class III lesions have additional deficiency of the superior and lateral portions of the acetabulum.[27]

Pathologic fracture healing occurs in only 35% of all cases, although higher percentages are noted for both breast and prostate cancer with life expectancy greater than 6 months. Internal fixation and local radiation less than 30 Gy increase the likelihood of healing.

TREATMENT AND FOLLOW-UP

Treatment options for skeletal metastasis are varied. Medical options include pain management, various chemotherapy regimens, and bisphosphonates, which reduce osteoclastic activity and prevent further lytic bone destruction. strontium-89, phosphorus-32, and hormone therapies have been used for diffuse bone pain palliation. External beam radiation therapy can be used for focal painful bony lesions, although the exact regimen is in debate. Interventional radiology options include procedures, such as embolization of vascular metastatic lesions, vertebroplasty and kyphoplasty, and increasing use of radiofrequency or thermal ablation. Surgical options are also available.

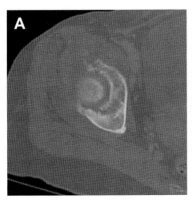 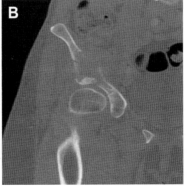

Fig. 13. An 81-year-old woman with metastatic meningioma with Harrington class III acetabular lesion. Axial (*A*) and coronal (*B*) reformatted images show extensive destruction of the roof, medial, and lateral cortices.

MULTIPLE MYELOMA

Myeloma is the most common malignant primary bone tumor, accounting for approximately 10% of all hematologic malignancies. The median age at diagnosis is 65 years. The disease has higher incidence in men and in African Americans. Its etiology is still unclear but the pathologic basis is clonal duplication of B lymphocytes (ie, plasma cells).

Myeloma often is suspected initially on the basis of laboratory screening tests. As myelomatous cells displace normal hematopoietic bone marrow elements, anemia, leucopenia, and thrombocytopenia may occur. Secreted monoclonal paraprotein can be detected with electrophoresis or by measuring Bence Jones protein from urine samples. As the disease progresses, renal insufficiency and hypercalcemia can occur. Osteolytic lesions, pathologic fractures, and vertebral fractures resulting in cord compression are other possible complications.

Bone marrow biopsy or at least aspirate is essential in diagnosis. A diagnosis must fulfill 3 criteria: (1) greater than 10% atypical marrow plasma cells and/or biopsy-proved plasmacytoma, (2) monoclonal paraprotein, and (3) myeloma-related organ dysfunction.[28] The widely used original Durie-Salmon staging system[29] accounts for various laboratory markers as well as conventional radiographic findings (**Box 2**). More recently, the important roles of MR imagnig and/or PET/CT were recognized and new consensus agreement is available with the new Durie-Salmon PLUS staging system (**Box 3**).[30]

IMAGING APPEARANCE

Multiple myeloma first involves the active red marrow tissue and then destroys the bone secondarily. Common sites of myelomatous involvement are the skull, spine, pelvis, ribs, and proximal long bones (humeri and femora). The typical radiographic appearances include focal circumscribed osteolytic lesions or diffuse inhomogeneous osteopenia due to osteoclast stimulation and osteoblast suppression.[31] In the skull, multiple similar-sized punched-out lesions are characteristic. Long bone lesions are typically central in location and display endosteal cortical scalloping with increasing size (**Fig. 14**). In larger lesions, a soft tissue component may be present. Rib involvement typically presents as osteolysis or circumscribed expansion with central inhomogeneity.[32]

Multislice helical CT is more sensitive than radiographs in detecting myeloma. Sagittal and

---

Box 2
Durie-Salmon staging system (1975)

Stage I

    All criteria need to be fulfilled:

       Hemoglobin >10 g/dL

       Serum calcium <12 mg/dL

       Radiographs: normal or single osteolytic lesion

       M-gradient IgG <5 g/dL

       IgA <3 g/dL

       Bence Jones protein excretion <4 g/24 h

Stage II

    Neither fitting stage I or stage II

Stage III

    One criterion at minimum:

       Hemoglobin <8.5 g/dL

       Serum calcium >12 mg/dL

       Radiographs: extensive osteolytic lesions

       M-gradient IgG >7 g/dL

       IgA >5 g/dL

       Bence Jones protein excretion >12 g/24 h

Adapted from Durie BG, Salmon SE. A clinical staging system of multiple myeloma: correlation of measured myeloma cell mass with presenting clinical features, response to treatment and survival. Cancer 1975; 36:842–54; with permission.

---

coronal reconstructions in addition to axial planes are especially helpful (**Fig. 15**). As expected from its pathophysiology, the osseous destruction involves the cancellous bone first before involving the cortical bone or manifesting as a soft tissue mass. The lesion is usually well circumscribed with a narrow zone of transition and is typically similar to soft tissue in attenuation (40–80 HU).

With both conventional radiography and multidetector CT, sclerotic lesions (or lytic lesions with a sclerotic border) are rare as is primarily diffuse skeletal sclerosis. These appearances can be seen after treatment, although a rare manifestation, such as polyneuropathy, organomegaly, endocrinopathy, monoclonal gammopathy, skin changes (POEMS) syndrome, is also a consideration. POEMS syndrome diagnosis is established by presence of 2 major criteria (polyneuropathy and monoclonal gammopathy) and any minor criteria.[33] Diffuse osteopenia due to myeloma and tumor-induced osteoclastic activity is difficult to distinguish from senile osteoporosis. MR

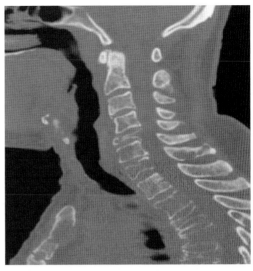

Fig. 15. A 56-year-old man with multiple myeloma. Reformatted sagittal CT image shows numerous lytic lesions and multiple compression fractures in the cervical and thoracic spine as well as the sternum.

imaging in these circumstances may be helpful in differential diagnosis.

Although conventional radiography plays a major role in the work-up of myeloma, it often yields false-negative results especially in the spine and in the pelvis (**Fig. 16**). In as many as one-third of patients, the disease is understaged without MR imaging.[34] Multiplanar T1-weighted and fat-saturated T2 or inversion recovery sequences can be used to detect various patterns of marrow infiltration with high degree of sensitivity (**Figs. 17** and **18**). Even in asymptomatic Durie-Salmon stage I patients with negative radiographs, MR imaging depicts diffuse or focal infiltration in 29% to 50% of patients.[35,36] One potential pitfall of MR imaging is due to granulocyte colony-stimulating factor therapy; in one series, 40% of treated patients showed marrow changes mimicking tumor infiltration on MR imaging that were attributable to red marrow reconversion.[37] One needs to know if patients are on long-acting or short-acting granulocyte colony-stimulating factor agents.

The increasing use of advanced imaging in management of multiple myeloma patients led to a consensus conference where an updated staging system was agreed on.[28] The resulting Durie-Salmon PLUS staging system incorporates MR imaging and PET/CT findings and is generally predictive of survival. Normal skeletal survey or just a single lesion on MR imaging or PET/CT imaging defines stage IA disease, whereas stage IB disease requires fewer than 5 focal lesions or

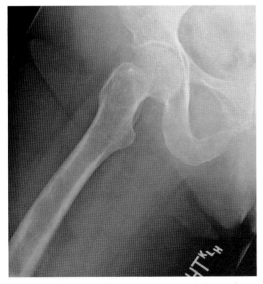

Fig. 14. An 83-year-old woman with multiple myeloma. Long central lytic lesion with endosteal cortical scalloping is noted in the right proximal femur.

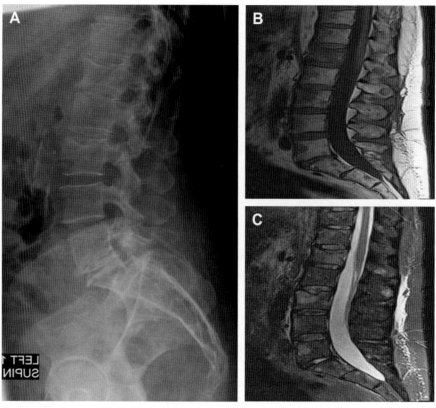

Fig. 16. A 66-year-old woman with multiple myeloma complicated with compression fractures of L1 and L3 vertebral bodies. Although the fractures were noted on the conventional radiograph (A), the radiograph did not show numerous other myelomatous deposits in the lumbar spine detected on subsequent T1-weighted (B) and T2 STIR (C) MR imaging.

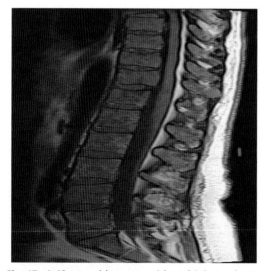

Fig. 17. A 48-year-old woman with multiple myeloma. T1-weighted MR imaging sequence shows severe diffuse infiltration of the lumbar spine as defined by the Durie-Salmon PLUS system.

mild diffuse disease in the spine. Diagnosis of more advanced stage disease depends on higher numbers of focal lesions, between 5 and 20 lesions for stage II and greater than 20 focal lesions for stage III disease. More extensive diffuse spinal involvement, defined by T1 signal intensity in relation to adjacent intervertebral disk, also can be used to diagnose stage II or III disease (see **Figs. 16** and **17**). Finally, renal function status was incorporated into this system and delineates stages IIA and IIIA from stages IIB and IIIB (see **Box 3**).

A salt-and-pepper pattern of spinal bone marrow can be seen in a few patients with MR imaging.[34] On both T1-weighted and T2-weighted sequences, the bone marrow signal is patchy and inhomogeneous but without a focal lesion on fat saturated sequences. Also, there is no significant enhancement noted in these cases. These patients usually have stage I disease and can be watched without requiring therapy. A recent study comparing the original Durie-Salmon staging system with the new Durie-Salmon PLUS staging system showed moderate

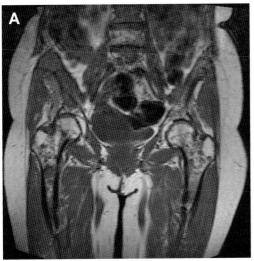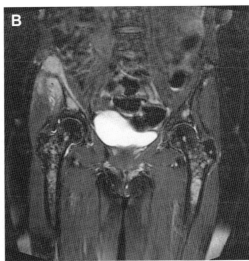

Fig. 18. A 69-year-old woman with multiple myeloma. Coronal MR images show numerous foci of bone marrow replacement, demonstrated by decreased T1 signal (*A*) and increased T2 STIR signal (*B*) in the lumbar spine, iliac wings, and the femurs.

concordance and suggests the newer criteria should not solely be the reason for initiating systemic therapy.[38]

FDG-PET can be used to detect multiple myeloma with good sensitivity and specificity. It has been shown superior to conventional radiography but less so compared with MR imaging.[39] Its ability to assess metabolic activity can be useful, especially when evaluating treatment response and monitoring relapse.

Survival from multiple myeloma varies widely, ranging from a few months to more than 10 years. The MR imaging appearance of myeloma has been shown to be a predictor of disease progression. In Durie-Salmon stage I disease, patients with pathologic MR imaging findings had significantly earlier progression of disease compared with patients with normal MR imaging.[36] In another study, patients showing pathologic MR imaging findings had a 5-year survival rate of 30% compared with 80% in patients with normal MR imaging.[40] Yet another study showed significantly longer survival in patients with normal looking or salt-and-pepper pattern of infiltration.[34] The number of focal lesions detected on MR imaging has significant prognostic as well as survival impact. Presence of more than 7 focal lesions is an independent adverse feature for survival.[41] Alternatively, resolution of focal lesions detected on MR imaging conferred superior survival.[41,42]

Primary differential considerations for patients with elevated paraprotein are monoclonal gammopathy of unknown significance (MGUS) and smoldering myeloma. MGUS is a common asymptomatic condition of the elderly. No focal osteolytic lesions should be present on radiographs or CT, and MR imaging should be negative. If MR imaging is done, it should be with a whole-body technique. Patients with MGUS merit monitoring as it can evolve to manifest various hematologic malignancies, including multiple myeloma. Smoldering myeloma is an intermediate category between MGUS and multiple myeloma. These patients may have mild organ dysfunction and the bone marrow contains between 10% and 30% of plasma cells by volume. Solitary plasmacytoma consists of a single lytic lesion (**Fig. 19**), commonly in the axial skeleton, especially in the thoracic spine. There may be an associated soft tissue component. Because some think of solitary plasmacytoma as multiple myeloma with only one of the lesions detected, further evaluation with a whole-body imaging technique (MR imaging or PET/CT) is strongly recommended for these patients (**Fig. 20**).

TREATMENT AND FOLLOW-UP

For those with early-stage multiple myeloma without any detectable lesions, a watchful waiting strategy may be used. High-dose chemotherapy after stem cell transplant in patients with stage II and III disease has significantly increased survival duration. Bisphosphonate therapy has been shown to reduce incidence of fractures and increase the quality of life. Recently, bisphosphonate

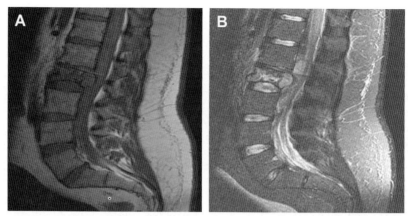

Fig. 19. A 33-year-old man with a plasmacytoma in lumbar spine. Only the L2 vertebral body was involved in this patient with pathologic fracture noted on T1 (*A*) and fat-suppressed T2 (*B*) MR images. Subsequent skeletal survey did not yield additional lesions.

therapy has been linked with osteonecrosis of the jaw. This condition was preceded by dental procedures in approximately half the cases whereas patients with spontaneous cases had a higher risk of nonhealing and recurrence. The osteonecrosis healed in 75% of patients in one series.[43] Additionally, bisphosphonate therapy may be associated with atypical subtrochanteric femoral fracture.[44] These have a characteristic radiographic appearance (**Fig. 21**). Potential risks related to bisphosphonate therapy must be balanced with the benefits of fracture and pain reduction. The treatment of complications and pain management become more important in advanced stage disease.

Much of assessment of pathologic fracture risk and treatment was discussed previously. The particular need for radiologists to assimilate information from all available imaging studies when assessing pathologic fracture risk is further illustrated by recent research which shows that the combination of a high standardized uptake value of greater than 3.5 on FDG-PET and extensive vertebral body signal abnormality on MR imaging (diffuse or multifocal) is highly suggestive of an impending vertebral body fracture.[45]

Percutaneous vertebroplasty is a valuable interventional technique that can be used to treat acute or subacute fractures in patients who are not eligible for surgery and whose pain is not controlled

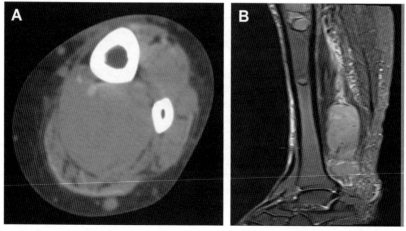

Fig. 20. A 44-year-old man with a plasmacytoma shown in flexor hallucis longus muscle on axial CT (*A*). Subsequent MR imaging showed multiple marrow replacing myelomatous lesions in the proximal tibia (*B*) in addition to the soft tissue plasmacytoma.

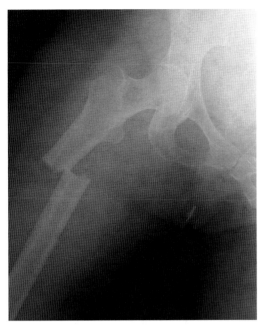

Fig. 21. A 67-year-old woman with transverse subtrochanteric fracture. The fracture occurred following minor trauma and represents a typical fracture related to bisphosphonate therapy showing focal lateral cortical thickening.

by conservative means. Prophylaxis and extreme pain due to osteolysis are other potential indications. Adjunct radiation therapy and radiofrequency ablation of tumor elements may also be applied. Patient selection is of paramount importance, especially given recent controversy surrounding this technique. Relative contraindications include marked posterior vertebral wall defect and soft tissue mass extension into the epidural space.

Only a few MR imaging studies have examined bone marrow signal changes after treatment of multiple myeloma. In one study, patients with complete clinical response showed either normalization of bone marrow signal or absent or only peripheral enhancement of the lesions.[46] Those changes were not detected, however, in all patients with clinical response to therapy in terms of complete remission. Patients with partial response to therapy showed an overall decrease in bone marrow alterations. In those patients, focal and diffuse pathologic contrast uptake was still present. Despite clinical remission, new compression fractures were frequently seen. These fractures were assumed to result from progressive osteoporosis. In patients with a diffuse infiltrative pattern, who responded to therapy, the bone marrow signal showed an increase on T1-

weighted sequences, indicating restitution of fat cells. Newer MR imaging techniques for early response assessment include dynamic contrast enhancement, arterial spin labeling, and diffusion-weighted imaging.[47–49]

FDG-PET may be a useful tool in monitoring relapse or response to therapy. Negative PET scans have been shown to reliably predict stable MGUS. The development of new FDG-positive sites in the skeleton after therapy has indicated relapse and a poor prognosis. Decreased tracer uptake has been reported in patients with good response.[12] A new high standardized uptake value lesion may represent a new clonal colony and should be biopsied for analysis.

LYMPHOMA

Primary lymphoma of bone (PLB) is uncommon, accounting for approximately 5% of malignant primary bone tumors. Nearly all cases are non-Hodgkin lymphoma with only 6% represented by Hodgkin disease in one large case series with 237 patients.[50] Peak incidence is in the fourth through sixth decades of life and is rare in patients younger than 10 years. The distal femur is the most commonly involved site (25%) with other affected sites, including other long bones, such as the proximal tibia and humerus, as well as the skull, vertebral column, and pelvis. Insidious and intermittent bone pain, weight loss, and fever are common clinical presentations. If the vertebrae are involved, patients may present with radicular symptoms and spinal cord compression. Pathologic fractures are also a common initial presentation (**Fig. 22**). Primary bone lymphoma has the best prognosis of all the primary malignant bone tumors. One recent article reported a 100% 5-year survival.[51]

Radiographic appearance of PLB typically shows a solitary permeative or moth-eaten pattern of bone destruction and highly aggressive interrupted single or double layer periosteal reaction. In long bones, the lesion is usually centered at the metadiaphyseal junction (**Fig. 23**). Soft tissue masses are frequently associated. A sequestrum is also a common finding[50] seen in up to 15% of cases (**Fig. 24**). Differential considerations include other so-called small blue cell tumors (eg, Ewing sarcoma and neuroblastoma in the young), myeloma, metastasis, and infection. Lymphoma is one of the causes of an ivory vertebral body. Multifocal involvement can occur, typically involving the skull, spine, femur, and tibia.

MR imaging appearance of lymphoma is often nonspecific, demonstrating a marrow replacement pattern, which can be focal or diffuse. Focal

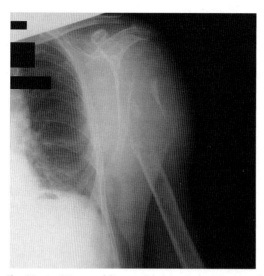

Fig. 22. An 85-year-old man with primary lymphoma of bone. Left shoulder radiograph shows a large lytic lesion in the proximal humerus with a pathologic fracture.

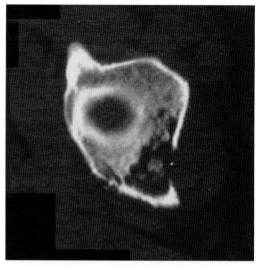

Fig. 24. A 20-year-old man with PLB shows a sequestrum in the posterior medial acetabulum.

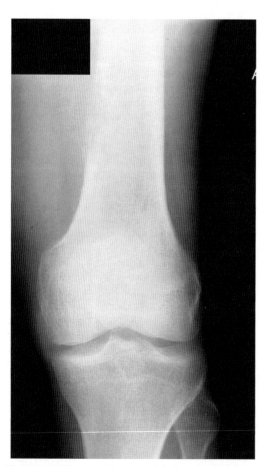

Fig. 23. A 73-year-old man with lymphoma shows a permeative lesion at the distal femoral metadiaphyseal junction with ill-defined borders. Its eccentric location is also a common feature of PLB.

marrow replacement, however, with surrounding soft tissue mass and absent cortical bone destruction is a typical pattern as is marked diffuse marrow signal abnormality with frequently normal-appearing radiographs.[50] Although signal intensity can vary (presumably due to fibrous tissue content in the affected marrow), the abnormal lesions are decreased in signal on T1-based sequences and increased in signal on T2-based sequences. Associated extraosseous soft tissue masses are most reliably detected with MR imaging. Involvement extending across joints is another distinct feature, which can be detected more easily using MR imaging.

LEUKEMIA

Chronic lymphocytic leukemia (CLL), a form of low-grade lymphocytic non-Hodgkin lymphoma, is the most common variety of leukemia in the elderly. Two-thirds of patients are older than 60 years whereas the peak incidence is in patients greater than 80 years of age. Monoclonal duplication of mature B lymphocytes is the underlying cause for this disorder. As these cells replace the bone marrow elements, anemia, leucopenia, and thrombocytopenia may occur manifesting clinically as weakness, bruising, and recurrent infections.

The marrow replacement process is seen radiographically as nonspecific diffuse osteopenia. Small osteolytic lesions can be seen as well as more mass like bony erosions due to the accumulation of leukemic cells (**Fig. 25**). These are termed,

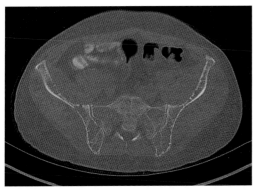

Fig. 25. A 44-year-old man with CLL. Multiple osteolytic lesions are seen on axial CT image through the sacrum and iliac wings. These represent accumulations of leukemic cells.

chloromas, because of their green-tinged appearance pathologically resulting from copper ions in myeloperoxidase. CLL can also affect the small bones of the hand, called *leukemic acropachy*. Bone destruction, clubbing, and soft tissue edema can occur, especially in the metacarpals and the terminal phalanges. Arthritis is present in approximately 12% of patients with CLL. Gout, osteonecrosis secondary to steroid therapy, and osteomyelitis are secondary complications of CLL.

The MR imaging appearance of leukemia is nonspecific; it may present as diffuse infiltration. Signal intensity of bone on T1-weighted sequences is diffusely decreased with corresponding increased signal intensity on T2-weighted sequences (Fig. 26). In patients with early-stage disease and abnormality on T1-weighted sequences, earlier therapeutic intervention was required because the disease was more severe in form in one study.[52] After gadolinium contrast administration, leukemic infiltrates show diffuse enhancement. As one potentially useful parameter, the dynamic contrast enhancement characteristics have been shown to be an indicator for outcome and survival in patients who are in complete remission from acute myeloid leukemia.[53]

LANGERHANS CELL HISTIOCYTOSIS

Proliferation of specific histiocytes (Langerhans cell histiocytes) can manifest in various forms. Localization to one or a few bones has been known as eosinophilic granuloma. Chronic dissemination with multiple bone lesions and with abdominal organ and lymph node involvement is known as Hand-Schüller-Christian disease. Acute or subacute dissemination with bone and abdominal organ involvement is known as Letterer-Siwe disease.

Localized forms of Langerhans cell histiocytosis account for the majority of the cases. These occur most frequently in the pediatric population and have an excellent long-term prognosis. Flat bones are the most commonly involved sites, characteristically affecting the skull, mandible, pelvis, and ribs (Fig. 27). Long bone involvement is also common, resulting in typical geographic lytic lesions with little or no surrounding sclerosis that are located centrally within the intramedullary space. Significant surrounding edema is a common finding on MR imaging (Fig. 28).[54] Although less common in the spine, a classic presentation is vertebra plana resulting from a collapsed vertebral body (Fig. 29). The classic type of eosinophilic granuloma may

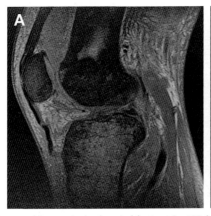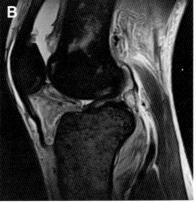

Fig. 26. A 31-year-old man in leukemic blast crisis. MR imaging shows diffuse marrow signal abnormality with decreased T1-weighted signal (*A*) and increased signal on T2 STIR sequence (*B*). There are round lesions within the distal femur replacing the bone marrow representing chloromas.

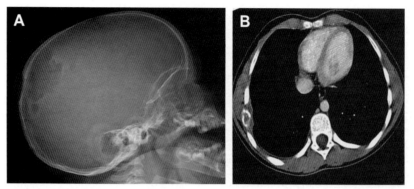

Fig. 27. (*A*) A 2-year-old boy with large geographic lytic lesions in the skull with beveled edges proved to be Langerhans cell histiocytosis. (*B*) A 10-year-old girl with right rib lesion. CT shows a lytic lesion with surrounding soft tissue and pleural thickening. This lesion on biopsy was shown to be Langerhans cell histiocytosis. (*Courtesy of* Gerald Behr, MD, New York, NY.)

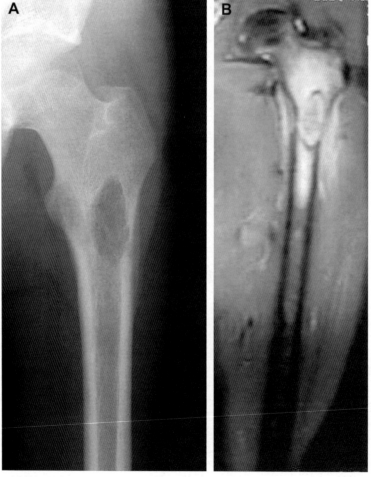

Fig. 28. A 16-year-old boy with 1-month history of left hip/thigh pain. AP hip radiograph (*A*) shows geographic lytic lesion with endosteal scalloping and thick, solid, smooth periosteal reaction laterally. Coronal STIR (*B*) MR image shows extensive bone marrow edema around the lesion and some edema in the surrounding soft tissues.

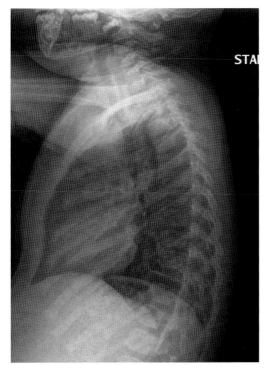

Fig. 29. A 2-year-old boy presents with back pain and vertebra plana due to Langerhans cell histiocytosis. (*Courtesy of* Gerald Behr, MD, New York, NY.)

resolve spontaneously, with no clinical or surgical intervention.[55] If spinal lesions are symptomatic, CT-guided corticosteroid injection has been reported to result in complete resolution of pain and healing of lesions in 90% of patients.[56]

SUMMARY

This review explores in depth the most common malignant process involving the bone, namely metastatic disease, as well as some of the more common proliferative forms of hematopoietic disease of bone marrow. These are commonly encountered pathologic processes that often have vague nonspecific symptoms. Imaging findings are frequently subtle on initial radiographs; however, advanced imaging techniques, including CT, MR, and PET, allow for accurate diagnosis, staging, and follow-up in most cases.

REFERENCES

1. Mundy GR. Metastasis to bone: causes, consequences and therapeutic opportunities. Nat Rev Cancer 2002;2:584–93.
2. Coleman RE. Clinical features of metastatic bone disease and risk of skeletal morbidity. Clin Cancer Res 2006;12:6243s–9s.
3. Batson OV. The function of the vertebral veins and their role in the spread of metastases. Ann Surg 1940;112:138–49.
4. Kitazawa S, Maeda S. Development of skeletal metastases. Clin Orthop Relat Res 1995;312:45–50.
5. Simon MA, Bartucci EJ. The search for the primary tumor in patients with skeletal metastases of unknown origin. Cancer 1986;58:1088–95.
6. Sherry MM, Greco FA, Johnson DH, et al. Metastatic breast cancer confined to the skeletal system. An indolent disease. Am J Med 1986;81:381–6.
7. Disler DG, McCauley TR, Ratner LM, et al. In-phase and out-of-phase MR imaging of bone marrow: prediction of neoplasia based on the detection of coexistent fat and water. Am J Roentgenol 1997;169:1439–47.
8. Tumeh SS, Beadle G, Kaplan WD. Clinical significance of solitary rib lesions in patients with extraskeletal malignancy. J Nucl Med 1985;26:1140–3.
9. Corcoran RJ, Thrall JH, Kyle RW, et al. Solitary abnormalities in bone scans of patients with extraosseous malignancies. Radiology 1976;121:663–7.
10. Taira AV, Herfkens RJ, Gambhir SS, et al. Detection of bone metastases: assessment of integrated FDG PET/CT imaging. Radiology 2007;243:204–11.
11. Reske S, Blumstein N, Neumaier B, et al. Imaging prostate cancer with 11C-choline PET/CT. J Nucl Med 2006;47:1249–54.
12. Bredella MA, Steinbach L, Caputo G, et al. Value of FDG PET in the assessment of patients with multiple myeloma. Am J Roentgenol 2005;184:1199–204.
13. Edelstyn GA, Gillespie PJ, Grebbell FS. The radiological demonstration of osseous metastases: experimental observations. Clin Radiol 1967;18:158–62.
14. Chen WT, Shih TT, Chen RC, et al. Blood perfusion of vertebral lesions evaluated with gadolinium-enhanced dynamic MRI: in comparison with compression fracture and metastasis. J Magn Reson Imaging 2002;15:308–14.
15. Sartoris DJ, Clopton P, Nemcek A, et al. Vertebral-body collapse in focal and diffuse disease: patterns of pathologic processes. Radiology 1986;160:479–83.
16. Algra PR, Heimans JJ, Valk J, et al. Do metastases in vertebrae begin in the body or the pedicles? Imaging study in 45 patients. Am J Roentgenol 1992;158:1275–9.
17. Cuénod CA, Laredo JD, Chevret S, et al. Acute vertebral collapse due to osteoporosis or malignancy: appearance on unenhanced and gadolinium-enhanced MR images. Radiology 1996;199:541–9.
18. Baur A, Stäbler A, Brüning R, et al. Diffusion-weighted MR imaging of bone marrow: differentiation of benign versus pathologic compression fractures. Radiology 1998;207:349–56.
19. Dennis JM. The solitary dense vertebral body. Radiology 1961;77:618–21.

20. Coury C. Hippocration fingers and hypertrophic osteoarthropathy. A study of 350 cases. Br J Dis Chest 1960;54:202–9.

21. Deutsch A, Resnick D, Niwayama G. Case report 145. Bilateral, almost symmetrical skeletal metastases (both femora) from bronchogenic carcinoma. Skeletal Radiol 1981;6:144–8.

22. Tubiana-Hulin M. Incidence, prevalence and distribution of bone metastases. Bone 1991;12:S9–10.

23. Saad F, Lipton A, Cook R, et al. Pathologic fractures correlate with reduced survival in patients with malignant bone disease. Cancer 2007;110:1860–7.

24. Van der Linden YM, Dijkstra PD, Kroon HM, et al. Comparative analysis of risk factors for pathological fracture with femoral metastases. J Bone Joint Surg Br 2004;86:566–73.

25. Beals RK, Lawton GD, Snell WE. Prophylactic internal fixation of the femur in metastatic breast cancer. Cancer 1971;28:1350–4.

26. Mirels H. Metastatic disease in long bones. Clin Orthop Relat Res 1989;249:256–64.

27. Harrington KD. The management of acetabular insufficiency secondary to metastatic malignant disease. J Bone Joint Surg Am 1981;63:653–64.

28. Durie BG, Kyle RA, Belch A, et al. Myeloma management guidelines: a consensus report from the Scientific Advisors of the International Myeloma Foundation. Hematol J 2003;4:379–98.

29. Durie BG, Salmon SE. A clinical staging system for multiple myeloma. Correlation of measured myeloma cell mass with presenting clinical features, response to treatment, and survival. Cancer 1975; 36:842–54.

30. Dimopoulos M, Terpos E, Comenzo RL, et al. International myeloma working group consensus statement and guidelines regarding the current role of imaging techniques in the diagnosis and monitoring of multiple myeloma. Leukemia 2009;23:1545–56.

31. Tian E, Zhan F, Walker R, et al. The role of the Wnt-signaling antagonist DKK1 in the development of osteolytic lesions in multiple myeloma. N Engl J Med 2003;349:2483–94.

32. Mulligan M. Myeloma update. Semin Musculoskelet Radiol 2007;11:231–9.

33. Dispenzieri A. POEMS syndrome. Hematology Am Soc Hematol Educ Program 2005;360–7.

34. Baur A, Stäbler A, Nagel D, et al. Magnetic resonance imaging as a supplement for the clinical staging system of Durie and Salmon? Cancer 2002;95:1334–45.

35. Van de Berg BC, Lecouvet FE, Michaux L, et al. Stage I multiple myeloma: value of MR imaging of the bone marrow in the determination of prognosis. Radiology 1996;201:243–6.

36. Dimopoulos MA, Moulopoulos A, Smith T, et al. Risk of disease progression in asymptomatic multiple myeloma. Am J Med 1993;94:57–61.

37. Hartman RP, Sundaram M, Okuno SH, et al. Effect of granulocyte-stimulating factors on marrow of adult patients with musculoskeletal malignancies: incidence and MRI findings. Am J Roentgenol 2004; 183:645–53.

38. Fechtner K, Hillengass J, Delorme S, et al. Staging monoclonal plasma cell disease: comparison of the Durie-Salmon and the Durie-Salmon PLUS staging systems. Radiology 2010;257:195–204.

39. Breyer RJ, Mulligan ME, Smith SE, et al. Comparison of imaging with FDG PET/CT with other imaging modalities in myeloma. Skeletal Radiol 2006;35:632–40.

40. Kusumoto S, Jinnai I, Itoh K, et al. Magnetic resonance imaging patterns in patients with multiple myeloma. Br J Haematol 1997;99:649–55.

41. Walker R, Barlogie B, Haessler J, et al. Magnetic resonance imaging in multiple myeloma: diagnostic and clinical implications. J Clin Oncol 2007;25:1121–8.

42. Barlogie B, Anaissie E, van Rhee F, et al. The Arkansas approach to therapy of patients with multiple myeloma. Best Pract Res Clin Haematol 2007;20: 761–81.

43. Badros A, Terpos E, Katodritou E, et al. Natural history of osteonecrosis of the jaw in patients with multiple myeloma. J Clin Oncol 2008;26:5904–9.

44. Park-Wyllie LY, Mamdani MM, Juurlink DN, et al. Bisphosphonate use and the risk of subtrochanteric or femoral shaft fractures in older women. JAMA 2011; 305:783–9.

45. Mulligan M, Chirindel A, Karchevsky M. Characterizing and predicting pathologic spine fractures in myeloma patients with FDG PET/CT and MR imaging. Cancer Invest 2011;29(5):370–6.

46. Moulopoulos LA, Dimopoulos MA, Alexanian R, et al. Multiple myeloma: MR patterns of response to treatment. Radiology 1994;193:441–6.

47. Fenchel M, Konaktchieva M, Weisel K, et al. Early response assessment in patients with multiple myeloma during anti-angiogenic therapy using arterial spin labelling: first clinical results. Eur Radiol 2010;20:899–906.

48. Lin C, Luciani A, Belhadj K, et al. Multiple myeloma treatment response assessment with whole-body dynamic contrast-enhanced MR imaging. Radiology 2010;254:521–31.

49. Horger M, Weisel K, Horger W, et al. Whole-body diffusion-weighted MRI with apparent diffusion coefficient mapping for early response monitoring in multiple myeloma: preliminary results. Am J Roentgenol 2011;196:1373.

50. Mulligan ME, McRae GA, Murphey MD. Imaging features of primary lymphoma of bone. Am J Roentgenol 1999;173:1691–7.

51. Kirsch J, Ilaslan H, Bauer TW, et al. The incidence of imaging findings, and the distribution of skeletal lymphoma in a consecutive patient population seen over 5 years. Skeletal Radiol 2006;35:590–4.

52. Lecouvet FE, Vande Berg BC, Michaux L, et al. Early chronic lymphocytic leukemia: prognostic value of quantitative bone marrow MR imaging findings and correlation with hematologic variables. Radiology 1997;204:813–8.

53. Chen BB, Hsu CY, Yu CW, et al. Dynamic contrast-enhanced MR imaging measurement of vertebral bone marrow perfusion may be indicator of outcome of acute myeloid leukemia patients in remission. Radiology 2011;258:821–31.

54. Azouz EM, Saigal G, Rodriquez M, et al. Langerhans' cell histiocytosis: pathology, imaging and treatment of skeletal involvement. Pediatr Radiol 2005;35: 103–15.

55. Stull MA, Kransdorf MJ, Devaney KO. Langerhans cell histiocytosis of bone. Radiographics 1992;12: 801–23.

56. Rimondi E, Mavrogenis A, Rossi G, et al. CT-guided corticosteroid injection for solitary eosinophilic granuloma of the spine. Skeletal Radiol 2011;40:757–64.

The Clinical Evaluation of Soft Tissue Tumors

Tessa Balach, MD[a], G. Scott Stacy, MD[b], Rex C. Haydon, MD[c],*

KEYWORDS
- Soft tissue tumor • Benign • Malignant
- Evaluation • Extremity • Sarcoma

In 2010, the estimated incidence of soft tissue sarcomas was 10,520 with an associated 3920 deaths.[1] These numbers include not only sarcomas of the extremities, but also sarcomas of the trunk, retroperitoneum, and head and neck. It should be noted that approximately three-quarters of all soft tissue sarcomas occur in the extremities. Extremity tumors, benign and malignant, are the focus of this article.[2]

The vast majority of soft tissue masses that present to a physician are, in fact, benign lesions. The incidence of benign soft tissue tumors is estimated to outnumber malignant tumors by a factor of at least 100. For example, lipomas have an estimated incidence of 1/1000 annually, suggesting that 300,000 lipomas present for evaluation per year,[3] a striking contrast to the 10,000 soft tissue sarcomas reported.

When including both benign and malignant soft tissue tumors, a physician is likely to encounter several in his or her practice each year. Despite the enormous frequency of lipomas, other benign lesions or even sarcomas should be considered during evaluation of soft tissue masses, and this article will outline a clinical strategy for the diagnosis of these tumors.

DIAGNOSIS OF SOFT TISSUE TUMORS
History and Physical Examination

Classically, a patient with a soft tissue sarcoma presents with a painless soft tissue mass that is increasing in size. As part of any medical examination, a detailed history is the first step in the evaluation of a patient with a soft tissue tumor. Details elicited in the history should include information about how the patient noticed the lesion, how long the mass has been present, changes in its size over time, and symptoms associated with the lesion (eg, pain at rest, pain with activity, radiating pain when the lesion is touched). The clinician should also seek out a history of trauma. Many patients will associate the onset of the mass with minor trauma. Although this history of trauma is often circumstantial, it can play a role in the diagnosis of some masses, such as myositis ossificans, while excluding others as true tumors, such as an arm mass resulting from retracted musculature following a biceps tendon rupture. Information regarding whether or not the lesion fluctuates in size may be important for shaping a differential diagnosis. Inflammatory nodules and lymph nodes can fluctuate in size; hemangiomas routinely increase and decrease in size,

The authors have nothing to disclose.

[a] Department of Orthopaedic Surgery, New England Musculoskeletal Institute, University of Connecticut, 263 Farmington Avenue, Farmington, CT 06030-4037, USA

[b] Section of Musculoskeletal Imaging, Department of Radiology, University of Chicago Medical Center, 5841 South Maryland Avenue, MC 2026, Chicago, IL 60637, USA

[c] Section of Orthopaedic Surgery and Rehabilitation Medicine, University of Chicago, 5841 South Maryland Avenue, MC 3079, Chicago, IL 60637, USA

* Corresponding author.
E-mail address: rhaydon@surgery.bsd.uchicago.edu

Radiol Clin N Am 49 (2011) 1185–1196
doi:10.1016/j.rcl.2011.07.005
0033-8389/11/$ – see front matter © 2011 Published by Elsevier Inc.

often related to activity. In addition, information regarding the presence of constitutional symptoms, fevers, weight loss, and general health should be obtained.

A history of syndromes associated with increased risk of soft tissue tumors or sarcomas (eg, Li-Fraumeni syndrome, Gardner syndrome, neurofibromatosis) should be elicited. A history of cancer should also be sought, because although rare, malignant tumors, such as lung carcinoma, melanoma, and lymphoma, can metastasize to the soft tissues. A complete medical history can reveal other conditions associated with soft tissue masses, such as tumoral calcinosis in patients with renal failure on hemodialysis or heterotopic bone formation in patients with traumatic brain injury.

Physical examination should attempt to estimate the size of the mass, its location (whether superficial or deep), its mobility, and its consistency. The mass should be palpated to determine its location in relation to fascial boundaries and other anatomic landmarks. Tenderness of the lesion to palpation should be noted, as this may indicate an inflammatory lesion. Masses should be palpated and/or auscultated to determine if there is pulsatile flow through the lesion, suggesting the possibility of a pseudoaneurysm or vascular lesion.[4]

Masses should also be evaluated for the presence of a Tinel sign, which would suggest a nerve sheath tumor or a mass involving a sensory nerve. In addition, distal limb swelling and local skin changes should be observed and documented, as these could be signs of locoregional compression of venous or lymphatic drainage. Proximal lymph node basins should be evaluated for the presence or absence of lymphadenopathy. Signs of systemic illness should also be observed.

Unfortunately, a history and physical examination rarely help to meaningfully narrow the list of differential diagnoses, as many of the signs and symptoms of soft tissue tumors are nonspecific. Imaging of these lesions is, therefore, the next step toward establishing a diagnosis.

Radiologic Imaging

In general, magnetic resonance imaging (MR imaging) has become the modality of choice for the detection and characterization of soft tissue masses. However, radiographs can provide important information that can obviate or guide further imaging and therapy, and therefore continue to be recommended as an inexpensive first-line imaging study.[5] Radiographs can help to confirm that a palpable mass is arising from bone rather than soft tissue. Radiographs are also useful for

detecting mineralization in a mass. For example, peripheral mineralization of a mass that arises following a clear history of trauma supports the diagnosis of myositis ossificans. They may show phleboliths in a soft tissue mass, supporting the diagnosis of a benign vascular lesion. Articular and juxta-articular conditions that may present with masses, such as synovial (osteo)chondromatosis and tumoral calcinosis, may be more easily diagnosed with radiography than with MR imaging (Fig. 1). Further imaging following radiographs may be necessary to better delineate lesion extent, or to confirm or better define a nonvisible or nonspecific lesion on radiographs.

MR imaging has largely replaced computed tomography (CT) for soft tissue mass evaluation.[5] The superior soft tissue contrast of MR imaging allows for easier detection of soft tissue masses and better delineation of their extent.[6] Determination of involvement of neurovascular structures and medullary bone is also superior (Figs. 2 and 3). Therefore, MR imaging is preferred for staging most tumors. MR imaging is also best suited for providing a tissue-specific diagnosis, which can be established in up to one-third of cases based on imaging features.[7–9] Although a specific diagnosis cannot be reached in most cases, MR imaging can offer clues that may support malignancy, such as size and heterogeneity of signal intensity of the lesion, as well as involvement of bone and neurovascular structures.[5,10] It can also reveal non-neoplastic entities that may mimic tumors, such as hematoma, and is recommended for follow-up of spontaneous soft tissue hemorrhage, particularly in older adults.

The MR imaging protocol for evaluation of soft tissue tumors needs to be flexible, as it depends on the location and estimated anatomic extent of the lesion.[11] As a general rule, the mass should be imaged in at least 2 orthogonal planes, one of which should be the transverse plane.[7] T1-weighted and fat-suppressed T2-weighted pulse sequences are a standard part of most protocols. The use of intravenous gadolinium will depend on the clinical situation, but it is useful for differentiating solid components of the tumor from those that are cystic or necrotic; this can assist with assessment of aggressiveness of the lesion and help to guide biopsy.[5] As with bone tumors, special MR imaging techniques, such as dynamic contrast-enhanced MR imaging, MR spectroscopy, and diffusion-weighted MR imaging show potential for differentiating between some benign and malignant tumors, but further investigation is needed.[12–14]

CT may be preferred to MR imaging in certain circumstances, including the evaluation of soft

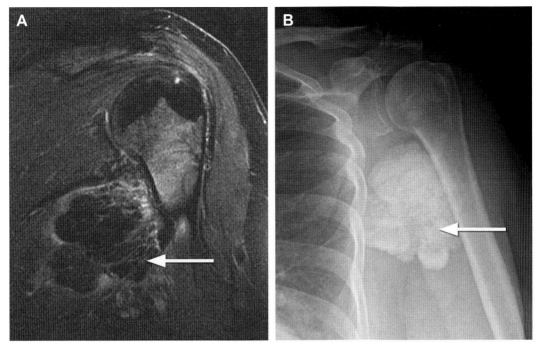

Fig. 1. A 64-year-old woman presented to her physician for evaluation of shoulder pain. Fat-suppressed T2-weighted coronal oblique image (*A*) of the shoulder shows a mass of low signal intensity medial to the proximal humeral diaphysis (*arrow*). The low signal intensity of the mass suggests either mineralization or dense fibrous tissue. Anteroposterior radiograph (*B*) revealed a large area of dense amorphous calcification (*arrow*) adjacent to the proximal humerus consistent with tumoral calcinosis. On further investigation, a diagnosis of underlying hyperparathyroidism was determined.

tissue masses arising in the abdominal or chest wall.[5] CT can also better demonstrate mineralization of soft tissue masses, and help confirm a diagnosis of myositis ossificans.[11] It is generally superior to MR imaging for depiction of fine bone detail, and hence may be preferred for demonstration of subtle cortical involvement. CT can also be sufficient for confirming lipoma. Finally, it is an

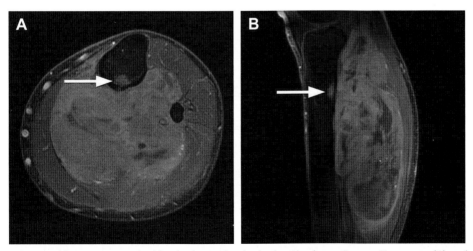

Fig. 2. A 40-year-old man presented with a leg mass that he had noticed over 2 years. Transverse (*A*) and sagittal (*B*) fat-suppressed T1-weighted MR images following intravenous administration of gadolinium-chelate demonstrate a large heterogeneously enhancing mass in the deep posterior compartment of the leg with extension into the intramedullary space of the tibia (*arrows*). In-office core needle biopsy demonstrated a high-grade pleomorphic sarcoma.

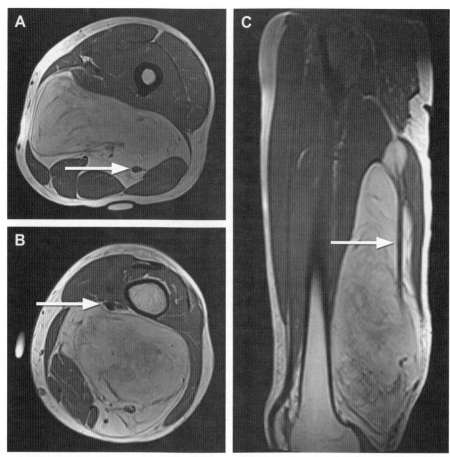

Fig. 3. These images demonstrate the utility of MR imaging for identifying vital anatomic structures in relation to tumor. The transverse T1-weighted image through the proximal thigh (*A*) shows a large lipomatous tumor surrounding the sciatic nerve (*arrow*), whereas distally (*B*) the tumor abuts the femoral vessels (*arrow*). The sagittal T1-weighted image (*C*) again shows the sciatic nerve (*arrow*) surrounded by the large lipomatous tumor.

appropriate imaging modality for those patients who cannot undergo MR imaging, for detecting pulmonary metastases, and for directing percutaneous biopsy. Administration of intravenous contrast may be necessary for better visualization of the primary tumor.

Sonography is gaining wider acceptance among experienced users as a suitable modality for evaluation of soft tissue masses, although MR imaging remains superior for characterizing pathology in most cases. Sonography is useful for confirming the presence of a mass and for differentiating solid from cystic lesions. Doppler imaging can be used to study vascularity of lesions. It is a viable substitute for MR imaging in certain cases, such as for detection of Morton neuroma or evaluation of suspected cysts, ganglia, and bursae near joints.[5,15]

The role of positron emission tomography (PET) scanning in the workup of soft tissue tumors has yet to be established.[5] It can be used as a problem-solving tool in certain cases. For example, it can provide an indication of metabolic activity of a lesion, and, with PET/CT fusion images, help guide biopsy to target areas that may result in a higher diagnostic yield. PET has also shown some promise in helping differentiate benign from malignant bone lesions; however, further research is needed, as there is overlap in standard uptake values between benign and malignant tumors.[16]

Biopsy

A correct histologic diagnosis of a soft tissue tumor is often not possible on the basis of imaging studies alone, making biopsy a requirement for diagnosis in most cases. The goal of any biopsy is to obtain adequate tissue for accurate diagnosis; however, this can be achieved through a variety of different methods. Biopsies can be broadly divided into 1 of 2 categories: open and closed. An open biopsy is commonly performed in the operating room and generally requires an incision, whereas a closed biopsy is performed percutaneously using a needle or core biopsy instrument.

Closed biopsies are associated with less local morbidity, but yield less tissue for diagnosis, and therefore, may be associated with lower accuracy. Closed biopsies can be performed with or without image guidance, and include both fine-needle aspiration (FNA) and core needle biopsy techniques.

FNA of soft tissue tumors provides the pathologist with a small sample of cells from the lesion. The cytopathologist examining the sample can usually distinguish benign from malignant cells with high accuracy and can even distinguish between sarcoma and carcinoma.[17,18] Accurate subtyping, however, is more difficult because of the limited nature of the specimen, and the inability to examine extracellular architecture. Furthermore, samples are often not large enough to perform an extended battery of stains or cytogenetic analyses.[17] FNA is often recommended for superficial masses for which there is a relatively narrow range of diagnoses based on clinical and/or radiographic evidence, or when local recurrence of a previously diagnosed tumor is suspected.

Core needle biopsies, on the other hand, provide the pathologist with a larger sample of tissue that preserves the extracellular architecture between the cells, which can be an important part of making a specific histologic diagnosis.[19–22] Also, there is usually enough tissue for immunohistochemistry and cytogenetic analysis, if needed.

Superficial masses can typically be biopsied without image guidance. A successful closed biopsy is dependent on several factors: (1) the mass must be of sufficient size that it is easily palpable, (2) the area of the mass believed to have the most diagnostic tissue is easily identified (ie, nonfluid portions of a heterogeneous tumor), and (3) the mass should be far enough away from critical neurovascular bundles that risk of injury is minimal. When these criteria are not met, the physician should consider an image-guided biopsy. Image guidance decreases the risk of injury to neurovascular structures and can help to ensure that the most diagnostic portion of the mass is sampled.

The treating physician should plan the biopsy path with the radiologist according to the planned surgical resection so as to minimize contamination of multiple compartments, joint spaces, and neurovascular structures. Although controversy exists over the necessity of needle biopsy tract excision, it is safer to assume that the biopsy tract will need to be resected en bloc with the tumor specimen when planning the biopsy.[23–25]

Despite advances with closed biopsy techniques and improvement in diagnostic accuracy with small samples of tissue, open biopsy remains the gold standard. These biopsies, performed under an anesthetic in the operating room, can be incisional or excisional and offer the advantage of immediate frozen section analysis to ensure that diagnostic tissue has been obtained.

Incisional biopsy, which involves the surgical removal of a small portion of a mass, is reserved for large tumors for which treatment may require more than surgical resection depending on the exact diagnosis. Open biopsy is also performed when needle biopsies are nondiagnostic. An incisional biopsy should be performed by the treating surgeon to avoid potential contamination of normal tissue planes that can jeopardize surgical planning.[26,27] During the procedure, a small portion of biopsied tissue is examined with frozen section analysis. In selected cases, if the biopsy confirms a benign lesion, the mass can be resected under the same anesthetic. If the biopsy confirms a malignant lesion, surgery can proceed with wide resection to include the biopsy tract, or the surgical site can be closed and the patient referred for neoadjuvant therapy, as indicated. Biopsy incisions should always be longitudinal and as small as possible so they may be easily excised en bloc with the final tumor specimen. Meticulous hemostasis should be maintained throughout the biopsy to prevent hematoma formation and potential contamination of surrounding tissue.[4] The consequences of a poorly planned biopsy are significant and can alter surgical plans, local recurrence rates, and overall survival.[21,26,27]

For small (<5 cm) masses, excisional biopsy can be performed with little morbidity. For these tumors, resection of the entire mass is sufficient treatment, regardless of whether the mass is benign or malignant. If the surgeon suspects that the tumor is malignant on the basis of clinical and radiographic findings, the mass can be excised with a margin of normal tissue, as there are few data to support the use of neoadjuvant chemotherapy or radiation for small soft tissue sarcomas.

Tumors that are uniformly isointense with normal adipose tissue on all MR imaging sequences, regardless of their size and depth, are often treated with excisional biopsy. Although some of these may be atypical lipomas on final pathologic review, the surgery for atypical lipomas is generally the same as that for lipomas.

TREATMENT OF SOFT TISSUE TUMORS
Benign Tumors

Benign soft tissue tumors can be treated with excision or observation depending on their location, propensity for progression, risk for malignant transformation, and associated symptoms.

Small benign lesions that are painful, such as schwannomas, can be excised for symptomatic relief (**Fig. 4**). Small superficial or subcutaneous lesions that are asymptomatic can often be observed. Masses that are smaller than 5 cm in maximum dimension and superficial to fascia are highly likely to be benign. These lesions are easily monitored through physical examination and can be safely watched in most circumstances. They include diagnoses ranging from lipomas to hemangiomas to nodular fasciitis. These tumors have a very limited potential to progress locally, and when they are minimally symptomatic, do not require further intervention. We recommend the patient be evaluated 6 to 12 weeks after initial presentation, and then every 3 to 6 months thereafter for approximately 1 year to document a lack of growth of the mass. Should the mass begin to increase in size, change in character, or become symptomatic, further imaging or biopsy may be warranted.

Deep, large (eg, >5 cm), benign lesions can be observed or excised, depending on the criteria listed previously. Deep lipomas or myxomas are often treated with marginal excision, in part because they can be mistaken for low-grade malignancies, and biopsy may miss the malignant portions of the overall mass (**Fig. 5**). Furthermore, certain benign tumors are known to progress locally, such as desmoid tumors or aggressive fibromatosis. Although these tumors exhibit a variable degree of local progression, they are usually excised before they involve a critical structure.

Furthermore, some benign tumors, such as neurofibromas, can undergo malignant transformation. For nerve sheath tumors that have unusual imaging characteristics or that are increasing in size, surgical excision should be considered. If the benign nature of the mass can be ensured on the basis of biopsy and clinical/radiographic findings, and if the mass has a low risk of local progression or malignant transformation, then observation with serial imaging studies is a reasonable option.

Malignant Tumors

Malignant soft tissue tumors represent a large group of heterogeneous cancers with variable behaviors both locally and with respect to distant disease. These tumors are staged according to the Enneking/Musculoskeletal Tumor Society staging system or the American Joint Committee on Cancer staging system (**Tables 1 and 2**).[28–30] We present the general treatment strategies and guidelines that are used to treat soft tissue sarcomas in the extremities, but one should bear in mind that these principles do not necessarily apply to other soft tissue malignancies that can occur in the extremities, such as lymphoma, melanoma, or myoepithelial tumors.

A patient diagnosed with a soft tissue sarcoma should be staged before further treatment is planned to understand the systemic extent of the disease, as this may have significant effect on the planned treatment.[31] For most of these sarcomas,

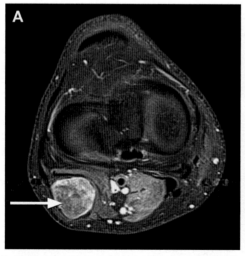 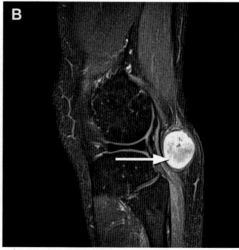

Fig. 4. A 58-year-old man presented with a painful posterior knee mass. Transverse fat-suppressed proton density–weighted (*A*) and sagittal fat-suppressed T2-weighted (*B*) MR images demonstrate a small (<5 cm), relatively superficial mass (*arrow*) in the posterior knee, which, based on the clinical and imaging presentation, was suggestive of a peripheral nerve sheath tumor. Excisional biopsy was performed and pathologic analysis confirmed a benign schwannoma.

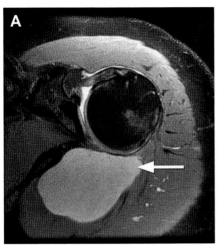 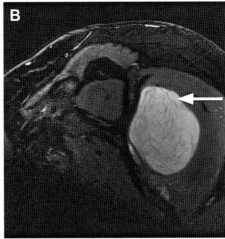

Fig. 5. A 60-year-old man presented for evaluation of a painless posterior shoulder mass. Transverse fat-suppressed proton density–weighted (*A*) and sagittal fat-suppressed T2-weighted (*B*) MR images demonstrate a large, deep mass (*arrow*) of uniform high signal intensity within the infraspinatus muscle, suggestive of a myxomatous tumor. Ultrasound-guided needle biopsy confirmed a benign myxoma and a marginal excision was performed.

MR imaging of the involved area with and without contrast enhancement should be performed. In addition, a CT scan of the chest is performed to examine for pulmonary metastases, the most common site of distant disease for these tumors. In the case of myxoid liposarcoma, CT of the abdomen and pelvis should be included, as these tumors have the potential for spread to the retroperitoneum.[32] Although uncommon, regional lymph node metastases can occur with certain soft tissue sarcomas, such as rhabdomyosarcoma, angiosarcoma, epithelioid sarcoma, clear cell sarcoma, and synovial sarcoma. Lymphadenopathy noted on physical examination should, therefore, be imaged and biopsied, if clinically indicated.

The treatment plan takes into account data from the staging studies in addition to information about tumor grade and size. Small lesions, regardless of tumor grade and patient age, are treated with surgery alone, as neither chemotherapy nor radiation therapy result in significant improvement in local control or overall survival.[33–35] Resection with a wide margin of normal issue is considered appropriate therapy for these sarcomas.

Large, high-grade, deep soft tissue sarcomas are associated with a worse prognosis, and surgery alone is often not sufficient for these patients. Radiation is commonly used to improve local control rates with or without chemotherapy. Chemotherapy remains controversial, as most soft tissue sarcomas are relatively chemoresistant, and reductions in event-free and overall survival appear to be modest. As such, decisions regarding chemotherapy for high-grade, deep, large soft tissue sarcomas are based on the specific clinical context and the perceived risk-benefit ratio.

The goal of radiation therapy in the treatment of soft tissue sarcomas is to improve local control in the setting of limb salvage surgery. The use of radiation in the preoperative or postoperative setting

Table 1
Enneking/MSTS staging system for soft tissue sarcomas

Stage	Histologic Grade	Primary Tumor Site	Distant Metastasis
I_A	G_1	T_1	M_0
I_B	G_1	T_2	M_0
II_A	G_2	T_1	M_0
II_B	G_2	T_2	M_0
III_A	Any G	T_1	M_1
III_B	Any G	T_2	M_1
Definitions			
Histologic Grade	G1: Low grade G2: High grade		
Primary Tumor	T1: Intracompartmental T2: Extracompartmental		
Distant Metastasis	M0: No distant metastasis M1: Distant metastasis		

Data from Enneking WF. A system of staging musculoskeletal neoplasms. Clin Orthop Relat Res 1986;(204): 9–24; and Enneking WF, Spanier SS, Goodman MA. A system for the surgical staging of musculoskeletal sarcoma. Clin Orthop Relat Res 1980;(153):106–20.

Table 2
American Joint Committee on Cancer staging system for soft tissue sarcomas

Stage	Primary Tumor	Regional Lymph Nodes	Distant Metastasis	Histologic Grade
IA	T1a, T1b	N0	M0	G1, GX
IB	T2a, T2b	N0	M0	G1, GX
IIA	T1a, T1b	N0	M0	G2, G3
IIB	T2a, T2b	N0	M0	G2
III	T2a, T2b	N0	M0	G3
	Any T	N1	M0	Any G
IV	Any T	N1	M1	Any G

Definitions	
Primary tumor	T1: Tumor ≤5 cm in greatest dimension T1a: superficial tumor T1b: deep tumor T2: Tumor >5 cm in greatest dimension T2a: superficial tumor T2b: deep tumor
Regional lymph nodes	NX: Lymph nodes cannot be assessed N0: No regional lymph node metastasis N1: Regional lymph node metastasis
Distant metastasis	M0: No distant metastasis M1: Distant metastasis
Histologic grade	GX: Grade cannot be assessed G1: Well differentiated – low grade G2: Moderately differentiated – low grade G3: Poorly differentiated – high grade

From Edge SB, Byrd DR. AJCC cancer staging manual. 7th edition. New York: Springer; 2010; with permission.

has been shown to reduce the rate of local recurrence, but radiation has no effect on long-term survival rate in patients with large, high-grade tumors.[36–38] Controversy still exists regarding whether preoperative or postoperative radiation is superior, as local recurrence rates are similar in several series. Preoperative radiation therapy offers several advantages, including a smaller treatment volume on average that allows for more targeted treatment of the tumor and improved shielding of normal tissue.[37,39] Furthermore, the blood supply to the tumor and surrounding reactive tissues is intact compared with the postoperative setting, which may increase the effectiveness of radiation and allow for administration of lower doses. The major disadvantage is the significant risk of wound-healing complications compared with postoperative radiation therapy.[37] These wound-healing problems can have significant consequences to the patient, including the need for additional surgeries, soft tissue transfers to cover the defects, and in the worst cases, loss of the limb. Postoperative radiation therapy, on the other hand, adds no additional risk to wound healing over the baseline operative risk[37]; however, the treatment volumes are often larger with a higher dose of radiation administered to achieve local control. The late effects of radiation therapy, including edema and fibrosis, are more common with postoperative radiation therapy.[40,41] Regardless of whether preoperative or postoperative radiation therapy is chosen, its addition to the treatment of large, high-grade soft tissue sarcomas is recommended.

The role of chemotherapy is less clearly defined. Some studies have demonstrated improvements in survival, whereas others have found no significant benefit.[42–48] The use of chemotherapy in either the neoadjuvant or adjuvant settings, therefore, remains controversial.[47–49] Despite the current debate, chemotherapy is strongly considered in patients with soft tissue sarcoma known to be at high risk of local recurrence and/or metastatic spread (ie, large, high-grade tumors), or in patients who present with metastatic disease.[43,50]

The goal of surgical resection is to perform a wide en bloc resection of the tumor and biopsy tract ideally with a 2-cm margin of uninvolved tissue. The limiting factor in achieving ideal margins is often adjacent major neurovascular structures or bone (**Fig. 6**). Closer margins are

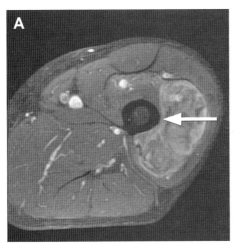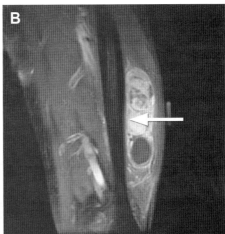

Fig. 6. A 65-year-old man presented for evaluation of a painless, enlarging mass in his lateral thigh. Transverse (*A*) and coronal (*B*) fat-suppressed T1-weighted MR images of the thigh following intravenous administration of gadolinium-chelate, demonstrate a large, heterogeneous, enhancing mass abutting the femur (*arrows*). In-office needle biopsy demonstrated a pleomorphic high-grade sarcoma. Resection with ideal 2-cm margins was not possible because of the tumor's proximity to the femur. Preoperative radiation was administered to decrease local recurrence in the setting of anticipated close margins.

accepted when the tumor abuts vital structures as a means of accomplishing limb salvage, but the use of radiation should be considered to decrease local recurrence rates.

As a result of radiation therapy, improvements in imaging, and a greater understanding of the factors underlying local recurrence and overall survival, the use of amputation to treat soft tissue sarcomas has decreased and most patients are able to safely undergo limb salvage surgeries. Data regarding overall survival rates support this shift in surgical treatment, as studies have demonstrated no difference in long-term survival between patients who undergo amputation and those who undergo limb salvage.[45,51,52] It must be acknowledged, however, that local recurrence rates are higher in the limb salvage groups when compared with amputation.[51] Therefore, although the most reliable way to achieve long-term local control is through amputation, this is reserved for tumors than cannot otherwise be resected with adequate margins (eg, a tumor that surrounds popliteal neurovascular structures).[53] Malignant tumors that have been incompletely or marginally excised are treated with wide reexcision and possible adjuvant radiation.[54,55]

FOLLOW-UP OF SOFT TISSUE TUMORS

Soft tissue sarcomas, even after wide resection, have local recurrence rates of up to 15% in some studies, with most recurrences in the first 2 years postoperatively.[54–57] These data support the

need for long term follow-up in these patients. Postoperative surveillance at our institution includes physical examination of the operative site to evaluate for palpable recurrence, regular chest radiography, and intermittent chest CT. The American College of Radiology recommends periodic nonenhanced CT of the chest for evaluation of metastatic disease to the lungs postoperatively, acknowledging that a cost-benefit analysis does not necessarily support the use of CT scans over good-quality conventional chest radiography.[58] The optimal modality and frequency of postoperative imaging evaluation of the chest has not been clearly established. MR imaging is regarded as the modality of choice for detection of local recurrence; however, the timing and frequency of MR imaging is less well established. The American College of Radiology recommends a relatively aggressive approach in which MR imaging is obtained at 3-month to 6-month intervals for the first 5 years following surgery, and then annually for the next 5 years, acknowledging that physical examination may preclude the need for imaging, particularly in low-risk patients.[58] The timing and frequency of imaging, however, is tailored to the individual patient, and is generally more aggressive for higher risk patients or for patients with deeper central tumors. Patients are seen and evaluated in the office 2, 6, and 12 weeks postoperatively, then every 3 months for the first year, every 4 months for the second postoperative year, every 6 months for the third postoperative year, and annually thereafter for at least 5 years.

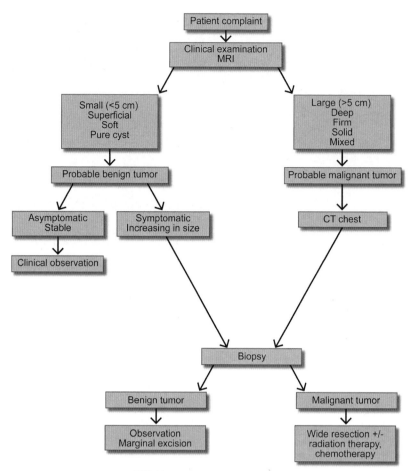

MRI: Magnetic resonance imaging of whole mass
CT: Computed tomography

Fig. 7. An algorithm for the clinical evaluation of soft tissue tumors.

One exception to this surveillance routine is the follow-up of patients with a diagnosis of myxoid liposarcoma. These tumors are known to metastasize not only to the lungs, but to the retroperitoneum. In light of this unusual pattern of metastasis, CT of the chest, abdomen, and pelvis should be performed in lieu of only chest radiography or only chest CT, in addition to routine clinical evaluations.

Benign tumors that have been excised should be followed on a similar schedule for up to 1 year. Benign tumors that are being observed should be followed for a minimum of 1 year every 3 to 6 months to document a lack of progression of the tumors and the need for further imaging or treatment.

SUMMARY

Soft tissue tumors are a wide and heterogeneous group of neoplasms, the treatment of which can vary based on specific diagnosis. We present an algorithm for approaching, diagnosing, and treating these tumors (**Fig. 7**).

REFERENCES

1. SEER Cancer Stat Fact Sheets. [SEER Web Site]. 2011. Available at: http://www.seer.cancer.gov/statfacts/index.html. Accessed April 4, 2011.

2. Fletcher CD, Rydholm A, Singer C, et al. Pathology and genetics of tumours of soft tissue and bone. In: Fletcher CD, Unni KK, Mertens F, et al, editors. World Health Organisation classification of tumours; 4. Lyon (France): Oxford: IARC Press; Oxford University Press (distributor); 2002. p. 12–8.

3. Rydholm A, Berg NO. Size, site and clinical incidence of lipoma. Factors in the differential diagnosis of lipoma and sarcoma. Acta Orthop Scand 1983; 54(6):929–34.

4. Sim FH, Frassica FJ, Frassica DA. Soft-tissue tumors: diagnosis, evaluation, and management. J Am Acad Orthop Surg 1994;2(4):202–11.

5. Morrison WB, Zoga AC, Daffner RH, et al. Soft-Tissue Masses. American College of Radiology. ACR Appropriateness Criteria® 2009. Available at: http://www.acr.org/SecondaryMainMenuCategories/quality_safety/app_criteria/pdf/ExpertPanelonMusculoskeletalImaging/SoftTissueMassesDoc19.aspx. Accessed April 13, 2011.

6. Weekes RG, Berquist TH, McLeod RA, et al. Magnetic resonance imaging of soft-tissue tumors: comparison with computed tomography. Magn Reson Imaging 1985;3(4):345–52.

7. Walker EA, Song AJ, Murphey MD. Magnetic resonance imaging of soft-tissue masses. Semin Roentgenol 2010;45(4):277–97.

8. Crim JR, Seeger LL, Yao L, et al. Diagnosis of soft-tissue masses with MR imaging: can benign masses be differentiated from malignant ones? Radiology 1992;185(2):581–6.

9. Kransdorf MJ, Jelinek JS, Moser RP Jr, et al. Soft-tissue masses: diagnosis using MR imaging. AJR Am J Roentgenol 1989;153(3):541–7.

10. Berquist TH, Ehman RL, King BF, et al. Value of MR imaging in differentiating benign from malignant soft-tissue masses: study of 95 lesions. AJR Am J Roentgenol 1990;155(6):1251–5.

11. De Schepper AM, Bloem JL. Soft tissue tumors: grading, staging, and tissue-specific diagnosis. Top Magn Reson Imaging 2007;18(6):431–44.

12. van Rijswijk CS, Geirnaerdt MJ, Hogendoorn PC, et al. Soft-tissue tumors: value of static and dynamic gadopentetate dimeglumine-enhanced MR imaging in prediction of malignancy. Radiology 2004;233(2):493–502.

13. Wang CK, Li CW, Hsieh TJ, et al. Characterization of bone and soft-tissue tumors with in vivo 1H MR spectroscopy: initial results. Radiology 2004;232(2):599–605.

14. van Rijswijk CS, Kunz P, Hogendoorn PC, et al. Diffusion-weighted MRI in the characterization of soft-tissue tumors. J Magn Reson Imaging 2002;15(3):302–7.

15. Adler RS, Bell DS, Bamber JC, et al. Evaluation of soft-tissue masses using segmented color Doppler velocity images: preliminary observations. AJR Am J Roentgenol 1999;172(3):781–8.

16. Shin DS, Shon OJ, Han DS, et al. The clinical efficacy of (18)F-FDG-PET/CT in benign and malignant musculoskeletal tumors. Ann Nucl Med 2008;22(7):603–9.

17. Wakely PE Jr, Kneisl JS. Soft tissue aspiration cytopathology. Cancer 2000;90(5):292–8.

18. Ng VY, Thomas K, Crist M, et al. Fine needle aspiration for clinical triage of extremity soft tissue masses. Clin Orthop Relat Res 2010;468(4):1120–8.

19. Adams SC, Potter BK, Pitcher DJ, et al. Office-based core needle biopsy of bone and soft tissue malignancies: an accurate alternative to open biopsy with infrequent complications. Clin Orthop Relat Res 2010;468(10):2774–80.

20. Mitsuyoshi G, Naito N, Kawai A, et al. Accurate diagnosis of musculoskeletal lesions by core needle biopsy. J Surg Oncol 2006;94(1):21–7.

21. Skrzynski MC, Biermann JS, Montag A, et al. Diagnostic accuracy and charge-savings of outpatient core needle biopsy compared with open biopsy of musculoskeletal tumors. J Bone Joint Surg Am 1996;78(5):644–9.

22. Strauss DC, Qureshi YA, Hayes AJ, et al. The role of core needle biopsy in the diagnosis of suspected soft tissue tumours. J Surg Oncol 2010;102(5):523–9.

23. Kaffenberger BH, Wakely PE Jr, Mayerson JL. Local recurrence rate of fine-needle aspiration biopsy in primary high-grade sarcomas. J Surg Oncol 2010;101(7):618–21.

24. Kilpatrick SE, Ward WG, Chauvenet AR, et al. The role of fine-needle aspiration biopsy in the initial diagnosis of pediatric bone and soft tissue tumors: an institutional experience. Mod Pathol 1998;11(10):923–8.

25. Schwartz HS, Spengler DM. Needle tract recurrences after closed biopsy for sarcoma: three cases and review of the literature. Ann Surg Oncol 1997;4(3):228–36.

26. Mankin HJ, Lange TA, Spanier SS. The hazards of biopsy in patients with malignant primary bone and soft-tissue tumors. J Bone Joint Surg Am 1982;64(8):1121–7.

27. Mankin HJ, Mankin CJ, Simon MA. The hazards of the biopsy, revisited. Members of the Musculoskeletal Tumor Society. J Bone Joint Surg Am 1996;78(5):656–63.

28. Edge SB, Byrd DR. AJCC cancer staging manual. 7th edition. New York: Springer; 2010.

29. Enneking WF. A system of staging musculoskeletal neoplasms. Clin Orthop Relat Res 1986;(204):9–24.

30. Enneking WF, Spanier SS, Goodman MA. A system for the surgical staging of musculoskeletal sarcoma. Clin Orthop Relat Res 1980;(153):106–20.

31. Peabody TD, Simon MA. Principles of staging of soft-tissue sarcomas. Clin Orthop Relat Res 1993;(289):19–31.

32. DeVita VT, Hellman S, Rosenberg SA. Cancer: principles and practice of oncology. 7th edition. Philadelphia; London: Lippincott Williams & Wilkins; 2005.

33. Gibbs CP, Peabody TD, Mundt AJ, et al. Oncological outcomes of operative treatment of subcutaneous soft-tissue sarcomas of the extremities. J Bone Joint Surg Am 1997;79(6):888–97.

34. Pisters PW, Pollock RE, Lewis VO, et al. Long-term results of prospective trial of surgery alone with selective use of radiation for patients with T1 extremity and trunk soft tissue sarcomas. Ann Surg 2007;246(4):675–81 [discussion: 681–2].

35. Rydholm A, Gustafson P, Rooser B, et al. Subcutaneous sarcoma. A population-based study of 129 patients. J Bone Joint Surg Br 1991;73(4):662–7.

36. Mendenhall WM, Indelicato DJ, Scarborough MT, et al. The management of adult soft tissue sarcomas. Am J Clin Oncol 2009;32(4):436–42.

37. O'Sullivan B, Davis AM, Turcotte R, et al. Preoperative versus postoperative radiotherapy in soft-tissue sarcoma of the limbs: a randomised trial. Lancet 2002;359(9325):2235–41.

38. O'Sullivan B, Wylie J, Catton C, et al. The local management of soft tissue sarcoma. Semin Radiat Oncol 1999;9(4):328–48.

39. Pollack A, Zagars GK, Goswitz MS, et al. Preoperative vs. postoperative radiotherapy in the treatment of soft tissue sarcomas: a matter of presentation. Int J Radiat Oncol Biol Phys 1998;42(3):563–72.

40. Davis AM, O'Sullivan B, Bell RS, et al. Function and health status outcomes in a randomized trial comparing preoperative and postoperative radiotherapy in extremity soft tissue sarcoma. J Clin Oncol 2002;20(22):4472–7.

41. Davis AM, O'Sullivan B, Turcotte R, et al. Late radiation morbidity following randomization to preoperative versus postoperative radiotherapy in extremity soft tissue sarcoma. Radiother Oncol 2005;75(1):48–53.

42. Cormier JN, Huang X, Xing Y, et al. Cohort analysis of patients with localized, high-risk, extremity soft tissue sarcoma treated at two cancer centers: chemotherapy-associated outcomes. J Clin Oncol 2004;22(22):4567–74.

43. Fernberg JO, Hall KS. Chemotherapy in soft tissue sarcoma. The Scandinavian Sarcoma Group experience. Acta Orthop Scand Suppl 2004;75(311):77–86.

44. Frustaci S, Gherlinzoni F, De Paoli A, et al. Adjuvant chemotherapy for adult soft tissue sarcomas of the extremities and girdles: results of the Italian randomized cooperative trial. J Clin Oncol 2001; 19(5):1238–47.

45. Rosenberg SA, Tepper J, Glatstein E, et al. Prospective randomized evaluation of adjuvant chemotherapy in adults with soft tissue sarcomas of the extremities. Cancer 1983;52(3):424–34.

46. Zalupski MM, Baker LH. Systemic adjuvant chemotherapy for soft tissue sarcomas. Hematol Oncol Clin North Am 1995;9(4):787–800.

47. Blay JY, Le Cesne A. Adjuvant chemotherapy in localized soft tissue sarcomas: still not proven. Oncologist 2009;14(10):1013–20.

48. Bramwell VH. Adjuvant chemotherapy for adult soft tissue sarcoma: Is there a standard of care? J Clin Oncol 2001;19(5):1235–7.

49. Benjamin RS. Evidence for using adjuvant chemotherapy as standard treatment of soft tissue sarcoma. Semin Radiat Oncol 1999;9(4):349–51.

50. King JJ, Fayssoux RS, Lackman RD, et al. Early outcomes of soft tissue sarcomas presenting with metastases and treated with chemotherapy. Am J Clin Oncol 2009;32(3):308–13.

51. Potter DA, Kinsella T, Glatstein E, et al. High-grade soft tissue sarcomas of the extremities. Cancer 1986;58(1):190–205.

52. Williard WC, Hajdu SI, Casper ES, et al. Comparison of amputation with limb-sparing operations for adult soft tissue sarcoma of the extremity. Ann Surg 1992; 215(3):269–75.

53. Pisters PW, O'Sullivan B, Maki RG. Evidence-based recommendations for local therapy for soft tissue sarcomas. J Clin Oncol 2007;25(8):1003–8.

54. Zagars GK, Ballo MT, Pisters PW, et al. Surgical margins and reresection in the management of patients with soft tissue sarcoma using conservative surgery and radiation therapy. Cancer 2003;97(10): 2544–53.

55. Potter BK, Adams SC, Pitcher JD Jr, et al. Local recurrence of disease after unplanned excisions of high-grade soft tissue sarcomas. Clin Orthop Relat Res 2008;466(12):3093–100.

56. Cool P, Grimer R, Rees R. Surveillance in patients with sarcoma of the extremities. Eur J Surg Oncol 2005;31(9):1020–4.

57. Trovik CS. Local recurrence of soft tissue sarcoma. A Scandinavian Sarcoma Group Project. Acta Orthop Scand Suppl 2001;72(300):1–31.

58. Fitzgerald JJ, Roberts CC, Daffner RH, et al. Follow-up of malignant or aggressive musculoskeletal tumors. American College of Radiology. ACR Appropriateness Criteria® 2011. Available at: http://www.acr.org/SecondaryMainMenuCategories/quality_safety/app_criteria/pdf/ExpertPanelonMusculoskeletalImaging/FollowUpofMalignantorAggressiveMusculoskeletalTumorsDoc11.aspx. Accessed April 13, 2011.

Magnetic Resonance Imaging of Benign Soft Tissue Neoplasms in Adults

Eric A. Walker, MD[a,b,*], Michael E. Fenton, MD[c],
Joel S. Salesky, MD[c], Mark D. Murphey, MD[b,c,d]

KEYWORDS

- Soft tissue tumor • Benign • MR imaging
- Soft tissue neoplasm

Benign soft tissue lesions outnumber their malignant counterparts by a factor of 100:1.[1,2] Many of these lesions are small and superficial and do not lead to imaging evaluation or biopsy; so precise estimates are unavailable. Magnetic resonance (MR) imaging is the favored modality for evaluation of soft tissue tumors and tumorlike conditions because of its superior soft tissue contrast, multiplanar imaging capability, and lack of radiation exposure. MR imaging is valuable for lesion detection, diagnosis, and staging.

When planning an MR imaging study for evaluation of a soft tissue lesion, at least 2 orthogonal planes should be obtained. In our experience, lesions are typically best evaluated in the axial plane, and this plane is usually the most familiar to radiologists. The secondary plane of imaging for an anterior or posterior lesion is typically the sagittal plane. Coronal sequences are optimal for evaluation of medial or lateral masses.

T1-weighted (T1W) and T2-weighted (T2W) sequences should be obtained because most soft tissue lesions have been described with their spin echo (SE) T1W and T2W signal characteristics. Fast-spin echo sequences in place of SE sequences can reduce scanning time and patient motion artifacts. Gradient echo sequences can be useful for demonstrating hemosiderin with "blooming" and also are subject to artifact caused by metal, hemorrhage, and air. Short tau inversion recovery and chemical shift–selective fat saturation T2W images increase sensitivity to abnormal tissue containing increased water content. However, in our opinion, these techniques also reduce information concerning various tissue consistencies and should be used in the secondary, not the primary, plane of imaging. The smallest diagnostic field of view is preferable when evaluating these lesions.

The use of intravenous contrast for lesion evaluation is controversial but appropriate in certain circumstances. Gadolinium contrast agents increase the T1W signal intensity of many soft tissue tumors, allowing distinction between tumor and muscle or tumor and edema, but the surrounding area of edema may enhance as well. Information about tumor vascularity is also obtained.[3,4] Comparing precontrast and postcontrast T1W fat

---

Disclaimer: The opinions or assertions contained herein are the private views of the authors and are not to be construed as official or as reflecting the views of the Departments of the Army, Navy, or Defense.

[a] Department of Radiology, H066, Milton S. Hershey Medical Center, 500 University Drive, P.O. Box 850, Hershey, PA 17033, USA

[b] Department of Radiology and Nuclear Medicine, Uniformed Services University of the Health Sciences, 4301 Jones Bridge Road, Bethesda, MD 20814, USA

[c] American Institute for Radiologic Pathology, 1010 Wayne Avenue, Suite 320, Silver Spring, MD 20910, USA

[d] Department of Radiology, Walter Reed Army Medical Center, Washington, DC, USA

* Corresponding author. Department of Radiology, H066, Milton S. Hershey Medical Center, 500 University Drive, P.O. Box 850, Hershey, PA 17033.

E-mail address: ewalker@hmc.psu.edu

Radiol Clin N Am 49 (2011) 1197–1217

doi:10.1016/j.rcl.2011.07.007

saturation sequences is useful to distinguish true enhancement from a high T1W signal process such as lesion hemorrhage or a proteinaceous fluid collection.

Many investigators have evaluated the use of dynamic enhancement with gadolinium to aid in differentiating benign from malignant soft tissue lesions.[3,5,6] High soft tissue vascularity and perfusion result in an increased rate of enhancement. Benign lesions usually reveal less enhancement overall and a delayed rate of enhancement.[7] There is a significant overlap between the rate of enhancement of benign and malignant lesions.[8] In our opinion and experience, dynamic enhancement does not obviate biopsy of the otherwise indeterminate solid soft tissue mass.

Studies are conflicting regarding the use of tumor margins, homogenous versus heterogeneous signal intensity, and lesion size to distinguish benign from malignant lesions. The most optimistic report suggests the distinction can be made in more than 90% of cases.[9] Other investigators note that malignant lesions can appear smoothly marginated and homogenous and MR appearance cannot accurately separate benign and malignant processes.[3,10–14] Only a minority (5%) of soft tissue tumors are larger than 5 cm in diameter, and about 1% of benign lesions are deep.[15,16] In general, well-defined smooth margins, homogenous signal intensity, and small size are seen with benign lesions. Unless a specific diagnosis can be determined, a lesion should be considered indeterminate and biopsy performed, with an appropriate biopsy path discussed with the orthopedic oncologist or treating surgeon.[17,18]

Lesion location is important for limiting the differential diagnosis. MR imaging with its excellent soft tissue contrast is superior for determining lesion location. Descriptions of lesion location include intramuscular, intermuscular, subcutaneous, and intra-articular/periarticular. A multifocal or an extensive lesion also limits diagnostic considerations to include angiomatous lesions, neurofibromatosis (NF), fibromatosis, lipomatosis, and myxoma (in cases of Mazabraud syndrome). In contradistinction to other organ locations, metastases and lymphoma are less likely considerations. Specific anatomic location may also aid in diagnosis, such as elastofibroma occurring deep to the scapular tip.

Lesions discussed in this review are included because of their frequency, location, or unique imaging characteristics, allowing a specific diagnosis or limited differential diagnosis. For common but nonspecific lesions, a reasonable differential diagnosis requires knowledge of lesion prevalence, anatomic distribution, and age range.

Lesions that predominantly affect pediatric patients (see the article by Navarro and colleagues elsewhere in this issue for further exploration of this topic), malignant soft tissue tumors (see the article by Walker and colleagues elsewhere in this issue for further exploration of this topic), and tumorlike conditions (see the article by Stacy and colleagues elsewhere in this issue for further exploration of this topic) are discussed in separate articles within this issue.

NODULAR FASCIITIS

Nodular fasciitis (**Fig. 1**) is a benign soft tissue lesion composed of proliferating fibroblasts. The lesion may grow rapidly and show high mitotic activity, simulating a more aggressive lesion. It is the most common tumor or tumorlike condition of fibrous tissue.[19] Nodular fasciitis typically affects patients aged between 20 and 40 years, with no sex predilection.[19–22] Lesions typically present as a rapidly growing painless mass that may cause mild pain or tenderness in approximately 50% of cases.[19] The upper extremity is involved in 46% of cases, particularly the volar forearm. Other common locations include the head/neck (20%), the trunk (18%) and the lower extremity (16%).[23] The size of this lesion can vary from 0.5 to 10 cm, but most (71%) are 2 cm or smaller.[24] Nodular fasciitis has 3 common locations: subcutaneous, fascial, and intramuscular.[22] Lesions are subcutaneous between 3 and 10 times more frequently than other sites. The fascial form is the second most common, and the least frequent is the intramuscular type. The deeper intramuscular form is usually larger and is the most likely to be mistaken for sarcoma.[22,25,26] Recurrence of nodular fasciitis is rare even after partial resection.[24]

Calcification or ossification is rarely seen on radiograph.[27] On T1W images, nodular fasciitis has a signal intensity similar to or slightly higher than skeletal muscle.[25,28] With T2W sequences, the condition most often has a high signal intensity (> subcutaneous fat) but may demonstrate intermediate signal intensity.[26] Lesions are frequently homogeneous on T1W sequences and heterogeneous on longer repetition time (TR) acquisitions.[28] This lesion, as well as ancient schwannoma, is one of the few benign lesions that may demonstrate central necrosis, which may contribute to lesion heterogeneity.[23] Contrast enhancement was present in all cases in a series of 8 patients with a diffuse enhancement pattern in 63% of cases and peripheral enhancement in approximately 25%.[26] Linear extension along the fascia (fascial tail sign) may suggest the diagnosis, and mild surrounding edema may also be present.[23]

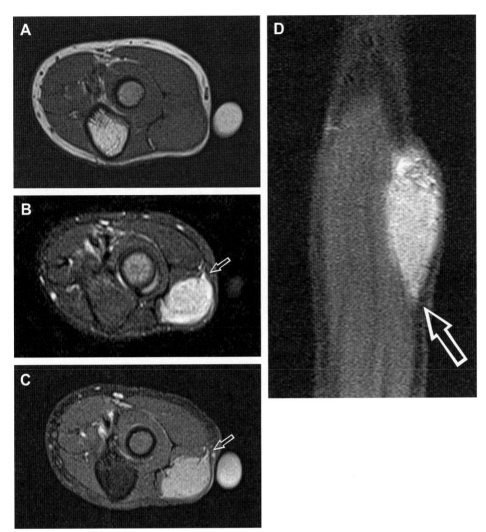

Fig. 1. Nodular fasciitis. Nodular fasciitis in a 5-year-old boy who presented with a palpable elbow mass. (*A*) Axial T1W (repetition time/echo time [TR/TE], 501/15) MR image demonstrates a subcutaneous soft tissue mass, which is isointense to mildly hyperintense compared with muscle. This mass is hyperintense on (*B*) axial short tau inversion recovery (STIR) image (TR/TE, 4700/35). Axial (*C*) and sagittal (*D*) T1W, postcontrast, fat-suppressed (TR/TE, 704/15) MR images reveal relatively homogenous diffuse enhancement. Mild linear fascial extension (fascial tail sign, *white arrows*) is demonstrated on STIR and postcontrast imaging.

The differential diagnosis on MR imaging includes benign fibrous histiocytoma, extra-abdominal desmoid tumor, neurofibroma, and malignant fibrous histiocytoma (MFH) or fibrosarcoma.

SUPERFICIAL FIBROMATOSIS: PALMAR AND PLANTAR FIBROMA

Palmar fibromatosis (Dupuytren disease) (**Fig. 2**A, B) is the most common of the superficial fibromatoses, affecting 1% to 2% of the population.[23] These lesions occur 3 to 4 times more commonly in men and most frequently in patients older than 65 years (up to 20%).[29,30] Bilateral lesions are present in 40% to 60% of cases.[23] The lesions are painless slow-growing palmar nodules, which may cause a flexion contracture most commonly affecting the flexor tendons of the fourth finger.[31] Patients with palmar fibromatosis commonly have other types of fibromatoses, including plantar fibromatosis (5%–20%), Peyronie disease (2%–4%), and knuckle pad fibromatosis.[23,30]

MR imaging typically shows multiple nodular or cordlike superficial soft tissue masses, which involve the aponeurosis of the volar aspect of the hand, extending superficially in parallel to the flexor tendons. Nodules may progress slowly (months to years) into fibrous cords, which attach

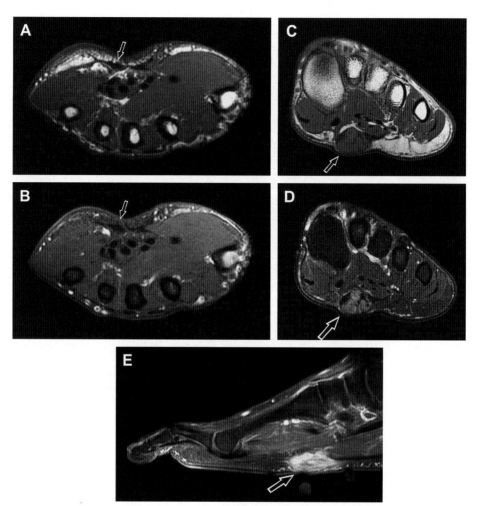

Fig. 2. Superficial fibromatosis. Palmar fibromatosis in a 44-year-old man with palmar pain at the midhypothenar eminence (*A*, *B*). (*A*) Axial T1W and (*B*) axial fat-suppressed T1W postcontrast (TR/echo time [TR/TE], 500/21) images reveal low-signal nodular thickening of the palmar fascia (*arrows*). (*C–E*) Plantar fibromatosis in a 54-year-old man with left foot pain for 1 year. MR images demonstrate a well-defined mass (*arrows*) in the medial aspect of the plantar aponeurosis (*C*). Short-axis T1W (TR/TE, 568.5/15) sequence reveals the mass with lesion signal intensity similar to skeletal muscle. There is heterogeneity with several foci of low signal within the lesion. The signal intensity of the mass is intermediate to hyperintense relative to skeletal muscle and heterogeneous on (*D*) short-axis T2W image with fat saturation (TR/TE, 2693.7/60), and there is marked heterogeneous enhancement on (*E*) sagittal fat-suppressed T1W postcontrast (TR/TE, 539.5/15) image with linear extension along the plantar aponeurosis.

to and cause traction on the underlying flexor tendons, resulting in flexion contractures of the digits (Dupuytren contractures).[32] The lesion size is reported to range from 10 to 55 mm. Lesion signal intensity on T1W and T2W images is low (similar to tendon), reflecting hypocellularity and dense collagen. MR imaging can be helpful for surgical planning because relatively immature lesions demonstrate intermediate to higher signal on T1W and T2W images, reflecting the high cellularity, and have a higher local recurrence rate after local resection. Mature lesions with low T1W and T2W signal intensity are less likely to locally

recur.[31,33,34] Lesions show diffuse enhancement, which is more prominent in lesions with higher cellularity.

Plantar fibromatosis (Ledderhose disease) (see **Fig. 2**C–E) occurs less frequently than the palmar lesion, with an incidence of 0.23%.[35] In our experience, Ledderhose disease is more frequently imaged than Dupuytren disease. Similar to palmar fibromatosis, incidence increases with advancing age, but 44% of patients were younger than 30 years in a large Armed Forces Institute of Pathology study (501 patients).[30,36] Men are affected twice as often as women, and lesions are bilateral in 20% to 50% of cases.[37,38] Patients present with one or more subcutaneous nodules, which most frequently affect the medial aspect of the plantar arch (78%)[39] and can extend to the skin or deep structures of the foot. Nodules may be multiple in 33% of cases.[39] The lesions are typically painless, but patients may have pain with prolonged standing or walking.

With MR imaging, well- or ill-defined superficial lesions along the deep plantar aponeurosis typically blend with the adjacent plantar musculature. Lesions typically show heterogeneous signal (92%), which is isointense to hypointense to skeletal muscle on T1W (100%) and T2W (78%) sequences. The degree of enhancement has been reported as marked in approximately 60% and mild in 33% of cases.[39] Linear tails of extension (fascial tail sign) along the aponeurosis are frequent and best seen after intravenous contrast administration.[23,32]

DEEP FIBROMATOSIS

The World Heath Organization in April 2002 designated the term desmoid-type fibromatosis for all the deep fibromatoses. Desmoid tumor is a descriptive term from the Greek word *desmos* (meaning band or tendon). The biological behavior of fibromatosis is intermediate between fibroma and fibrosarcoma, although they do not metastasize.[23] Deep or musculoaponeurotic fibromatoses include extra-abdominal fibromatosis (aggressive fibromatosis, desmoid tumor, musculoaponeurotic fibromatosis) (**Fig. 3**), abdominal fibromatosis, and intra-abdominal fibromatosis. Intra-abdominal fibromatosis arises within the pelvis and mesentery and is the type most commonly associated with Gardner syndrome.[40,41] Abdominal fibromatosis tends to occur in women during or immediately after pregnancy or with oral contraceptive use. Estrogen seems to be a stimulatory growth factor.[42] The rectus abdominis and internal oblique muscles of the anterior abdominal wall are most frequently affected.[30] The most common locations of extra-abdominal fibromatosis are the shoulder/upper arm (28%), chest wall/paraspinal region (17%), thigh (12%), and head and neck (10%–23%). These fibromatoses are most common in the second and third decades, with a peak incidence in the ages between 25 and 40 years.[23,43] Around 2 to 4 people per million are affected with this lesion, and less than 5% are seen in the pediatric age group.[30] There is a female predilection in younger patients, which equalizes in older patients. Desmoid-type fibromatosis presents as a deep, firm, and poorly circumscribed soft tissue mass, which is usually slow growing and painless.[23,30] Lesions may be multicentric in 10% to 15% of cases and may insinuate about vital neurovascular structures.[23,44] A skeletal dysplasia has been reported

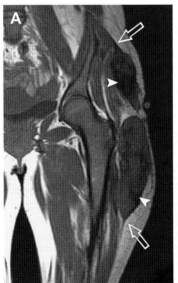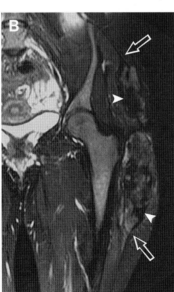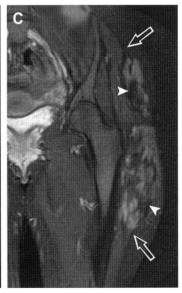

Fig. 3. Deep fibromatosis. Deep fibromatosis in a 31-year-old woman with a slowly enlarging thigh mass. (*A*) Coronal T1W (TR/echo time [TR/TE], 500/15), (*B*) T2W fat-suppressed (TR/TE, 500/15), and (*C*) T1W postcontrast fat-suppressed (TR/TE, 4800/70) MR images demonstrate a bilobed heterogeneous thigh mass with intermediate T1 and intermediate T2 signal, with diffuse patchy enhancement. Fascial linear extension can be seen at the proximal and distal aspect (*arrows*). Areas of bandlike nonenhancing low T1 and T2 signal correspond with hypocellular areas of collagen (*arrowheads*).

in 19% of patients with multicentric desmoid-type fibromatosis.

MR imaging is the optimal modality for evaluation of deep fibromatosis because of its superior soft tissue contrast. Lesions are usually centered intermuscularly with a rim of fat (split fat sign). Invasion of the surrounding muscle is frequent. Lesion borders are equally distributed between well-defined (49%–54%) or irregular infiltrative margins (45%–51%).[21,32,45] Linear extension along fascial planes (fascial tail sign) is a common manifestation (80%–83% of cases).[21,32] The signal intensity of desmoid-type fibromatosis is quite variable, reflecting the relative amounts of collagen and degree of cellularity of the lesion. Immature lesions with marked cellularity reveal higher signal intensity on long TR images. In our experience, these immature lesions are also associated with a higher local recurrence rate after resection. Relatively mature hypocellular areas with abundant collagen reveal lower signal intensity on T1W and T2W sequences often in a bandlike morphology.[21,46] Large studies of patients have shown that the most common appearance of desmoid-type fibromatosis on MR imaging is intermediate signal intensity on both T1W (similar to muscle, 83%–95% of cases) and T2W images (lower than fat but higher than muscle on images without fat suppression, 46%–77% of cases).[21,45,47–49] T1W and T2W sequences commonly show significant heterogeneity. Postcontrast MR imaging reveals moderate to marked heterogeneous enhancement, with less than 10% of lesions lacking significant enhancement.[50] Although low-signal T2W areas are not specific for desmoid-type fibromatosis (see suggested differential diagnosis later), the bandlike morphology of some areas of low signal intensity suggests this diagnosis, seen in 62% to 91% of cases.[21,45] These low-signal bands are best observed on T2W or T1W fat-saturated images after intravenous gadolinium administration (the hypocellular collagenized bands do not enhance).

The differential diagnosis for soft tissue lesions with prominent areas of low signal intensity on T1W and T2W sequences includes desmoid-type fibromatosis, densely calcified masses, pigmented villonodular synovitis (PVNS)/giant cell tumor of the tendon sheath (GCTTS), elastofibroma, granular cell tumor, desmoplastic fibroblastoma, and MFH/fibrosarcoma.

ELASTOFIBROMA

Elastofibroma (**Fig. 4**) is not a neoplasm but rather a slowly growing fibroelastic reactive pseudotumor, likely resulting from mechanical friction between the scapula and the chest wall.[51,52] These lesions were noted in 24% of women and 11% of men in an autopsy series of patients older than 55 years.[53] A review of 258 chest computed tomographic (CT) examinations revealed an incidence of 2% of elastofibroma.[54] Most patients are older adults with peak incidence in the sixth and seventh decades. Lesions may be bilateral in 10% to 66% of cases.[23] There is a 2:1 female predominance. Most patients are asymptomatic (>50%), but the most common symptom is stiffness, present in 25% of cases.[55] The lesion is found between the inferior scapula tip and the chest wall in 95% to 99% of cases.[55] T1W and T2W images show a crescentic heterogeneous lesion with signal similar to adjacent skeletal muscle and streaks of tissue often at the periphery isointense to fat. T2W hypointensity is likely related to low cellularity of the fibrous tissue and elastic fibers. Heterogeneous enhancement is common.[23,56] A key imaging feature is entrapped fat within the lesion, which is well seen with CT or MR imaging. The characteristic lesion location along with demonstration of entrapped fat is pathognomonic of elastofibroma.

LIPOMA

A lipoma is a benign neoplasm composed of mature adipose tissue. It is the most common soft tissue neoplasm and represents about 50% of all soft tissue tumors. The incidence is approximately 2.1 per 100 people.[15,57] Lipoma is more common than liposarcoma by a ratio of 100:1.[15,58,59] Most lipomas are discrete masses categorized by anatomic location as superficial (subcutaneous) or deep. Deep lesions are much less common and account for approximately 1% of lipomas but are imaged more frequently.[15] Lipoma is rare in the first 2 decades of life.[60]

Superficial lipomas (**Fig. 5**A) typically present in the fifth to seventh decades, with 80% of lesions in patients aged 27 to 85 years.[61] Both men and women have been reported as more commonly affected, but there is no clear-cut sex predilection.[59,62,63] Lesions are typically small, with 80% measuring less than 5 cm.[59] Superficial lipomas are most commonly located in the trunk, shoulders, upper arm, and neck and are unusual in the hand or foot.[59] The local recurrence rate is approximately 4%.[63] Superficial lipoma is often difficult to distinguish from the surrounding subcutaneous tissue, particularly if the lesion is nonencapsulated. For this reason, we prefer placing a fiducial marker over superficial lesions, position the patient so the lesion is not compressed, and

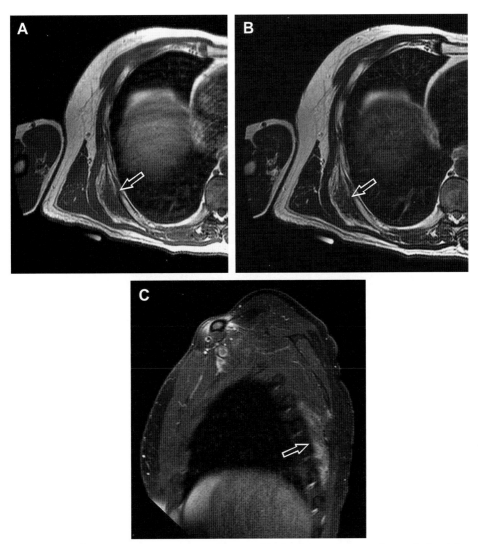

Fig. 4. Elastofibroma. Elastofibroma in a 61-year-old man with slowly growing mass beneath the right scapular tip. (*A*) Axial T1W (TR/echo time [TR/TE], 500/20) and (*B*) T2W (TR/TE, 3500/96) images without fat suppression demonstrate a lenticular mass (*white arrow*) with signal similar to skeletal muscle and hyperintense peripheral linear streaks of entrapped fat. Heterogeneous enhancement (*white arrow*) is noted in (*C*) sagittal T1W image after gadolinium enhancement (TR/TE, 505/7).

compare the area with the contralateral unaffected side.

Deep lipomas (including the intramuscular and intermuscular lipomatous tumors) (see **Fig. 5**B, C) occur most commonly in patients aged 20 to 60 years. Men are affected more frequently than women, and lesions commonly affect the large muscles of the lower extremity (45%), trunk (17%), shoulder (12%), and upper extremity (10%).[61] Lipomas of the retroperitoneum are rare, and a lipomatous lesion in this location should be treated as a liposarcoma until proven otherwise.[58,64] The size range of lipoma is large, and

some lesions can measure up to 20 cm.[15,58,59] Both superficial and deep lipomas often present with a painless slow-growing soft tissue mass.[63] Lipomas may be multiple in 5% to 15% of patients.[15,23,59,62] Weiss and colleagues[60] separate deep lipomas from the intramuscular and intermuscular lipomatous tumors, but we group all lipomatous lesions found beneath the superficial fascia together as deep lipomas. In our experience, deep lipomas involving the extremity are most commonly intramuscular.[61]

Diffuse lipomatosis is overgrowth of mature adipose tissue infiltrating through the soft tissues

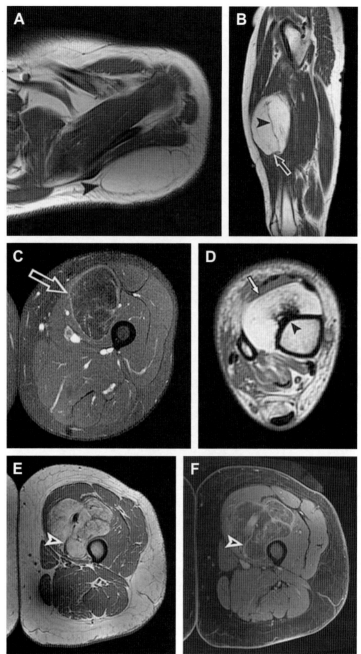

Fig. 5. Benign lipomatous lesions. Encapsulated lipoma in a 20-year-old man with enlarging shoulder mass (*A*). Axial T1W (TR/echo time [TR/TE], 500/11) image demonstrates a well-encapsulated (*black arrowhead*) subcutaneous lesion with signal isointense to subcutaneous fat. Intramuscular lipoma in a 38-year-old woman with slowly growing thigh mass for 6 years (*B, C*). (*B*) Sagittal T1W (TR/TE, 470.7/20) and (*C*) axial T1W fat-saturated postcontrast (TR/TE, 625/22) images demonstrate an intramuscular lesion (*arrows*) with signal identical to subcutaneous fat and thin fibrous septa (*black arrowhead*). Parosteal lipoma in a 41-year-old man with ankle mass (*D*). Axial T1W (TR/TE, 621.5/7) sequence reveals a fatty lesion (*arrow*) with high signal along the bone surface with an osseous excrescence (*arrowhead*) arising from the tibia. Note the absence of cortical and medullary continuity. Hibernoma in a 40-year-old woman with enlarging thigh mass for 5 months (*E, F*). (*E*) Axial T1W (TR/TE, 966.7/14) and (*F*) spoiled gradient recalled echo (TR/TE, 200/1.2) fat-saturated postcontrast sequences demonstrate an intramuscular lesion with signal intensity similar to, but not identical to, mature adult fat with prominent vessels (*arrowheads*). Unlike lipoma, serpentine vessels and prominent septa result in a lesion of greater complexity than normal subcutaneous tissue (compare with [*A*]).

of an affected extremity or the trunk. It is identical to lipoma microscopically.[65] Diffuse lipomatosis may be associated with osseous overgrowth and deformity.

Radiologic evaluation is diagnostic in up to 71% of cases.[61] Lipomas most commonly demonstrate signal isointense to subcutaneous fat on all pulse sequences with high signal on T1W and T2W sequences and thin (<2 mm) septations; however, 28% to 30% may have thick septa or nodularity similar to liposarcoma.[66] We also find it useful to compare the degree of lesion septation to adjacent normal subcutaneous fat. Lipomas typically reveal septations of no greater thickness or number than this normal tissue. Intramuscular lipomas may have irregular margins, which interdigitate with the adjacent skeletal muscle referred to as infiltrating lipoma. In a 2003 study of 58 lipomatous lesions, lipomas showed no enhancement of septa in 58% of cases and moderate enhancement of the septa in 37%.[67] The fibrous capsule often enhances. Calcifications are reported in 11% of benign fatty tumors but are more common in malignant lesions.[68]

The differential diagnosis for a lipomatous lesion with mild complexity includes lipoma, angiolipoma, myolipoma, chondroid lipoma, lipoblastoma, spindle cell/pleomorphic lipoma, hibernoma, and well-differentiated liposarcoma.

LIPOMA ARBORESCENS

Lipoma arborescens is the infiltration of subsynovial tissue by mature adipocytes. It is thought to be a reactive process frequently associated with degenerative joint disease, chronic rheumatoid arthritis, or prior trauma.[60] Clinical symptoms include painless synovial thickening and intermittent effusions.[23] Men are affected more frequently, and the age range is 9 to 66 years. The most common location is the knee.[69] The MR imaging appearance is that of a large villous frondlike mass in the suprapatellar bursa with signal similar to subcutaneous fat on all sequences and an associated joint effusion. Enhancement may be noted about these fatty fronds secondary to inflamed synovium, although typically mild.[23]

HIBERNOMA

Hibernoma (see **Fig. 5**E, F) is a rare tumor of brown fat. These lesions usually occur between the ages of 20 and 40 years, with a peak in the third decade.[60] Hibernomas show a mild female predilection and are commonly seen in the thigh (30%), subcutaneous regions of the back (particularly the periscapular and interscapular region),

neck, axilla, shoulder, thorax, and retroperitoneum.[70,71] The clinical presentation is usually a slow-growing painless mass that most often arises in the subcutaneous tissue, but 10% are intramuscular.[60] MR imaging features are similar to those of lipoma with prominent septations that largely represent serpentine vessels including a feeding vascular pedicle. Identification of these vascular structures by MR imaging excludes lipoma or well-differentiated liposarcoma and, in our experience, is pathognomonic of the diagnosis. Care should be taken to avoid this vascularity when these lesions are biopsied.[23] Intense uptake is reported with fludeoxyglucose F 18 positron emission tomographic scanning, which is not typically noted with lipoma or well-differentiated liposarcoma and reflects the hypervascularity and increased cellular activity of hibernoma.[72,73]

PAROSTEAL LIPOMA

Parosteal lipoma (see **Fig. 5**D) represents 0.3% of all lipomas.[74] Patients are usually adults with an average age of 50 years. Parosteal lipoma shows a slight predilection for men. Lesions are usually adjacent to the diaphysis or metadiaphysis of the femur, humerus, or bones of the leg and forearm.[74] The most frequent clinical presentation is a painless nontender mass that gradually increases in size.[75] An osseous excrescence extending into a lipomatous mass or cortical thickening is noted in more than two-thirds of cases.[23,76] MR imaging demonstrates signal identical to subcutaneous fat on all sequences. Fibrovascular septa may demonstrate high signal on long TR sequences and mild enhancement.[75,77]

PVNS AND GCTTS

Benign proliferative lesions of the synovium, bursa, and tendon sheath represent a family of abnormalities. These lesions are believed to be benign neoplasms rather than secondary to a reactive process.[78,79] They are divided based on their location (intra-articular vs extra-articular) and their pattern of growth (localized vs diffuse).[23] The localized or focal form of PVNS is usually extra-articular, involving the synovium about tendon sheaths or bursae. This form is often referred to as GCTTS. The diffuse form of PVNS is a monoarticular process but affects the entire synovium of a single joint.

Localized disease is approximately 7 times more common than the diffuse form of PVNS. It is typically seen in adults, in the third to fifth decades of life, with a slight female predominance.[80–83] Localized disease most commonly occurs in the hand and wrist (65%–89%) and clinically presents as a soft tissue swelling or a painless mobile soft tissue nodule, most frequently volar in location. It is second only to the ganglion in its frequency to cause a soft tissue mass of the hand and wrist.[81,84] Radiographs may reveal a nonspecific soft tissue mass but are normal in 20% of patients.[81–83] Pressure erosions of bone occur in approximately 15% of cases.[80,83] MR imaging shows a well-defined mass intimately involving the tendon with nonspecific intrinsic signal characteristics. Lesions generally show intermediate T1W signal intensity equal to or less than muscle and T2W signal intensity equal to or

less than fat.[85] Gadolinium enhancement is noted in most cases.[86] Local recurrence after complete resection is rare.[87–89]

The diffuse type of PVNS (**Fig. 6**) is most commonly seen in the third and fourth decades of life with an equal male and female distribution.[90] This type most commonly affects large joints, with knee involvement in 75% to 80% of patients. Less commonly, in decreasing order of frequency, the hip, ankle, shoulder, and elbow are affected.[91–93] Involvement of more than 1 joint is rare. Patients often present with mechanical pain, swelling, and decreased range of motion because of a slow-growing mass, which worsens with activity and

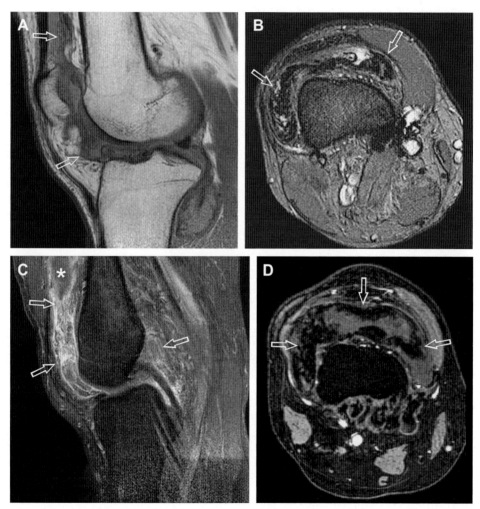

Fig. 6. PVNS. Diffuse PVNS in a 37-year-old woman with pain and swelling of right knee for 1 year. (*A*) Sagittal proton density–weighted (TR/echo time [TR/TE], 2000/21.3) and (*B*) axial fat-saturated T2W (TR/TE; 3800/105) MR images show diffuse low–signal intensity thickening (*arrows*) of the synovium. (*C*) Sagittal fat-saturated T1W postcontrast image shows diffuse synovial enhancement (*arrows*) throughout the knee. Note the peripheral enhancement around the joint effusion (*asterisk*). (*D*) Axial gradient echo imaging (TR/TE, 50/12) in a 26-year-old man with chronic knee pain shows accentuation (blooming) of the low signal of the thickened synovium (*arrows*) resulting from hemosiderin deposition.

improves with rest.[94] In contrast to the localized form, tumor recurrence after surgical resection is common, approaching 50%.[95] Pressure erosions with sclerotic borders on both sides of the joint, reflecting a synovial-based lesion, are seen in 15% of patients, more commonly in smaller less capacious joints such as the hip (93%) and shoulder (75%).[91,92] Despite the erosions, the joint space and bone mineralization are usually preserved. On MR imaging, associated bone marrow edema may be noted at sights of osseous erosion. MR imaging characteristically shows a diffuse, heterogeneous, synovial-based thickening extending along the joint surface. On T1W imaging, the signal intensity of the mass is similar to, or slightly less than, that of skeletal muscle. Predominantly low signal intensity on T2W imaging is generally seen owing to the shortening of T2 relaxation times because of hemosiderin deposition.[90,96,97] This low signal intensity also causes susceptibility (blooming) artifact on gradient echo imaging, helping to distinguish PVNS from other entities that may cause diffuse synovial thickening.[98] PVNS typically shows prominent enhancement after the administration of gadolinium contrast.[99,100] Coexistent joint effusions are seen in up to 50% of cases and are usually surrounded by thickened, low–signal intensity, hemosiderin-laden synovium.[101]

BENIGN PERIPHERAL NERVE SHEATH TUMOR

Benign peripheral nerve sheath tumors (BPNST) are typically divided into schwannoma (neurilemoma) and neurofibroma.[78] Both lesions contain cells closely related to the normal Schwann cell.

Schwannoma is slightly less common than neurofibroma and comprises approximately 5% of all benign soft tissue tumors.[58] Schwannoma is most commonly seen in patients aged between 20 and 50 years with an equal sex distribution.[102,103] Schwannoma is usually a slow-growing nonaggressive lesion that presents as a painless mass smaller than 5 cm. Pain may be associated with larger lesions or schwannomatosis.[23,102] Common sites of involvement include the cutaneous nerves of the head, neck, and flexor surface of the extremities. The posterior mediastinum and retroperitoneum are frequent locations for deep-seated lesions.[102] Lesions are usually sporadic (90%) but may be plexiform or multiple in approximately 5% of cases; 3% occur with NF type 2 and 2% occur with schwannomatosis.[104,105] The lesion is typically separable from the adjacent nerve after incising the epineurium, and nerve function is thus preserved after resection.[23]

Neurofibroma (**Fig. 7**A, B) constitutes slightly more than 5% of benign soft tissue tumors.[58] Neurofibroma is most commonly seen in patients aged between 20 and 30 years and demonstrates no sex predilection.[102,103] Three types of neurofibroma are classically described, including localized (90%), diffuse, and plexiform lesions.[23,58] Superficial cutaneous or deep-seated nerves may be involved. Localized neurofibromas are usually slow-growing painless masses measuring less than 5 cm. The diffuse type primarily affects children and young adults and most frequently involves the subcutaneous tissue of the head and neck, and only 10% are associated with NF type 1 (NF1).[23,58] Neurofibroma, unlike schwannoma, cannot be separated from the nerve, and complete excision of the neoplasm requires sacrifice of the nerve.[106]

NF1 is seen in 1 in every 2500 to 3000 births.[107] Men are more commonly affected.[102] NF1 demonstrates multiple localized neurofibromas and frequently plexiform lesions. The localized form of neurofibroma is the most common type seen with NF1. These lesions occur anywhere in the body, both superficial and deep. Plexiform neurofibromas (see **Fig. 7**C) develop (or occur) in approximately 50% of patients with NF1.[108] Plexiform neurofibroma represents diffuse involvement of a long segment of nerve, giving a ropelike or bag-of-worms appearance, and is pathognomonic of NF1. The incidence of malignant transformation to malignant peripheral nerve sheath tumor (MPNST) is between 2% and 29% in patients with NF1.[102,109]

On MR imaging, the intrinsic appearance of localized lesions is nonspecific with signal intensity similar to or lower than muscle on T1W images and higher than fat on T2W images. Recognition of a well-defined fusiform shape of the lesion in a typical large nerve location can suggest that the lesion represents schwannoma, localized neurofibroma, or MPNST. The fusiform shape is caused by the tubular entering and exiting nerve.[23] With schwannoma, the entering and exiting nerve may be eccentric to the soft tissue mass. BPNST of the paraspinal region often demonstrates a dumbbell shape with extension into an enlarged neural foramina.[110] Diffuse neurofibroma may show predominant low T2W signal, which may be related to the high collage content. Heterogeneity of BPNST is variable, particularly with hemorrhage, necrosis, and areas of degeneration seen most commonly in the ancient schwannomas (see **Fig. 7**D, E).[23] The target sign is almost pathognomonic for neurofibroma (58%) but can be seen with schwannoma (15%). This sign refers to low to intermediate T2W signal centrally secondary to

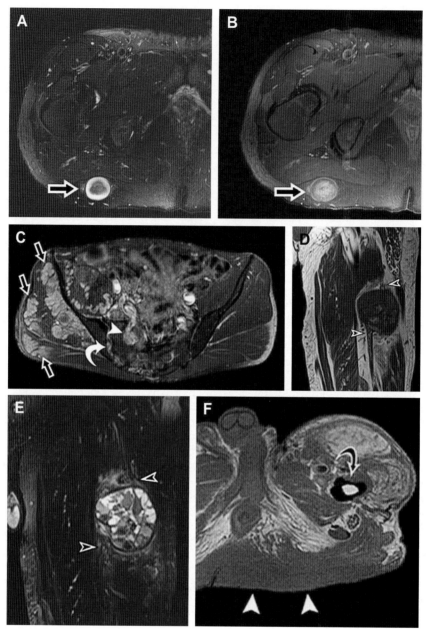

Fig. 7. Benign neural lesions. Neurofibroma in a 34-year-old man with NF1 and right buttock pain (*A, B*). (*A*) Axial T2W fat-saturated (TR/echo time [TR/TE], 4929/99) and (*B*) T1W fat-saturated postcontrast images (TR/TE, 750/12) demonstrate the target sign and central enhancement (*arrows*). The high peripheral signal on T2W images is secondary to myxoid stroma, and the fibrous center reveals marked enhancement. Plexiform neurofibromas in a 30-year-old man with NF1 (*C*). T1W fat-saturated postcontrast image (TR/TE; 645/14) shows plexiform neurofibromas between the gluteal muscles (*arrows*), in the right sacroiliac joint (*curved arrow*), and emerging from a right sacral foramen (*arrowhead*). An ancient schwannoma in a 60-year-old man with a painful left thigh mass for several months (*D, E*). (*D*) Coronal T1W (TR/TE, 560/10) and (*E*) T2W fat-saturated (TR/TE, 1700/25) images demonstrate a mass of the sciatic nerve with eccentric entering and exiting nerves (*arrowheads*). Note the marked heterogeneity from degeneration and cyst formation. Diffuse neurofibroma in a 53-year-old man with NF1 and left thigh mass for many years (*F*). Axial T1W image (TR/TE, 787/07) reveals replacement of the subcutaneous fat with plaquelike intermediate signal lesion (*arrowheads*). Also note osseous changes from mesodermal dysplasia in this patient with NF1 (*curved arrow*).

fibrous tissue with a higher collagen content and high T2W signal peripherally likely related to myxoid (high water content) tissue.[111] The central fibrous areas reveal contrast enhancement in neurofibroma (75%) and less frequently in schwannoma (8%).[112] The fascicular sign manifests as multiple ringlike structures seen on T2W or proton density-weighted images and is seen in superficial and deep-seated lesions.[23] The fascicular appearance is noted in 25% of neurofibromas and 63% of schwannomas.[112] A rim of fat (split fat sign) is often seen with deep-seated BPNSTs but is nonspecific and can be seen in many intermuscular lesions.[113] Diffuse neurofibromas (see **Fig. 7**F) demonstrate a reticulated linear branching or plaquelike pattern within the subcutaneous tissue replacing the fat.[114]

MORTON NEUROMA

Morton neuroma (**Fig. 8**) is a nonneoplastic perineural fibrosis about the plantar digital nerve. The lesion is likely related to chronic injury. It is most commonly encountered between the third and fourth heads followed by the second and third metatarsal heads.[102,115] The lesion exhibits a strong predilection for women (18:1) usually between the fourth and sixth decades of life and may be related to pointed and high-heeled shoe wear.[23,116] The usual clinical presentation is paroxysmal pain often elicited by exercise and relieved by rest. The lesion is almost always unilateral. Pain may radiate proximally or distally.[102,116] Asymptomatic lesions are common and usually smaller than lesions causing symptoms.[117,118]

The typical appearance is a fusiform enlargement of the plantar digital nerve plantar to the transverse metatarsal ligament, at the level of the metatarsophalangeal joint. The lesion is best imaged with MR imaging or ultrasonography. On MR imaging, Morton neuroma is best identified on the short-axis T1W sequence and is similar in signal to skeletal muscle within the intermetatarsal space on the plantar side of the transverse metatarsal ligament. T2W sequences demonstrate lesion signal less than fat, and differentiation from the surrounding muscle and fat may be difficult. Fat suppression of the fluid-sensitive sequence increases conspicuity. Enhancement of lesions is variable, occurring in 36% to 50% of lesions as reported in the literature.[119,120] Associated intermetatarsal bursal fluid occurs in up to 67% of cases.[121] Prone imaging may improve detection of Morton neuroma.[122]

BENIGN VASCULAR LESIONS: HEMANGIOMA AND VASCULAR MALFORMATION

Hemangiomas and vascular malformations (**Fig. 9**) comprise 7% of benign soft tissue tumors and are the most common tumor in children.[23] A common classification system by Weiss and colleagues[123] refers to hemangioma in its broadest sense based

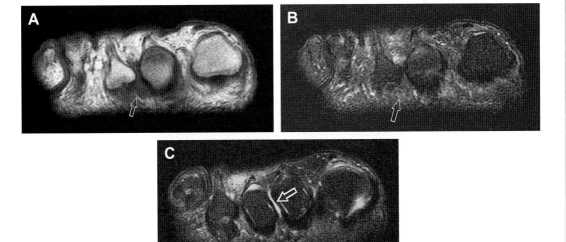

Fig. 8. Morton neuroma. Morton neuroma in a 60-year-old woman with foot pain. (*A*) Short-axis T1W (TR/echo time [TR/TE], 500/20) and (*B*) T2W (TR/TE, 2500/70) fat-suppression images demonstrate a 6-mm lesion of intermediate T1W and low T2W signal just plantar to the interspace of the second and third metatarsal heads (*arrows*). (*C*) Also note the intermetatarsal bursal fluid (*arrow*) revealed slightly more proximal in the forefoot on this fat-suppressed T2W image.

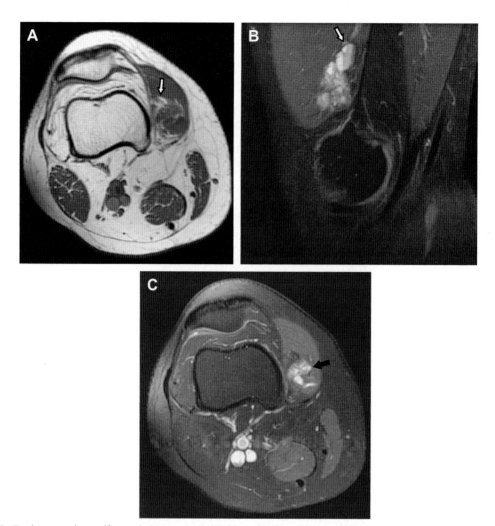

Fig. 9. Benign vascular malformation. Hemangioma (slow-flow vascular malformation) within the vastus medialis muscle. (*A*) Axial T1W image (TR/echo time [TR/TE], 500/20) and (*B*) sagittal T2W (TR/TE; 2500/70) image with fat suppression show heterogeneous signal intensity from fat hypertrophy (*arrow [A]*) and slow-flow vessels. T2W image reveals fluid levels (*arrow [B]*) from layering blood in slow-flow vascular channels. (*C*) Axial T1W (TR/TE, 570/16.7) postcontrast image shows enhancement of vascular channels (*arrow*).

on the common pathologic feature of a benign nonreactive lesion with an increase in the number of normal- or abnormal-appearing vessels; subdivision is based on the predominant type of vascular channel (capillary, cavernous, arteriovenous, or venous). Another classification system by Mulliken and Glowacki defines hemangiomas as true neoplasms and vascular malformations as an error in the formation of the vascular system[124,125]; this classification system was originally based on cutaneous lesions which frequently spontaneously involute and have diagnostic clinical features and therefore are often not imaged.

Both classification systems have advantages and disadvantages regarding their use that are beyond the scope of discussion for this article. The Mulliken/Glowacki classification is useful for clinicians and allows accurate diagnosis of neoplasm versus malformation based on history and physical examination. As it is based on lesions of infancy and childhood, it is discussed in detail in Dr Navarro's article "Soft Tissue Masses in Children" in this issue. In the typical adult patient, we find that the system proposed by Weiss and Goldblum is most applicable for benign vascular lesions occurring in deeper soft tissues such as muscles and joints. We henceforth refer to these lesions as hemangiomas, acknowledging that the distinction between hemangioma and vascular malformation is not always straightforward and that therefore some hemangiomas may represent true malformations (eg, venous malformations as described by Mulliken and Glowacki) rather than tumors.[126]

Of the nonregressing vascular lesions, cavernous hemangiomas (as defined by Weiss and colleagues) are the most common. These lesions may be superficial or deep. Superficial lesions may cause bluish skin discoloration. Deep lesions are more commonly intramuscular, have nonspecific clinical features, and are usually referred for radiologic evaluation. These lesions are often considered congenital in origin and grow at the same rate as normal tissues. Occurrence is more common in women than men by a ratio of 3:1, and growth may occur during pregnancy.[123] Clinical presentation depends on location, and the lesion may be painful and may change size with engorgement. Intramuscular lesions may be painful with exercise, presumably because of local muscle ischemia.

These lesions are commonly imaged when symptomatic and because they do not involute. Radiographs may be normal or may show a soft tissue mass and phleboliths (20%–67% of cases).[23] Reactive and pressure changes of bone may occur, particularly when lesions are adjacent to bone, and include benign periosteal reaction (23%), cortical scalloping, and linear lucencies (31%).[127] Nonenhanced CT shows a soft tissue density mass with or without phleboliths. MR imaging features are often characteristic. The lesion may be well defined or infiltrative. Lesions show low to intermediate signal intensity on T1W images. Associated fatty overgrowth due to chronically ischemic muscle is common in deep-seated lesions and follows subcutaneous adipose signal. Intralesional hemorrhage may occur, showing areas of high T1 signal and rarely fluid levels. Vascular elements show high signal intensity on T2W images and are typically serpentine in morphology, and thus lesions are often prominently heterogeneous. Enhancement is prominent, and feeding vessels may be evident. In our experience, approximately 90% of deep hemangiomas reveal these pathognomonic features of serpentine vascular channels and fat overgrowth and do not require biopsy for diagnosis.

Angiomatosis represents diffuse infiltration by hemangiomas and/or lymphangiomas. Imaging characteristics are similar to solitary lesions except for the distribution with involvement of multiple soft tissue planes and prominent longitudinal extension. Many angiomatous syndromes have been described. Most of these syndromes are without malignant potential with the exception of Maffucci syndrome.

GLOMUS TUMOR

Glomus tumor (**Fig. 10**) is a neoplasm that develops from the neuromyoarterial glomus

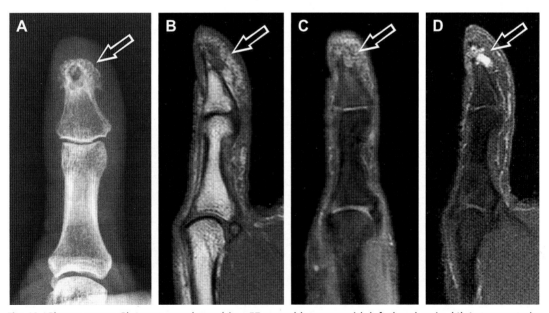

Fig. 10. Glomus tumor. Glomus tumor (*arrow*) in a 57-year-old woman with left thumb pain. (*A*) Anteroposterior radiograph of the thumb demonstrates prominent bone erosion of the terminal tuft. (*B*) Sagittal T1W (TR/echo time [TR/TE], 760/16.7) MR image demonstrates an intermediate-signal 6-mm mass on the volar aspect of the terminal tuft. The lesion is intermediate signal on (*C*) coronal proton density–weighted (TR/TE, 1500/10) fat-saturated image and demonstrates avid contrast enhancement on (*D*) sagittal T1W (TR/TE, 570/16.7) image with fat saturation.

body.[23,128] The estimated incidence is 1.6% of soft tissue tumors. There is no gender predilection overall, but there is a 3:1 female predominance for subungual lesions.[129] Multiple glomus tumors (nearly 10% of patients) may be present in NF1.[130,131] The lesion is most frequently diagnosed between 20 and 40 years of age. The most common site is the subungual location (65%)[132] in the finger, but other locations include the palm, wrist, forearm, and foot.[133] The average lesion size is approximately 7 mm in the upper extremity and 13 mm in the lower extremity in a recent series.[132] The most frequent clinical presentation is a small red-blue nodule causing paroxysms of pain radiating away from the lesion, which is often elicited by cold or pressure. The classic clinical triad of pain, point tenderness, and cold sensitivity is present in approximately 30% of cases.[134]

Imaging reveals a small mass related to the nail bed, with erosion of bone in 22% to 82% of cases.[23] MR imaging reveals a small mass with homogeneous high signal on T2W[135,136] and intermediate to low signal intensity noted on T1W images.[128] Rarely, glomus tumors may show cystic change.[137] Enhancement is typically prominent and diffuse. A high-resolution surface coil has proven useful to demonstrate cortical bone erosion.[134]

MYXOMA

Myxoma is a mesenchymal neoplasm composed of undifferentiated stellate cells in a myxoid stroma.[138] The lesion is most frequently seen in adults aged between 40 and 70 years, with a female predilection (67%).[43,139] Patients typically present with a painless soft tissue mass. Intramuscular myxomas (**Fig. 11**) are usually solitary. Multiple myxomas are almost always associated with monostotic or polyostotic fibrous dysplasia (Mazabraud syndrome).[140] In a study of 200 myxomas from various sites, 17% were noted to be intramuscular.[141] Most musculoskeletal myxomas are intramuscular (82%), with the thigh (51%), upper arm (9%), calf (7%), and buttock (7%) being the most frequent locations. A small number of lesions are intermuscular (9%), subcutaneous (9%), or juxta-articular (7%).[142] Myxomas show low (81%–100%) to intermediate (0%–19%) signal intensity on T1W images. On T2W sequences, all myxomas demonstrate high signal intensity. Lesions are homogeneous or only mildly heterogeneous and are well defined in 60% to 80% of cases. In 65% to 89% of cases, a thin rim of fat is noted most prominent at the superior and inferior aspects of the lesion, representing atrophy of the adjacent muscle. Perilesional high signal may be noted on fluid-sensitive sequences in 79% to 100% of myxomas caused by leakage of the myxomatous tissue into the surrounding muscle causing edema. Myxomas reveal mild (76%) to moderate (24%) contrast enhancement in a diffuse (57%) or thick peripheral and septal (43%) enhancement pattern. Cystic areas may be noted in slightly more than 50% of all myxomas.[142–145] The MR imaging appearance of an intramuscular lesion with low T1W signal

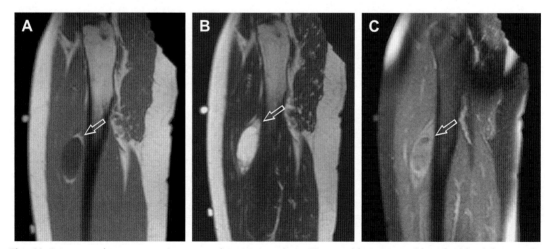

Fig. 11. Intramuscular myxoma. Intramuscular myxoma in a 49-year-old woman with palpable right anterior thigh mass. (*A*) Sagittal T1W (TR/echo time [TR/TE], 596/13) and (*B*) sagittal T2W (TR/TE, 5080/100) images demonstrate a well-defined cystlike mass with low T1 signal and high T2 signal. Note the surrounding edema on the T2 sequence most prominent at the superior and inferior poles of the lesion. Sagittal T1W (*C*) fat-saturated image after gadolinium enhancement (TR/TE, 500/13) reveals mild diffuse enhancement of the lesion.

and high signal intensity on fluid-sensitive sequences demonstrating a peripheral rim of fat and edema is highly suggestive if not pathognomonic for myxoma.

The differential diagnosis for a predominantly myxoid-appearing soft tissue lesion includes myxoid liposarcoma, myxofibrosarcoma (myxoid MFH), myxoid chondrosarcoma, myxoma, ganglion, synovial cyst, and peripheral nerve sheath tumor.

This has been a limited review of common benign soft tissue tumors in the adult population. In general, small-sized (<5 cm) well-defined margins and homogeneous MR imaging signal favor a benign lesion. When a specific diagnosis is not possible, a solid lesion should be considered indeterminant (even one with all the benign features mentioned earlier) and the appropriate biopsy path planned with the treating surgeon.

ACKNOWLEDGMENTS

We gratefully acknowledge the residents who attend the American Institute for Radiologic Pathology courses (past, present, and future) for their contribution of interesting cases to our series of patients, which allow our continued educational outreach.

REFERENCES

1. Hajdu SI. Benign soft tissue tumors: classification and natural history. CA Cancer J Clin 1987;37(2):66–76.
2. Walker EA, Song AJ, Murphey MD. Magnetic resonance imaging of soft-tissue masses. Semin Roentgenol 2010;45(4):277–97.
3. Beltran J, Chandnani V, McGhee RA Jr, et al. Gadopentetate dimeglumine-enhanced MR imaging of the musculoskeletal system. AJR Am J Roentgenol 1991;156(3):457–66.
4. Verstraete KL, De Deene Y, Roels H, et al. Benign and malignant musculoskeletal lesions: dynamic contrast-enhanced MR imaging–parametric "first-pass" images depict tissue vascularization and perfusion. Radiology 1994;192(3):835–43.
5. Benedikt RA, Jelinek JS, Kransdorf MJ, et al. MR imaging of soft-tissue masses: role of gadopentetate dimeglumine. J Magn Reson Imaging 1994; 4(3):485–90.
6. Erlemann R, Reiser MF, Peters PE, et al. Musculoskeletal neoplasms: static and dynamic Gd-DTPA–enhanced MR imaging. Radiology 1989;171(3): 767–73.
7. van Rijswijk CS, Geirnaerdt MJ, Hogendoorn PC, et al. Soft-tissue tumors: value of static and dynamic gadopentetate dimeglumine-enhanced MR imaging in prediction of malignancy. Radiology 2004;233(2): 493–502.
8. Mirowitz SA, Totty WG, Lee JK. Characterization of musculoskeletal masses using dynamic Gd-DTPA enhanced spin-echo MRI. J Comput Assist Tomogr 1992;16(1):120–5.
9. Berquist TH, Ehman RL, King BF, et al. Value of MR imaging in differentiating benign from malignant soft-tissue masses: study of 95 lesions. AJR Am J Roentgenol 1990;155(6):1251–5.
10. Sundaram M, McGuire MH, Herbold DR. Magnetic resonance imaging of soft tissue masses: an evaluation of fifty-three histologically proven tumors. Magn Reson Imaging 1988;6(3):237–48.
11. Moulton JS, Blebea JS, Dunco DM, et al. MR imaging of soft-tissue masses: diagnostic efficacy and value of distinguishing between benign and malignant lesions. AJR Am J Roentgenol 1995; 164(5):1191–9.
12. Totty WG, Murphy WA, Lee JK. Soft-tissue tumors: MR imaging. Radiology 1986;160(1):135–41.
13. Kransdorf MJ, Jelinek JS, Moser RP Jr, et al. Soft-tissue masses: diagnosis using MR imaging. AJR Am J Roentgenol 1989;153(3):541–7.
14. Crim JR, Seeger LL, Yao L, et al. Diagnosis of soft-tissue masses with MR imaging: can benign masses be differentiated from malignant ones? Radiology 1992;185(2):581–6.
15. Myhre-Jensen O. A consecutive 7-year series of 1331 benign soft tissue tumours. Clinicopathologic data. Comparison with sarcomas. Acta Orthop Scand 1981;52(3):287–93.
16. Rydholm A. Management of patients with soft-tissue tumors. Strategy developed at a regional oncology center. Acta Orthop Scand Suppl 1983; 203:13–77.
17. Mankin HJ, Lange TA, Spanier SS. The hazards of biopsy in patients with malignant primary bone and soft-tissue tumors. J Bone Joint Surg Am 1982; 64(8):1121–7.
18. Mankin HJ, Mankin CJ, Simon MA. The hazards of the biopsy, revisited. Members of the Musculoskeletal Tumor Society. J Bone Joint Surg Am 1996; 78(5):656–63.
19. Weiss SW, Goldblum JR, Enzinger FM. Benign fibroblastic/myofibroblastic proliferations. In: Weiss SW, Goldblum JR, editors. Enzinger and Weiss' soft tissue tumors. 5th edition. Philadelphia: Mosby Elsevier; 2008. p. 175–225.
20. Meister P, Buckmann FW, Konrad E. Nodular fasciitis (analysis of 100 cases and review of the literature). Pathol Res Pract 1978;162(2): 133–65.
21. Dinauer PA, Brixey CJ, Moncur JT, et al. Pathologic and MR imaging features of benign fibrous soft-tissue tumors in adults. Radiographics 2007; 27(1):173–87.

22. Shimizu S, Hashimoto H, Enjoji M. Nodular fasciitis: an analysis of 250 patients. Pathology 1984;16(2):161–6.

23. Kransdorf MJ, Murphey MD. Imaging of soft tissue tumors. 2nd edition. Philadelphia: Lippincott Williams & Wilkins; 2006.

24. Bernstein KE, Lattes R. Nodular (pseudosarcomatous) fasciitis, a nonrecurrent lesion: clinicopathologic study of 134 cases. Cancer 1982;49(8):1668–78.

25. Leung LY, Shu SJ, Chan AC, et al. Nodular fasciitis: MRI appearance and literature review. Skeletal Radiol 2002;31(1):9–13.

26. Wang XL, De Schepper AM, Vanhoenacker F, et al. Nodular fasciitis: correlation of MRI findings and histopathology. Skeletal Radiol 2002;31(3):155–61.

27. Broder MS, Leonidas JC, Mitty HA. Pseudosarcomatous fasciitis: an unusual cause of soft-tissue calcification. Radiology 1973;107(1):173–4.

28. Meyer CA, Kransdorf MJ, Jelinek JS, et al. MR and CT appearance of nodular fasciitis. J Comput Assist Tomogr 1991;15(2):276–9.

29. Mikkelsen OA. Dupuytren's disease—initial symptoms, age of onset and spontaneous course. Hand 1977;9(1):11–5.

30. Weiss SW, Goldblum JR, Enzinger FM. Fibromatoses. In: Weiss SW, Goldblum JR, editors. Enzinger and Weiss' soft tissue tumors. 5th edition. Philadelphia: Mosby Elsevier; 2008. p. 227–8.

31. Yacoe ME, Bergman AG, Ladd AL, et al. Dupuytren's contracture: MR imaging findings and correlation between MR signal intensity and cellularity of lesions. AJR Am J Roentgenol 1993;160(4):813–7.

32. Murphey MD, Ruble CM, Tyszko SM, et al. From the archives of the AFIP: musculoskeletal fibromatoses: radiologic-pathologic correlation. Radiographics 2009;29(7):2143–73.

33. Robbin MR, Murphey MD, Temple HT, et al. Imaging of musculoskeletal fibromatosis. Radiographics 2001;21(3):585–600.

34. Rombouts JJ, Noel H, Legrain Y, et al. Prediction of recurrence in the treatment of Dupuytren's disease: evaluation of a histologic classification. J Hand Surg Am 1989;14(4):644–52.

35. Yost J, Winters T, Fett HC, et al. Dupuytren's contracture; a statistical study. Am J Surg 1955;90(4):568–71.

36. Fetsch JF, Laskin WB, Miettinen M. Palmar-plantar fibromatosis in children and preadolescents: a clinicopathologic study of 56 cases with newly recognized demographics and extended follow-up information. Am J Surg Pathol 2005;29(8):1095–105.

37. Lee TH, Wapner KL, Hecht PJ. Plantar fibromatosis. J Bone Joint Surg Am 1993;75(7):1080–4.

38. Aviles E, Arlen M, Miller T. Plantar fibromatosis. Surgery 1971;69(1):117–20.

39. Morrison WB, Schweitzer ME, Wapner KL, et al. Plantar fibromatosis: a benign aggressive neoplasm with a characteristic appearance on MR images. Radiology 1994;193(3):841–5.

40. Clark SK, Phillips RK. Desmoids in familial adenomatous polyposis. Br J Surg 1996;83(11):1494–504.

41. Jones IT, Jagelman DG, Fazio VW, et al. Desmoid tumors in familial polyposis coli. Ann Surg 1986;204(1):94–7.

42. Pritchard DJ, Nascimento AG, Petersen IA. Local control of extra-abdominal desmoid tumors. J Bone Joint Surg Am 1996;78(6):848–54.

43. Fletcher CDM, Unni KK, Mertens F. World Health Organization pathology and genetics of tumors of soft tissue and bone. 3rd edition. Lyon (France): IARC Press; 2006.

44. Rock MG, Pritchard DJ, Reiman HM, et al. Extra-abdominal desmoid tumors. J Bone Joint Surg Am 1984;66(9):1369–74.

45. Lee JC, Thomas JM, Phillips S, et al. Aggressive fibromatosis: MRI features with pathologic correlation. AJR Am J Roentgenol 2006;186(1):247–54.

46. Sundaram M, McGuire MH, Schajowicz F. Soft-tissue masses: histologic basis for decreased signal (short T2) on T2-weighted MR images. AJR Am J Roentgenol 1987;148(6):1247–50.

47. Kransdorf MJ, Jelinek JS, Moser RP Jr, et al. Magnetic resonance appearance of fibromatosis. A report of 14 cases and review of the literature. Skeletal Radiol 1990;19(7):495–9.

48. Feld R, Burk DL Jr, McCue P, et al. MRI of aggressive fibromatosis: frequent appearance of high signal intensity on T2-weighted images. Magn Reson Imaging 1990;8(5):583–8.

49. Quinn SF, Erickson SJ, Dee PM, et al. MR imaging in fibromatosis: results in 26 patients with pathologic correlation. AJR Am J Roentgenol 1991;156(3):539–42.

50. Romero JA, Kim EE, Kim CG, et al. Different biologic features of desmoid tumors in adult and juvenile patients: MR demonstration. J Comput Assist Tomogr 1995;19(5):782–7.

51. Jarvi O, Saxen E. Elastofibroma dorse. Acta Pathol Microbiol Scand Suppl 1961;51(Suppl 144):83–4.

52. Jarvi OH, Saxen AE, Hopsu-Havu VK, et al. Elastofibroma—a degenerative pseudotumor. Cancer 1969;23(1):42–63.

53. Jarvi OH, Lansimies PH. Subclinical elastofibromas in the scapular region in an autopsy series. Acta Pathol Microbiol Scand A 1975;83(1):87–108.

54. Brandser EA, Goree JC, El-Khoury GY. Elastofibroma dorsi: prevalence in an elderly patient population as revealed by CT. AJR Am J Roentgenol 1998;171(4):977–80.

55. Nagamine N, Nohara Y, Ito E. Elastofibroma in Okinawa. A clinicopathologic study of 170 cases. Cancer 1982;50(9):1794–805.

56. Faccioli N, Foti G, Comai A, et al. MR imaging findings of elastofibroma dorsi in correlation with pathological features: our experience. Radiol Med 2009;114(8):1283–91.

57. Ronan SJ, Broderick T. Minimally invasive approach to familial multiple lipomatosis. Plast Reconstr Surg 2000;106(4):878–80.

58. Kransdorf MJ. Benign soft-tissue tumors in a large referral population: distribution of specific diagnoses by age, sex, and location. AJR Am J Roentgenol 1995;164(2):395–402.

59. Rydholm A, Berg NO. Size, site and clinical incidence of lipoma. Factors in the differential diagnosis of lipoma and sarcoma. Acta Orthop Scand 1983;54(6):929–34.

60. Weiss SW, Goldblum JR, Enzinger FM. Benign lipomatous tumors. In: Weiss SW, Goldblum JR, editors. Enzinger and Weiss' soft tissue tumors. 5th edition. Philadelphia: Mosby Elsevier; 2008. p. 429–76.

61. Murphey MD, Carroll JF, Flemming DJ, et al. From the archives of the AFIP: benign musculoskeletal lipomatous lesions. Radiographics 2004;24(5):1433–66.

62. Kransdorf MJ, Moser RP Jr, Meis JM, et al. Fat-containing soft-tissue masses of the extremities. Radiographics 1991;11(1):81–106.

63. Leffert RD. Lipomas of the upper extremity. J Bone Joint Surg Am 1972;54(6):1262–6.

64. Kransdorf MJ. Malignant soft-tissue tumors in a large referral population: distribution of diagnoses by age, sex, and location. AJR Am J Roentgenol 1995;164(1):129–34.

65. Ha TV, Kleinman PK, Fraire A, et al. MR imaging of benign fatty tumors in children: report of four cases and review of the literature. Skeletal Radiol 1994;23(5):361–7.

66. Murphey MD, Arcara LK, Fanburg-Smith J. From the archives of the AFIP: imaging of musculoskeletal liposarcoma with radiologic-pathologic correlation. Radiographics 2005;25(5):1371–95.

67. Ohguri T, Aoki T, Hisaoka M, et al. Differential diagnosis of benign peripheral lipoma from well-differentiated liposarcoma on MR imaging: is comparison of margins and internal characteristics useful? AJR Am J Roentgenol 2003;180(6):1689–94.

68. Kransdorf MJ, Bancroft LW, Peterson JJ, et al. Imaging of fatty tumors: distinction of lipoma and well-differentiated liposarcoma. Radiology 2002;224(1):99–104.

69. Armstrong SJ, Watt I. Lipoma arborescens of the knee. Br J Radiol 1989;62(734):178–80.

70. Evers LH, Gebhard M, Lange T, et al. Hibernoma—case report and literature review. Am J Dermatopathol 2009;31(7):685–6.

71. Furlong MA, Fanburg-Smith JC, Miettinen M. The morphologic spectrum of hibernoma: a clinicopathologic study of 170 cases. Am J Surg Pathol 2001;25(6):809–14.

72. Nishida J, Ehara S, Shiraishi H, et al. Clinical findings of hibernoma of the buttock and thigh: rare involvements and extremely high uptake of FDG-PET. Med Sci Monit 2009;15(7):CS117–22.

73. Smith CS, Teruya-Feldstein J, Caravelli JF, et al. False-positive findings on 18F-FDG PET/CT: differentiation of hibernoma and malignant fatty tumor on the basis of fluctuating standardized uptake values. AJR Am J Roentgenol 2008;190(4):1091–6.

74. Goldman AB, DiCarlo EF, Marcove RC. Case report 774. Coincidental parosteal lipoma with osseous excrescence and intramuscular lipoma. Skeletal Radiol 1993;22(2):138–45.

75. Murphey MD, Johnson DL, Bhatia PS, et al. Parosteal lipoma: MR imaging characteristics. AJR Am J Roentgenol 1994;162(1):105–10.

76. Bui-Mansfield LT, Myers CP, Chew FS. Parosteal lipoma of the fibula. AJR Am J Roentgenol 2000;174(6):1698.

77. Yu JS, Weis L, Becker W. MR imaging of a parosteal lipoma. Clin Imaging 2000;24(1):15–8.

78. Weiss SW, Goldblum JR, Enzinger FM. Benign tumors and tumor-like lesions of synovial tissue. In: Enzinger and Weiss's soft tissue tumors. 4th edition. St Louis (MO): Mosby; 2001. p. 1037–62.

79. Jaffe HL, Lichtenstein L, Sutro CJ. Pigmented villonodular synovitis, bursitis and tenosynovitis. Arch Pathol Lab Med 1941;31:731–65.

80. Ushijima M, Hashimoto H, Tsuneyoshi M, et al. Giant cell tumor of the tendon sheath (nodular tenosynovitis). A study of 207 cases to compare the large joint group with the common digit group. Cancer 1986;57(4):875–84.

81. Savage RC, Mustafa EB. Giant cell tumor of tendon sheath (localized nodular tenosynovitis). Ann Plast Surg 1984;13(3):205–10.

82. Oyemade GA, Abioye AA. A clinicopathologic review of benign giant cell tumors of tendon sheaths in Ibadan, Nigeria. Am J Surg 1977;134(3):392–5.

83. Karasick D, Karasick S. Giant cell tumor of tendon sheath: spectrum of radiologic findings. Skeletal Radiol 1992;21(4):219–24.

84. Bogumill GP, Sullivan DJ, Baker GI. Tumors of the hand. Clin Orthop Relat Res 1975;(108):214–22.

85. Jelinek JS, Kransdorf MJ, Shmookler BM, et al. Giant cell tumor of the tendon sheath: MR findings in nine cases. AJR Am J Roentgenol 1994;162(4):919–22.

86. Kitagawa Y, Ito H, Amano Y, et al. MR imaging for preoperative diagnosis and assessment of local tumor extent on localized giant cell tumor of tendon sheath. Skeletal Radiol 2003;32(11):633–8.

87. Huang GS, Lee CH, Chan WP, et al. Localized nodular synovitis of the knee: MR imaging appearance and clinical correlates in 21 patients. AJR Am J Roentgenol 2003;181(2):539–43.

88. Fraire AE, Fechner RE. Intra-articular localized nodular synovitis of the knee. Arch Pathol 1972;93(5):473–6.

89. Rao AS, Vigorita VJ. Pigmented villonodular synovitis (giant-cell tumor of the tendon sheath and

synovial membrane). A review of eighty-one cases. J Bone Joint Surg Am 1984;66(1):76–94.

90. Al-Nakshabandi NA, Ryan AG, Choudur H, et al. Pigmented villonodular synovitis. Clin Radiol 2004;59(5):414–20.

91. Dorwart RH, Genant HK, Johnston WH, et al. Pigmented villonodular synovitis of the shoulder: radiologic-pathologic assessment. AJR Am J Roentgenol 1984;143(4):886–8.

92. Dorwart RH, Genant HK, Johnston WH, et al. Pigmented villonodular synovitis of synovial joints: clinical, pathologic, and radiologic features. AJR Am J Roentgenol 1984;143(4):877–85.

93. Pimpalnerkar A, Barton E, Sibly TF. Pigmented villonodular synovitis of the elbow. J Shoulder Elbow Surg 1998;7(1):71–5.

94. Cotten A, Flipo RM, Chastanet P, et al. Pigmented villonodular synovitis of the hip: review of radiographic features in 58 patients. Skeletal Radiol 1995;24(1):1–6.

95. Byers PD, Cotton RE, Deacon OW, et al. The diagnosis and treatment of pigmented villonodular synovitis. J Bone Joint Surg Br 1968;50(2):290–305.

96. Hughes TH, Sartoris DJ, Schweitzer ME, et al. Pigmented villonodular synovitis: MRI characteristics. Skeletal Radiol 1995;24(1):7–12.

97. Kottal RA, Vogler JB 3rd, Matamoros A, et al. Pigmented villonodular synovitis: a report of MR imaging in two cases. Radiology 1987;163(2):551–3.

98. Spence LD, Adams J, Gibbons D, et al. Rice body formation in bicipito-radial bursitis: ultrasound, CT, and MRI findings. Skeletal Radiol 1998;27(1):30–2.

99. Dale K, Smith HJ, Paus AC, et al. Dynamic MR-imaging in the diagnosis of pigmented villonodular synovitis of the knee. Scand J Rheumatol 2000; 29(5):336–9.

100. Jamieson TW, Curran JJ, Desmet AA, et al. Bilateral pigmented villonodular synovitis of the wrists. Orthop Rev 1990;19(5):432–6.

101. Jelinek JS, Kransdorf MJ, Utz JA, et al. Imaging of pigmented villonodular synovitis with emphasis on MR imaging. AJR Am J Roentgenol 1989;152(2): 337–42.

102. Weiss SW, Goldblum JR, Enzinger FM. Benign tumors of peripheral nerves. In: Weiss SW, Goldblum JR, editors. Enzinger and Weiss' soft tissue tumors. 5th edition. Philadelphia: Mosby Elsevier; 2008. p. 825–901.

103. Miettinen M. Diagnostic soft tissue pathology. New York: Churchhill Livingstone; 2003.

104. Sheikh S, Gomes M, Montgomery E. Multiple plexiform schwannomas in a patient with neurofibromatosis. J Thorac Cardiovasc Surg 1998;115(1):240–2.

105. Ogose A, Hotta T, Morita T, et al. Multiple schwannomas in the peripheral nerves. J Bone Joint Surg Br 1998;80(4):657–61.

106. Kehoe NJ, Reid RP, Semple JC. Solitary benign peripheral-nerve tumours. Review of 32 years' experience. J Bone Joint Surg Br 1995;77(3):497–500.

107. Brasfield RD, Das Gupta TK. Von Recklinghausen's disease: a clinicopathological study. Ann Surg 1972;175(1):86–104.

108. Jett K, Friedman JM. Clinical and genetic aspects of neurofibromatosis 1. Genet Med 2010;12(1):1–11.

109. Evans DG, Baser ME, McGaughran J, et al. Malignant peripheral nerve sheath tumours in neurofibromatosis 1. J Med Genet 2002;39(5):311–4.

110. Li MH, Holtas S. MR imaging of spinal neurofibromatosis. Acta Radiol 1991;32(4):279–85.

111. Banks KP. The target sign: extremity. Radiology 2005;234(3):899–900.

112. Jee WH, Oh SN, McCauley T, et al. Extraaxial neurofibromas versus neurilemmomas: discrimination with MRI. AJR Am J Roentgenol 2004;183(3): 629–33.

113. Cohen LM, Schwartz AM, Rockoff SD. Benign schwannomas: pathologic basis for CT inhomogeneities. AJR Am J Roentgenol 1986;147(1):141–3.

114. Peh WC, Shek TW, Yip DK. Magnetic resonance imaging of subcutaneous diffuse neurofibroma. Br J Radiol 1997;70(839):1180–3.

115. Morton TS. VI. Metatarsalgia (Morton's painful affection of the foot), with an account of six cases cured by operation. Ann Surg 1893;17(6):680–99.

116. Wu KK. Morton's interdigital neuroma: a clinical review of its etiology, treatment, and results. J Foot Ankle Surg 1996;35(2):112–9 [discussion: 187–8].

117. Bencardino J, Rosenberg ZS, Beltran J, et al. Morton's neuroma: is it always symptomatic? AJR Am J Roentgenol 2000;175(3):649–53.

118. Zanetti M, Strehle JK, Zollinger H, et al. Morton neuroma and fluid in the intermetatarsal bursae on MR images of 70 asymptomatic volunteers. Radiology 1997;203(2):516–20.

119. Williams JW, Meaney J, Whitehouse GH, et al. MRI in the investigation of Morton's neuroma: which sequences? Clin Radiol 1997;52(1):46–9.

120. Zanetti M, Weishaupt D. MR imaging of the forefoot: Morton neuroma and differential diagnoses. Semin Musculoskelet Radiol 2005;9(3):175–86.

121. Erickson SJ, Canale PB, Carrera GF, et al. Interdigital (Morton) neuroma: high-resolution MR imaging with a solenoid coil. Radiology 1991;181(3):833–6.

122. Weishaupt D, Treiber K, Kundert HP, et al. Morton neuroma: MR imaging in prone, supine, and upright weight-bearing body positions. Radiology 2003;226(3):849–56.

123. Weiss SW, Goldblum JR, Enzinger FM. Benign tumors and tumor-like lesions of blood vessels. In: Weiss SW, Goldblum JR, editors. Enzinger and Weiss' soft tissue tumors. 5th edition. Philadelphia: Mosby Elsevier; 2008. p. 633–702.

124. Mulliken JB, Glowacki J. Hemangiomas and vascular malformations in infants and children: a classification based on endothelial characteristics. Plast Reconstr Surg 1982;69(3):412–22.

125. Mulliken JB, Young AE. Vascular birthmarks: hemangiomas and malformations. Philadelphia: Saunders; 1988.

126. Kransdorf MJ, Murphey MD, Fanburg-Smith JC. Classification of benign vascular lesions: history, current nomenclature, and suggestions for imagers. Am J Roentgenol 2011;197:1–4.

127. Ly JQ, Sanders TG, Mulloy JP, et al. Osseous change adjacent to soft-tissue hemangiomas of the extremities: correlation with lesion size and proximity to bone. AJR Am J Roentgenol 2003;180(6):1695–700.

128. Baek HJ, Lee SJ, Cho KH, et al. Subungual tumors: clinicopathologic correlation with US and MR imaging findings. Radiographics 2010;30(6):1621–36.

129. Shugart RR, Soule EH, Johnson EW Jr. Glomus tumor. Surg Gynecol Obstet 1963;117:334–40.

130. Sawada S, Honda M, Kamide R, et al. Three cases of subungual glomus tumors with von Recklinghausen neurofibromatosis. J Am Acad Dermatol 1995; 32(2 Pt 1):277–8.

131. Okada O, Demitsu T, Manabe M, et al. A case of multiple subungual glomus tumors associated with neurofibromatosis type 1. J Dermatol 1999; 26(8):535–7.

132. Park EA, Hong SH, Choi JY, et al. Glomangiomatosis: magnetic resonance imaging findings in three cases. Skeletal Radiol 2005;34(2):108–11.

133. Weiss SW, Goldblum JR, Enzinger FM. Perivascular tumors. In: Weiss SW, Goldblum JR, editors. Enzinger and Weiss' soft tissue tumors. 5th edition. Philadelphia: Mosby Elsevier; 2008. p. 751–67.

134. Drape JL, Idy-Peretti I, Goettmann S, et al. Subungual glomus tumors: evaluation with MR imaging. Radiology 1995;195(2):507–15.

135. Kneeland JB, Middleton WD, Matloub HS, et al. High resolution MR imaging of glomus tumor. J Comput Assist Tomogr 1987;11(2):351–2.

136. Matloub HS, Muoneke VN, Prevel CD, et al. Glomus tumor imaging: use of MRI for localization of occult lesions. J Hand Surg Am 1992;17(3): 472–5.

137. Tachibana R, Hatori M, Hosaka M, et al. Glomus tumors with cystic changes around the ankle. Arch Orthop Trauma Surg 2001;121(9): 540–3.

138. Stout AP. Myxoma, the tumor of primitive mesenchyme. Ann Surg 1948;127(4):706–19.

139. Weiss SW, Goldblum JR, Enzinger FM. Enzinger and Weiss' soft tissue tumors. 5th edition. Philadelphia: Mosby Elsevier; 2008.

140. Kransdorf MJ, Murphey MD. Diagnosis please. Case 12: Mazabraud syndrome. Radiology 1999; 212(1):129–32.

141. Enzinger FM. Intramuscular myxoma; a review and follow-up study of 34 cases. Am J Clin Pathol 1965; 43:104–13.

142. Murphey MD, McRae GA, Fanburg-Smith JC, et al. Imaging of soft-tissue myxoma with emphasis on CT and MR and comparison of radiologic and pathologic findings. Radiology 2002; 225(1):215–24.

143. Bancroft LW, Kransdorf MJ, Menke DM, et al. Intramuscular myxoma: characteristic MR imaging features. AJR Am J Roentgenol 2002;178(5): 1255–9.

144. Luna A, Martinez S, Bossen E. Magnetic resonance imaging of intramuscular myxoma with histological comparison and a review of the literature. Skeletal Radiol 2005;34(1):19–28.

145. Iwasko N, Steinbach LS, Disler D, et al. Imaging findings in Mazabraud's syndrome: seven new cases. Skeletal Radiol 2002;31(2):81–7.

Magnetic Resonance Imaging of Malignant Soft Tissue Neoplasms in the Adult

Eric A. Walker, MD[a,b,*], Joel S. Salesky, MD[c],
Michael E. Fenton, MD[c], Mark D. Murphey, MD[b,c,d]

KEYWORDS

- Soft tissue tumor • Malignant • MR imaging
- Soft tissue neoplasm

Soft tissue sarcomas are estimated to represent 1% of malignant tumors.[1–3] The incidence of soft tissue sarcoma is estimated at 2.7 per 100,000[4] and increases significantly with age. In patients who are 80 years and older, the incidence is 8 per 100,000.[5] Magnetic resonance (MR) imaging is the favored modality for evaluation of soft tissue tumors and tumorlike conditions. Although advances in thin-section computed tomography (CT) have recently allowed detailed multiplanar reconstructions, MR imaging allows superior contrast resolution without radiation exposure.

Intravenous contrast administration may be useful for evaluation of malignant soft tissue tumors. Contrast may allow distinction of small tumor nodules (usually in the periphery) in a predominantly cystic lesion or a spontaneous hematoma. Malignant lesions may show increased vascularity at the periphery and high interstitial pressure at their center leading to a high rim to center differential enhancement ratio.[6] Negative features regarding the use of intravenous contrast include increased cost and length of time of the examination. Severe reactions to gadolinium and nephrogenic systemic fibrosis are rare but can occur.

Dynamic enhancement with gadolinium has been used in an attempt to differentiate benign from malignant soft tissue lesions.[7–9] High soft tissue vascularity and perfusion result in an increased rate of enhancement. Malignant lesions usually reveal greater enhancement and an increased rate of enhancement.[10] One difficulty with dynamic contrast-enhanced imaging is a significant overlap between the rate of enhancement of benign and malignant lesions.[11] We do not routinely perform dynamic enhancement sequences at our institutions and we believe significant overlap limits differentiation of benign from malignant solid soft tissue masses with otherwise nonspecific features.

Although MR imaging is excellent at delineating soft tissue lesions, a correct histologic diagnosis based on imaging studies alone is seen in only 25% to 30% of cases.[12–14] However, we believe that this percentage continues to increase and ultimately will approach the 75% to 90% range.[15] Most lesions are nonspecific with intermediate T1 and intermediate to high T2 signal; however, a specific diagnosis can be obtained in many instances by evaluating lesion signal intensity, location, growth pattern, and other unique intrinsic

Disclaimer: The opinions or assertions contained herein are the private views of the authors and are not to be construed as official nor as reflecting the views of the Departments of the Army, Navy, or Defense.

[a] Department of Radiology, H066, Milton S. Hershey Medical Center, 500 University Drive, P.O. Box 850, Hershey, PA 17033, USA
[b] Department of Radiology and Nuclear Medicine, Uniformed Services University of the Health Sciences, 4301 Jones Bridge Road, Bethesda, MD 20814, USA
[c] American Institute for Radiologic Pathology, 1010 Wayne Avenue, Suite 320, Silver Spring, MD 20910, USA
[d] Department of Radiology, Walter Reed Army Medical Center, Washington, DC, USA
* Corresponding author. Department of Radiology, H066, Milton S. Hershey Medical Center, 500 University Drive, P.O. Box 850, Hershey, PA 17033.
E-mail address: ewalker@hmc.psu.edu

Radiol Clin N Am 49 (2011) 1219–1234
doi:10.1016/j.rcl.2011.07.006

radiologic.theclinics.com

characteristics of the lesion. Unless a specific diagnosis can be determined, the lesion should be considered indeterminate, and an appropriate biopsy path should be discussed with the orthopedic oncologist or treating surgeon. A poorly selected biopsy path may violate compartments needed for reconstruction and necessitate amputation for definitive treatment.[16,17]

Some investigators have proposed that criteria such as tumor margins, homogenous versus heterogeneous signal intensity, and lesion size can distinguish a benign from a malignant lesion in more than 90% of cases.[12] Other reports note that malignant lesions can appear smoothly marginated and homogenous and MR imaging appearance cannot accurately separate benign and malignant processes.[9,13,14,18–20] Malignancies tend to grow pushing against adjacent structures and forming a pseudocapsule as they enlarge. The pseudocapsule consists of compressed fibrous connective tissue, normal tissue, vascularization, and inflammatory reaction. Malignant lesions tend to respect anatomic compartments and fascial borders until late in their course.[21] Heterogeneous signal may represent mixed tissue types, necrosis, or hemorrhage within the lesion. Only a minority (5%) of benign soft tissue tumors are larger than 5 cm in diameter, and about 1% of benign lesions are deep.[5,22] In general, irregular margins, heterogeneous signal, and large size are indicators of a malignant lesion. Unless a specific diagnosis can be determined, a lesion should be considered indeterminate and biopsy performed.

An intracompartmental lesion is one that has not crossed any natural anatomic boundaries such as cortical bone, articular cartilage, joint capsule, major fascial plane, tendon, or ligament. Identifying invasion of other compartments is important for tumor staging and is often apparent on MR imaging. Aggressive lesions more readily invade surrounding tissues and cross anatomic boundaries. Vascular channels and poorly planned biopsy paths may contribute to invasion of adjacent compartments.

Lesion location is important for restricting the differential diagnosis. MR imaging with its excellent soft tissue contrast is the most valuable modality for determining location. Potential lesion locations include intramuscular, intermuscular, subcutaneous, and intra-articular/periarticular locations. A multifocal or an extensive lesion also limits diagnostic considerations to include angiomatous lesions, neurofibromatosis (NF), fibromatosis, lipomatosis, myxoma (Mazabraud syndrome), metastases, or lymphoma.

Lesions discussed in the following sections are included because of their frequency or their specific location or unique imaging characteristics that allow for a specific diagnosis or a limited differential diagnosis. For the common but nonspecific lesions, a reasonable differential diagnosis requires knowledge of lesion prevalence, anatomic distribution, and age range. Lesions that predominantly affect pediatric patients (see the article by Navarro and colleagues elsewhere in this issue for further exploration), benign soft tissue tumors (see the article by Walker and colleagues elsewhere in this issue for further exploration), and tumorlike conditions (see the article by Stacy and colleagues elsewhere in this issue for further exploration) are discussed in separate articles within this issue.

DERMATOFIBROSARCOMA PROTUBERANS

Dermatofibrosarcoma protuberans (DFSP) (**Fig. 1**) constitutes approximately 6% of soft tissue sarcomas.[23] This lesion is an intermediate-grade malignancy, but fibrosarcomatous transformation representing a higher-grade component may occur in 17% to 20% of cases.[24–26] DFSP most commonly occurs in the third to fifth decades of life with occasional reports of pediatric involvement.[27,28] Men are affected more frequently than women.[29] The lesion presents as a slowly growing reddish brown to bluish superficial skin nodule. Large lesions may become painful. Surgery with an excision margin of greater than 3 cm is associated with a local recurrence rate of 20%.[30] Head and neck tumors have a higher local recurrence rate (50%–75%). The incidence of metastasis is approximately 5%.[31] The trunk is affected in up to 50% of cases followed in frequency by the proximal upper and lower extremities (35%–40%) and the head and neck (14%).[29,32] Lesions may be multiple with small nodules coalescing to form a plaque.[29] MR imaging demonstrates a lesion involving the skin and subcutaneous adipose tissue causing a focal protuberance of the skin with a lobular or nodular architecture. Involvement of the underlying muscle is uncommon. The signal characteristics of the lesion are nonspecific, with signal similar to skeletal muscle on T1-weighted (T1W) images and similar to or greater than fat on T2-weighted (T2W) sequences. Fat-suppressed T2W sequences or short tau inversion recovery images typically demonstrate high signal intensity. Moderate enhancement is seen after intravenous gadolinium administration. The lesion may show heterogeneous signal if hemorrhage or necrosis is present. Satellite nodules in the adjacent subcutaneous tissue may be present, and linear extensions along the skin are often detected.[33]

A differential diagnosis for a subcutaneous lesion includes cutaneous malignant fibrous histiocytoma

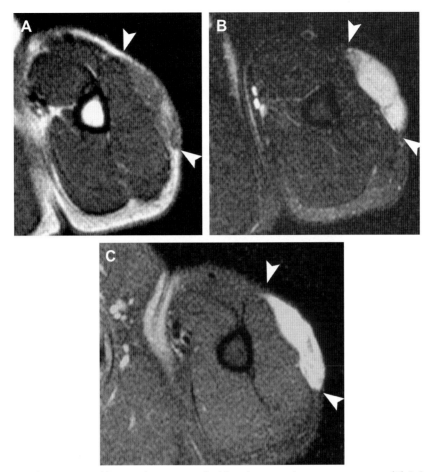

Fig. 1. DFSP. DFSP in a 21-year-old man who presented with a slow-growing upper arm mass. (*A*) Axial T1W (repetition time/echo time [TR/TE], 805/11) MR image demonstrates a superficial subcutaneous protuberant soft tissue mass arising from the skin of the upper arm. (*B*) Axial T2W image (TR/TE, 4284/70) and (*C*) axial T1W (TR/TE, 949/11) postcontrast image with fat saturation demonstrate linear extension along the skin (*white arrowheads*).

(MFH)/fibrosarcoma, DFSP, skin adnexal/appendage tumor, and metastasis.

FIBROSARCOMA/UNDIFFERENTIATED HIGH-GRADE PLEOMORPHIC SARCOMA OR MFH

The World Health Organization (WHO) significantly reorganized the nomenclature of malignant fibrous lesions of the soft tissue in April 2002. The WHO suggested replacing the term MFH with undifferentiated high-grade pleomorphic sarcoma (**Fig. 2**). Myxoid MFH is now myxofibrosarcoma. Giant cell MFH and inflammatory MFH are now called undifferentiated high-grade pleomorphic sarcoma with giant cells and undifferentiated high-grade pleomorphic sarcoma with prominent inflammation, respectively.[34] Having said this, most of our colleagues continue to use the term MFH either out of familiarity or because of convenience.

Fibrosarcoma is a malignant tumor of fibroblasts comprising 5% of soft tissue sarcomas.[33] It occurs primarily in adults with 60% of patients between the ages of 40 and 70 years.[35,36] There is a slight male predilection (61% of cases).[37] Fibrosarcoma most commonly involves the deep soft tissues of the extremities and trunk.[35,36,38] Patients usually present with a painless mass slowly enlarging over several months, and 30% of patients may have dull aching pain or tenderness.[35]

MFH/undifferentiated high-grade pleomorphic sarcoma is a high-grade lesion of fibroblasts, myofibroblasts, or undifferentiated mesenchymal cells.[33] Subtypes of MFH include storiform/pleomorphic (50%–60%), myxoid (25%), giant cell (5%–10%), and inflammatory (<5%) types.[34] MFH is the most common soft tissue sarcoma of adults, accounting for 20% to 30% of soft tissue sarcomas, and most occur in persons aged

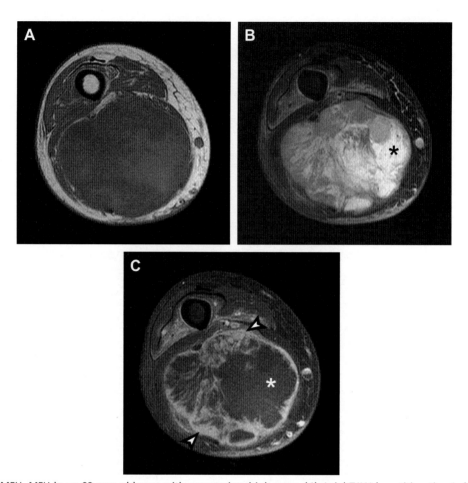

Fig. 2. MFH. MFH in an 82-year-old man with a posterior thigh mass. (*A*) Axial T1W (repetition time/echo time [TR/TE], 650/18) and (*B*) T2W fat-saturated (TR/TE, 4700/60) images demonstrate a large thigh lesion in an intramuscular location within the semimembranosus muscle. Note the significant necrosis (*asterisk*). (*C*) Irregular peripheral, septal, and nodular enhancing components are noted on a T1W fat-saturated postcontrast (TR/TE, 550/18) image (*arrowheads*). Postcontrast images are valuable to guide biopsy to areas of viable tissue. Asterisk denotes nonenhancing areas on (*C*) that correspond to high signal areas on (*B*) representing necrosis.

between 50 and 70 years.[39] MFH is the most frequent postradiation sarcoma.[40,41] There is a male predilection (70% of lesions). Patients usually present with an enlarging, painless soft tissue mass with an average size of 5 to 10 cm.[33] The most common locations are the lower extremity (50%), upper extremity (25%), retroperitoneum (15%), and head/neck (5%). Metastases at presentation are seen in up to 5% of patients.[42] Lesions are most common in deep intramuscular locations (70%), with 5% to 10% involving the subcutaneous tissue.[43]

Imaging features of adult fibrosarcoma and MFH are indistinguishable and similar to low-grade fibromyxoid sarcoma and sclerosing epithelioid fibrosarcoma; therefore, the MR imaging characteristics of these lesions are described together. Lesions are typically seen as an intramuscular mass with low to intermediate signal intensity on T1W and intermediate to high (>fat) signal on T2W images. The lesions are heterogeneous on all pulse sequences reflecting variable amounts of collagen, myxoid tissue, necrosis, and hemorrhage. Imaging of myxofibrosarcoma demonstrates low signal on T1W sequences and high signal intensity on long repetition time sequences reflecting the higher water content of the lesion.[34] Low-signal regions on T1W and T2W sequences may represent areas of high collagen content or calcification (present in 5%–20% pathologically).[33,43] The lesion margin is usually well defined because of a fibrous pseudocapsule. MFH and fibrosarcoma typically show enhancement, which may be heterogeneous if areas of necrosis or hemorrhage are present. Destruction of adjacent cortical bone may be present, similar to that which may be seen with synovial sarcoma.[43–46] In a patient with a history of spontaneous hematoma, suspicion of an underlying neoplasm (particularly MFH or synovial sarcoma) should be excluded with a diligent search for solid or nodular enhancing components, often peripherally located. Hematomas reveal variable thick nonnodular walls often containing hemosiderin. Edema is often seen surrounding a hematoma secondary to irritation from the bleeding, but a tumor that hemorrhages typically retains the blood inside the pseudocapsule and edema is not a prominent feature.[34,43]

Bone destruction by a soft tissue sarcoma is most commonly noted with undifferentiated pleomorphic sarcoma,[33] synovial sarcoma,[47] rhabdomyosarcoma,[48] and leiomyosarcoma.[49]

LIPOSARCOMA

The World Heath Organization reorganized the nomenclature of malignant lipomatous lesions of soft tissue in April 2002. Current subtypes of liposarcoma include well-differentiated liposarcoma, dedifferentiated liposarcoma, myxoid liposarcoma, pleomorphic liposarcoma, and mixed-type liposarcoma. The lesion previously referred to as round cell liposarcoma has been incorporated into the category of myxoid liposarcoma in recognition of the continuum of diagnosis.[34,42] Liposarcoma is the second most common soft tissue sarcoma after MFH.[23] The estimated annual incidence is 2.5 per million population.[50] Liposarcomas are extraordinarily rare in patients younger than 10 years. Most fatty masses in the pediatric population are lipoblastomas.[33]

WELL-DIFFERENTIATED LIPOSARCOMA

Well-differentiated liposarcoma (**Fig. 3**) is a low-grade malignancy that recurs locally but does not metastasize (unless there is a focus of dedifferentiation). It is the most common subtype representing about 50% of all liposarcomas. There is an equal sex distribution, although there is a male predominance for lesions of the groin. The peak prevalence is in the sixth and seventh decades.[51] Common lesion locations include the lower extremities (50%), retroperitoneum (20%–33%), upper extremity (14%), and trunk (12%).[51,52] Retroperitoneal lesions are typically large at presentation (often >20 cm) and have a local recurrence rate of up to 91% after resection. Lesions are frequently intramuscular but can occur in intermuscular and subcutaneous locations.[51,53] The most common clinical presentation of well-differentiated liposarcoma is a painless slow-growing (months–years) soft tissue

mass.[33,54] We use the term atypical lipomatous lesion to describe subcutaneous lesions because of their limited morbidity and lack of significant potential for dedifferentiation, although their histologic features are identical to well-differentiated liposarcoma.[51]

On MR imaging, well-differentiated liposarcoma is a mass composed of greater than 75% adipose tissue, and the significant nonadipose components are seen as prominent thick septa and focal nodular regions usually less than 2 cm in size.[54–58] The septations within a liposarcoma are almost always thicker and more numerous than the septa within the normal adjacent subcutaneous tissue. Nodular nonlipomatous components larger than 2 to 3 cm suggest a dedifferentiated liposarcoma.[51] Moderate to marked enhancement may be seen in the nonlipomatous thickened septa and nodular areas.[55] Statistical factors favoring the diagnosis of well-differentiated liposarcoma as opposed to lipoma include male sex, age greater than 66 years, lower percentage of fat in the lesion, mineralization, size larger than 10 cm, septa greater than 2 mm thick, or nonlipomatous nodular or globular foci.[58] Possibly, the most important task in the imaging of liposarcoma is to detect foci of dedifferentiation within the lesion because this significantly changes both treatment options and prognosis.

A differential diagnosis for soft tissue lesions with components of relatively high signal intensity (compared with skeletal muscle) on T1W images may include lipoma/well-differentiated liposarcoma, hemangioma (due to adjacent fat overgrowth), melanoma/clear cell sarcoma (perhaps due to melanin), subacute hemorrhage (due to methemoglobin), and neoplasms with a prominent hemorrhagic component.

MYXOID LIPOSARCOMA

Myxoid liposarcoma (**Fig. 4**) is an intermediate- to high-grade malignancy depending on the percentage of round cell component. It is the second most common type of liposarcoma, representing 20% to 50% of all liposarcomas.[51,59,60] Myxoid liposarcomas account for 10% of all soft tissue sarcomas.[61] Peak prevalence is about a decade younger than the other liposarcoma subtypes, usually from the forth to fifth decades of life. These lesions show no gender predilection[51] and predominantly affect the lower extremity (75%–80% of cases), particularly the popliteal region and medial thigh.[59] Extremity myxoid liposarcomas are most frequently intermuscular in location (70%–80% of cases). Intramuscular and subcutaneous lesions are less common.[50,53,60,62] Clinical

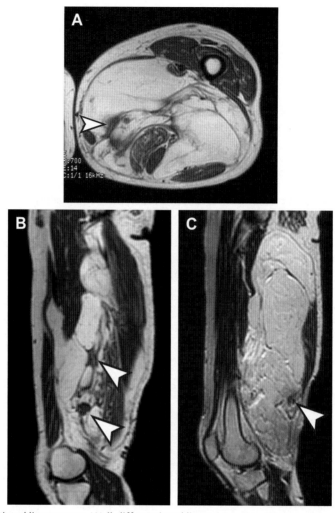

Fig. 3. Well-differentiated liposarcoma. Well-differentiated liposarcoma in a 65-year-old woman with thigh mass slowly growing over 3 years. (*A*) Axial T1W (repetition time/echo time [TR/TE], 700/14), (*B*) sagittal T1W (TR/TE, 650/14), and (*C*) sagittal T2W (TR/TE, 4500/98) images demonstrate a high–signal intensity intermuscular lipomatous lesion with predominantly fatty signal but thickened septa and nodularity (*arrowheads*).

presentation of myxoid liposarcoma is that of a painless soft tissue mass.[42] These lesions can be large at presentation (>15 cm), similar to well-differentiated liposarcoma.[51] They also have a high incidence of metastasis to extrapulmonary soft tissue (94%).[63]

On MR imaging, these lesions are typically large, well defined, and multilobulated. Low signal intensity on T1W images and marked high signal on T2W sequences reflect the high water content of the lesion, and these features may mimic a cyst. Sonography may be useful to demonstrate the solid nature of the lesion (hypoechoic rather than anechoic). On CT, the low attenuation of the lesion often simulates a cyst. Adipose tissue with high T1W signal typically constitutes a small volume

of the lesion (<10%) within the septa or as subtle small nodules. In our experience, approximately 90% of myxoid liposarcomas demonstrate fat on MR imaging, with only 10% more closely simulating a cyst and not containing visible fat. When confronted with a high water content mass in the soft tissues, a diligent search should be made for communication with a joint or tendon sheath suggesting a ganglion. Postcontrast images without thickened septae or nodular components also favor a cyst. Identification of the subtle fat component may require comparison of T1W and T2W images in the same plane (usually the axial plane).[51,64,65] Areas of intermediate T1W and T2W signal may represent foci of a round cell component. Myxoid liposarcoma may demonstrate

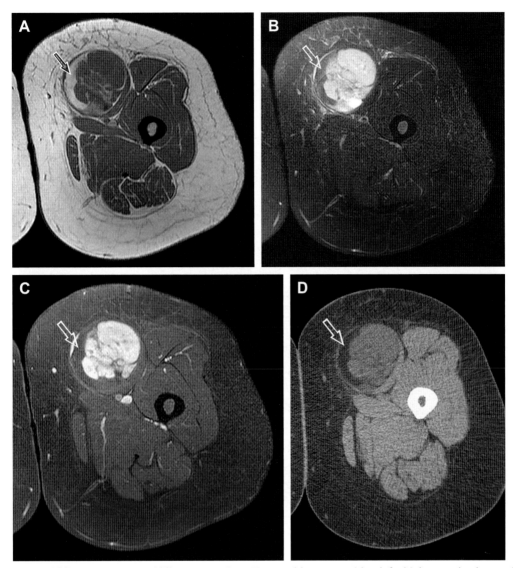

Fig. 4. Myxoid liposarcoma. Myxoid liposarcoma in a 48-year-old woman with a left thigh mass slowly growing over 1 year. (*A*) T1W (repetition time/echo time [TR/TE], 746/35) MR image demonstrates peripheral and septal areas of high signal (*arrow*). These regions correspond to areas of intermediate to low signal on both (*B*) T2W fat-suppressed (TR/TE, 5807/70), and (*C*) T1W postcontrast fat-suppressed (TR/TE, 638.3/7) images following the signal characteristics of fat. The lipid component is less than 10% of the total tumor volume. The pattern of enhancement (or imaging features on ultrasonography) can help differentiate myxomatous tumors from truly cystic lesions, which they can mimic on T2W and other fluid-sensitive MR images. (*D*) Axial CT demonstrates low-attenuation lipid component following the same pattern.

enhancement in a peripheral nodular (61% of cases), central nodular (44% of cases), or diffuse (17% of cases) pattern allowing differentiation from a cystic lesion. Round cell components may reveal more marked diffuse enhancement.[66]

Differential diagnosis for a predominantly myxoid-appearing soft tissue lesion includes myxoid liposarcoma, myxofibrosarcoma (or myxoid MFH), myxoid chondrosarcoma, myxoma, ganglion, synovial cyst/bursa, and peripheral nerve sheath tumor.

SYNOVIAL SARCOMA

Synovial sarcoma (**Fig. 5**) is a soft tissue malignancy typically occurring in young adults aged between 15 and 35 years, with the mean age of 32 years. It is a relatively common primary soft tissue malignancy, accounting for approximately 5% to 10% of soft tissue sarcomas with an equal male and female predominance.[23,67,68] The name synovial sarcoma is misleading given that the

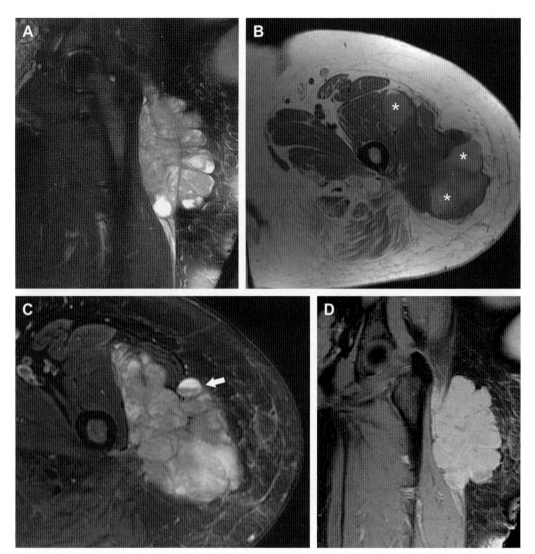

Fig. 5. Synovial sarcoma. Synovial sarcoma in a 47-year-old woman with slow-growing, painful, left lateral thigh mass. (*A*) Coronal fat-saturated T2W (repetition time/echo time [TR/TE], 4200/72.6), (*B*) axial T1W (TR/TE, 600/12), (*C*) axial fat-saturated T2W (TR/TE, 2800/68.1), and (*D*) coronal fat-saturated contrast-enhanced T1W (TR/TE, 225/1.8) MR images demonstrate a large, lobulated, heterogeneous mass centered at the iliotibial band. A combination of septations, hemorrhage (*asterisks*), and fluid level (*arrow*) account for the "bowl of grapes" appearance. Diffuse enhancement was noted in the solid components (see [*D*]).

lesion does not arise from the synovium or from an intra-articular location. In fact, the origin is likely from undifferentiated mesenchymal tissue.[69,70] Clinically, patients usually present with a slow-growing, palpable, and painful mass. The symptoms may be present from days to as long as 20 years before initial diagnosis.[71] Most tumors occur in the extremities, 60% to 70% in the lower limb, with the popliteal fossa being the most common location.[72] It is the most common soft tissue malignancy of the foot and ankle in patients aged between 6 and 35 years.[23] Other rare sites of involvement are the neck, pharynx, larynx, precoccygeal and paravertebral areas, thoracic and abdominal wall, and heart. Most synovial sarcomas are intermuscular in location and found within 5 cm of a joint. Synovial sarcoma centered in an intra-articular location is rare (<10%).[72] Lesions are intermediate- to high-grade neoplasms, and, as a result, metastases or local recurrence is common, seen in approximately 80% of patients. Metastases are present in 16% to 25% of cases at the time of diagnosis, with the lung most commonly affected.[73,74]

Radiographs are normal in approximately 50% of the cases; however, calcifications are seen in up to 30% of patients, often in a peripheral distribution. Adjacent bone involvement (periosteal reaction, osseous remodeling, or osseous invasion) is seen in 11% to 20% of cases.[67,71,75,76] MR imaging often shows a heterogeneous mass with areas that are hyperintense, isointense, and hypointense to fat on T2W imaging. This nonspecific triple sign (or triple signal) finding is seen in 30% to 50% of cases and represents the mixture of cystic (hemorrhage and necrosis) and solid components in the tumor.[77] A multiloculated appearance with numerous septa is commonly noted, with areas of hemorrhage and fluid levels demonstrating a "bowl of grapes" appearance.[72] Contrast enhancement is generally prompt and heterogeneous and is important to demonstrate areas of nodular enhancement in a predominantly cystic lesion. This procedure allows distinction from a truly cystic mass such as a ganglion or synovial cyst, and biopsy should be targeted at

these solid areas that harbor diagnostic tissue. Serpentine vascular channels within the tumor can be seen in 30% of cases.[72]

The differential diagnosis for neoplasms with serpentine vascular channels includes rhabdomyosarcoma, alveolar soft part sarcoma, synovial sarcoma, extraskeletal Ewing tumor/primitive neuroectodermal tumor, hemangioendothelioma, and hemangiopericytoma (HPC).

MALIGNANT PERIPHERAL NERVE SHEATH TUMOR

The previous nomenclature for malignant peripheral nerve sheath tumor (MPNST) (**Fig. 6**) includes malignant schwannoma and neurofibrosarcoma. MPNST accounts for 5% to 10% of soft tissue sarcomas. The condition usually affects patients aged 20 to 50 years, with a slight female predilection.[23,78] MPNST is associated with NF type 1 (NF1) in 25% to 70% of cases, where it presents at an average age of 29 to 36 years, with a male

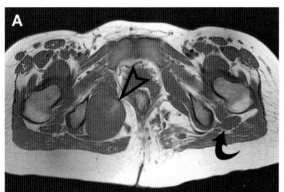
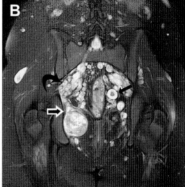
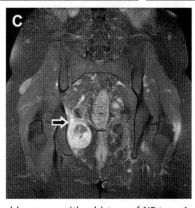

Fig. 6. MPNST. MPNST in an 18-year-old woman with a history of NF type 1 and pain in the right groin. (*A*) Axial T1W (repetition time/echo time [TR/TE], 448/12), (*B*) coronal T2W fat-saturated sequence (TR/TE, 4889/70), and (*C*) coronal T1W fat-saturated sequence postcontrast (TR/TE, 550/12) images demonstrate a heterogeneous intermuscular lesion with entering nerve (*white-outlined arrows*) and central necrosis. Also noted are plexiform neurofibroma of the sciatic nerves (*curved black arrows*) and target sign (*small black arrow*). T1W image reveals hemorrhage (*arrowhead*).

predilection (80%).[78] Patients present with pain and motor weakness more frequently than those with benign peripheral nerve sheath tumor (BPNST). A sudden increase in size of a previously stable lesion in a patient with NF1 should always raise suspicion for MPNST. MPNST usually affects medium to large deep-seated nerves, with the sciatic nerve, brachial plexus, and sacral plexus most commonly involved.[79] These lesions are typically larger than 5 cm in size, whereas BPNSTs are frequently smaller than 5 cm. Distinguishing MPNST and BPNST by imaging can be challenging because the lesions can appear very similar. There are some imaging features that may be helpful. The target sign and fascicular sign are uncommon in MPNST in comparison with BPNST. Lesion shape is fusiform, secondary to the entering and exiting nerve in both the BPNST and MPNST.[78] Margins of MPNST may be ill defined secondary to infiltrative growth. Because of this, a complete split fat sign is seen less frequently. An ill-defined margin on a deep-seated nonplexiform neural tumor is highly suggestive of MPNST.[33] Central necrosis and lesion heterogeneity are more common in malignant lesions but can also be seen with ancient schwannoma.[33] One study suggests that MPNST and BPNST cannot be adequately separated by evaluation of lesion heterogeneity.[80] When rhabdomyosarcoma elements are present, the lesion is called a Triton tumor. In general, enhancement of the benign neural tumor is variable, and prominent enhancement is more frequent in MPNST.[33] Fludeoxyglucose F 18 and 11C-methionine[81] positron emission tomographic imaging has been useful in identifying malignant change in plexiform neurofibromas[82,83] and predictive of patient survival.[84]

CLEAR CELL SARCOMA

Clear cell sarcoma (**Fig. 7**), also referred to as malignant melanoma of soft parts, is an uncommon neoplasm accounting for 1% of all soft tissue sarcomas.[85] It is a melanin-producing tumor in up to 75% of cases. The lesion commonly presents in young adults aged between 15 and 40 years age. There is a female predominance ratio of 3:2. Clear cell sarcoma often presents as a slowly enlarging mass, which is occasionally painful. The lesion is intimately associated with or within a tendon, ligament, aponeurosis, or fascial structure. There is a predilection for the lower extremity (75%), particularly the feet/ankle (43%) and knees (30%)[33,78,86] and a tendency for local recurrence and metastatic spread.[87] The lesion margins are indistinct with invasion of the adjacent muscles and no evident pseudocapsule. Clear cell sarcoma is often large at presentation, and determining the origin of the lesion from a particular tendon, ligament, or aponeurosis may be difficult in these lesions. An intratendinous location of origin is more apparent in smaller lesions.

Clear cell sarcoma typically demonstrates a slightly higher signal than muscle on T1W images (52%), although whether this is attributable to melanin is controversial.[33,87] T2W sequences may show signal greater than fat (70%) or low to intermediate signal (30%). There is typically

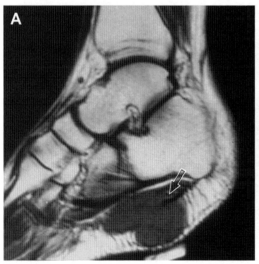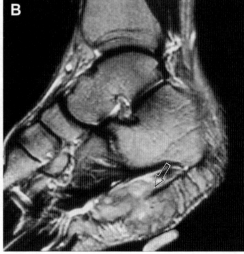

Fig. 7. Clear cell sarcoma. Clear cell sarcoma in a 20-year-old woman who noticed a bump on the plantar surface of her foot. (*A*) Sagittal T1W (repetition time/echo time [TR/TE], 450/25) and (*B*) T2W (TR/TE, 1800/90) images without fat suppression demonstrate a lesion emerging from the plantar fascia (*arrows*).

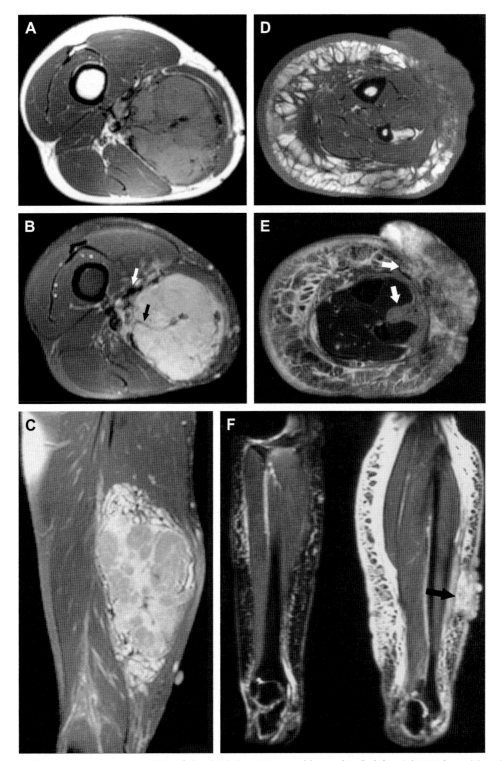

Fig. 8. Malignant vascular tumors. HPC of the thigh in a 35-year-old man (*A–C*). (*A*) Axial T1W (repetition time/echo time [TR/TE], 14/500), (*B*) axial fat-suppressed T2W (TR/TE, 52/3000), and (*C*) coronal T1 fat-suppressed post-contrast (TR/TE, 14/400) images show a soft tissue mass with prominent high-flow feeding and internal vessels (*arrows*). Characteristics are otherwise nonspecific with low to intermediate T1 and T2 signal intensity along with diffuse enhancement. Angiosarcoma of the lower leg in a 25-year-old man associated with chronic hereditary lymphangiectasia (*D–F*). (*D*) Axial T1W image (TR/TE, 544/7), (*E*) axial T2W (TR/TE, 2500/80) image with fat saturation, and (*F*) coronal T2W (TR/TE, 2500/80) image with fat suppression reveal a fungating mass with invasion of subcutaneous tissue and muscle (*arrows*) within a background of lymphedema shown by skin thickening and subcutaneous edema.

a homogeneous T1W signal and heterogeneity on T2W sequences. Prominent enhancement is frequently observed.[33]

Clear cell sarcoma, synovial sarcoma, and epithelioid sarcoma are often associated with tendons or aponeuroses.

AGGRESSIVE AND MALIGNANT VASCULAR TUMORS: HEMANGIOENDOTHELIOMA, HPC, AND ANGIOSARCOMA

Hemangioendothelioma is a rare tumor of vascular endothelial cells with intermediate aggressive behavior. This includes tumor infiltration, local recurrence (up to 15%), and metastasis (up to 30%).[33] This lesion affects soft tissue more often than bone and commonly involves superficial or deep soft tissues of the extremities, hands, feet, or the retroperitoneum.[33,88,89] A broad age range is observed from children to elderly.[33]

HPC (**Fig. 8**A–C) is a rare vascular tumor with intermediate aggressive behavior and benign and malignant forms. This tumor is closely related

and likely identical to extrapleural solitary fibrous tumor. HPC most frequently occurs during the fifth decade, with 80% occurring between ages 25 and 65 years, and there is an equal sex predilection.[33] Lesion location, in decreasing order of frequency, is within deep soft tissues of the thigh, retroperitoneum, head/neck, and upper extremity.[33] Clinical presentation is typically a painless slow-growing mass. Hypoglycemia occurs in 5%, which abates on tumor excision.[89]

Angiosarcoma (see **Fig. 8**D–F) is a malignant aggressive tumor of vascular endothelial cells with a propensity for local recurrence and metastasis. Predisposing factors include radiation and chronic lymphedema (eg, Stewart-Treves syndrome after mastectomy). Lesion location includes skin (33%); deep soft tissues (24%); and, less commonly, breast, liver, bone, spleen, heart, head, and neck.[33] Age distribution is broad and ranges from 22 to 91 years with a mean age of 65 years.[88]

Hemangioendothelioma, HPC, and angiosarcoma have similar imaging features. Morphology is of an aggressive infiltrative lesion. MR signal

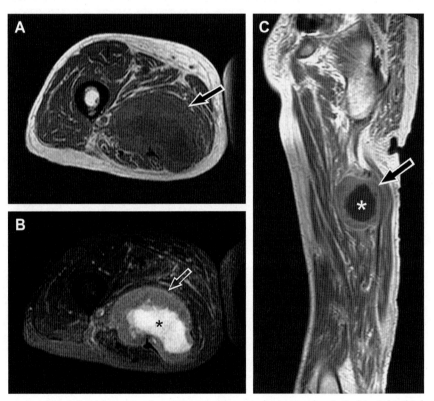

Fig. 9. Leiomyosarcoma. Leiomyosarcoma in a 77-year-old man who noticed pain in his right thigh region and experienced a 9.07-kg weight loss over several months. (*A*) Axial T1W image (repetition time/echo time [TR/TE], 544/7) and (*B*) axial T2W image with fat saturation (TR/TE, 2500/80) demonstrate a large heterogeneous lesion with intermediate signal (*arrows*) and central necrosis (*asterisk*). (*C*) Sagittal T1W image after gadolinium enhancement (TR/TE, 505/7) reveals thickened and irregular peripheral enhancing walls with a prominent central nonenhancing area (*asterisk*).

characteristics are nonspecific, with intermediate T1 and high T2 signal intensity. Hemorrhage may occur with areas of high T1 signal intensity. The most characteristic feature is the presence of serpentine vessels in an otherwise solid nonspecific soft tissue mass that is most commonly seen with HPC. These vessels are usually high-flow (low signal on T1 and T2) vascular structures.[90] Angiosarcoma may appear as a plaquelike subcutaneous mass in the background of an enlarged extremity with edema representing underlying lymphedema.

LEIOMYOSARCOMA

Leiomyosarcoma (**Fig. 9**) is a high-grade muscle tumor that represents approximately 9% of all soft tissue sarcomas[23,91] with approximately equal proportions in deep (both intramuscular and intermuscular in our experience) and subcutaneous locations.[42] Patients with soft tissue leiomyosarcoma have a median age in the fifth to sixth decades.[92–94] Retroperitoneal lesions (20% of cases) are more common in women by a ratio 2:1 to 7:1, and there is a male predilection for peripheral lesions (12% of cases).[94] Retroperitoneal lesions present clinically as an abdominal mass and swelling with pain in less than 10%.[93] The remainder of these tumors is located in the genitourinary and alimentary tracts. It is the second most common retroperitoneal tumor after liposarcoma.[95] Leiomyosarcoma is the predominant sarcoma to arise from larger blood vessels.[96,97] Extremity lesions present with a painless slowly enlarging mass most commonly affecting the thigh.[92] Metastases are most common to the lung followed by the liver.[93] Imaging of leiomyosarcoma is typically nonspecific. Mineralization on radiograph has been reported in 17% of cases.[98] Lesions are typically isointense to muscle on T1W images and variably hyperintense relative to muscle on T2W images, with prominent contrast enhancement.[98] Large lesions are usually more heterogeneous secondary to hemorrhage, necrosis, and cystic change.[95]

The most common cutaneous soft tissue sarcomas include Kaposi sarcoma (71.1%), DFSP (18.4%), MFH (5.3%), leiomyosarcoma (2.2%), and angiosarcoma (1.6%).[99]

SUMMARY

In this article, the MR imaging characteristics of several frequently encountered malignant soft tissue tumors in the adult were discussed. Many of these lesions have unique imaging characteristics that suggest a specific diagnosis. Often the imaging findings are indeterminate, and biopsy should be performed with the appropriate biopsy path discussed with the orthopedic oncologist or treating surgeon.

ACKNOWLEDGMENTS

We gratefully acknowledge the residents who attend the American Institute for Radiologic Pathology courses (past, present, and future) for their contribution of interesting cases to our series of patients, which allow our continued educational outreach.

REFERENCES

1. Hajdu SI. Soft tissue sarcomas: classification and natural history. CA Cancer J Clin 1981;31(5):271–80.
2. Jemal A, Siegel R, Ward E, et al. Cancer statistics, 2009. CA Cancer J Clin 2009;59(4):225–49.
3. Walker EA, Song AJ, Murphey MD. Magnetic resonance imaging of soft-tissue masses. Semin Roentgenol 2010;45(4):277–97.
4. Baldursson G, Agnarsson BA, Benediktsdottir KR, et al. Soft tissue sarcomas in Iceland 1955-1988. Analysis of survival and prognostic factors. Acta Oncol 1991;30(5):563–8.
5. Rydholm A. Management of patients with soft-tissue tumors. Strategy developed at a regional oncology center. Acta Orthop Scand Suppl 1983;203:13–77.
6. Ma LD, Frassica FJ, McCarthy EF, et al. Benign and malignant musculoskeletal masses: MR imaging differentiation with rim-to-center differential enhancement ratios. Radiology 1997;202(3):739–44.
7. Benedikt RA, Jelinek JS, Kransdorf MJ, et al. MR imaging of soft-tissue masses: role of gadopentetate dimeglumine. J Magn Reson Imaging 1994;4(3):485–90.
8. Erlemann R, Reiser MF, Peters PE, et al. Musculoskeletal neoplasms: static and dynamic Gd-DTPA–enhanced MR imaging. Radiology 1989;171(3):767–73.
9. Beltran J, Chandnani V, McGhee RA Jr, et al. Gadopentetate dimeglumine-enhanced MR imaging of the musculoskeletal system. AJR Am J Roentgenol 1991;156(3):457–66.
10. van Rijswijk CS, Geirnaerdt MJ, Hogendoorn PC, et al. Soft-tissue tumors: value of static and dynamic gadopentetate dimeglumine-enhanced MR imaging in prediction of malignancy. Radiology 2004;233(2):493–502.
11. Mirowitz SA, Totty WG, Lee JK. Characterization of musculoskeletal masses using dynamic Gd-DTPA enhanced spin-echo MRI. J Comput Assist Tomogr 1992;16(1):120–5.
12. Berquist TH, Ehman RL, King BF, et al. Value of MR imaging in differentiating benign from malignant

soft-tissue masses: study of 95 lesions. AJR Am J Roentgenol 1990;155(6):1251–5.

13. Crim JR, Seeger LL, Yao L, et al. Diagnosis of soft-tissue masses with MR imaging: can benign masses be differentiated from malignant ones? Radiology 1992;185(2):581–6.

14. Kransdorf MJ, Jelinek JS, Moser RP Jr, et al. Soft-tissue masses: diagnosis using MR imaging. AJR Am J Roentgenol 1989;153(3):541–7.

15. Murphey MD, Nomikos GC. Prospective diagnosis Q12 of soft tissue tumors. Presentation at the RSNA in 2001;221:473.

16. Mankin HJ, Lange TA, Spanier SS. The hazards of biopsy in patients with malignant primary bone and soft-tissue tumors. J Bone Joint Surg Am 1982; 64(8):1121–7.

17. Mankin HJ, Mankin CJ, Simon MA. The hazards of the biopsy, revisited. Members of the Musculoskeletal Tumor Society. J Bone Joint Surg Am 1996; 78(5):656–63.

18. Sundaram M, McGuire MH, Herbold DR. Magnetic resonance imaging of soft tissue masses: an evaluation of fifty-three histologically proven tumors. Magn Reson Imaging 1988;6(3):237–48.

19. Moulton JS, Blebea JS, Dunco DM, et al. MR imaging of soft-tissue masses: diagnostic efficacy and value of distinguishing between benign and malignant lesions. AJR Am J Roentgenol 1995;164(5):1191–9.

20. Totty WG, Murphy WA, Lee JK. Soft-tissue tumors: MR imaging. Radiology 1986;160(1):135–41.

21. Peabody TD, Simon MA. Principles of staging of soft-tissue sarcomas. Clin Orthop Relat Res 1993;(289):19–31.

22. Myhre-Jensen O. A consecutive 7-year series of 1331 benign soft tissue tumours. Clinicopathologic data. Comparison with sarcomas. Acta Orthop Scand 1981;52(3):287–93.

23. Kransdorf MJ. Malignant soft-tissue tumors in a large referral population: distribution of diagnoses by age, sex, and location. AJR Am J Roentgenol 1995; 164(1):129–34.

24. Connelly JH, Evans HL. Dermatofibrosarcoma protuberans. A clinicopathologic review with emphasis on fibrosarcomatous areas. Am J Surg Pathol 1992; 16(10):921–5.

25. Ding J, Hashimoto H, Enjoji M. Dermatofibrosarcoma protuberans with fibrosarcomatous areas. A clinicopathologic study of nine cases and a comparison with allied tumors. Cancer 1989;64(3):721–9.

26. Wrotnowski U, Cooper PH, Shmookler BM. Fibrosarcomatous change in dermatofibrosarcoma protuberans. Am J Surg Pathol 1988;12(4):287–93.

27. Taylor HB, Helwig EB. Dermatofibrosarcoma protuberans. A study of 115 cases. Cancer 1962;15:717–25.

28. Thornton SL, Reid J, Papay FA, et al. Childhood dermatofibrosarcoma protuberans: role of preoperative imaging. J Am Acad Dermatol 2005;53(1):76–83.

29. Weiss SW, Goldblum JR, Enzinger FM. Fibrohistiocytic tumors of intermediate malignancy. In: Weiss SW, Goldblum JR, editors. Enzinger and Weiss' soft tissue tumors. 5th edition. Philadelphia: Mosby Elsevier; 2008. p. 371–402.

30. Roses DF, Valensi Q, LaTrenta G, et al. Surgical treatment of dermatofibrosarcoma protuberans. Surg Gynecol Obstet 1986;162(5):449–52.

31. Rockley PF, Robinson JK, Magid M, et al. Dermatofibrosarcoma protuberans of the scalp: a series of cases. J Am Acad Dermatol 1989;21(2 Pt 1):278–83.

32. McPeak CJ, Cruz T, Nicastri AD. Dermatofibrosarcoma protuberans: an analysis of 86 cases—five with metastasis. Ann Surg 1967;166(5):803–16.

33. Kransdorf MJ, Murphey MD. Imaging of soft tissue tumors. 2nd edition. Philadelphia: Lippincott Williams & Wilkins; 2006.

34. Murphey MD. World Health Organization classification of bone and soft tissue tumors: modifications and implications for radiologists. Semin Musculoskelet Radiol 2007;11(3):201–14.

35. Pritchard DJ, Sim FH, Ivins JC, et al. Fibrosarcoma of bone and soft tissues of the trunk and extremities. Orthop Clin North Am 1977;8(4):869–81.

36. Pritchard DJ, Soule EH, Taylor WF, et al. Fibrosarcoma—a clinicopathologic and statistical study of 199 tumors of the soft tissues of the extremities and trunk. Cancer 1974;33(3):888–97.

37. Scott SM, Reiman HM, Pritchard DJ, et al. Soft tissue fibrosarcoma. A clinicopathologic study of 132 cases. Cancer 1989;64(4):925–31.

38. Ninane J, Gosseye S, Panteon E, et al. Congenital fibrosarcoma. Preoperative chemotherapy and conservative surgery. Cancer 1986;58(7):1400–6.

39. Weiss SW, Enzinger FM. Malignant fibrous histiocytoma: an analysis of 200 cases. Cancer 1978;41(6): 2250–66.

40. Weiss SW, Goldblum JR, Enzinger FM. Malignant fibrous histiocytoma (pleomorphic undifferentiated sarcoma). In: Weiss SW, Goldblum JR, editors. Enzinger and Weiss' soft tissue tumors. 5th edition. Philadelphia: Mosby Elsevier; 2008. p. 403–26.

41. Laskin WB, Silverman TA, Enzinger FM. Postradiation soft tissue sarcomas. An analysis of 53 cases. Cancer 1988;62(11):2330–40.

42. Fletcher CDM, Unni KK, Mertens F. World Health Organization Pathology and Genetics of tumors of soft tissue and bone. 3rd edition. Lyon (France): IARC Press; 2006.

43. Murphey MD, Gross TM, Rosenthal HG. From the archives of the AFIP. Musculoskeletal malignant fibrous histiocytoma: radiologic-pathologic correlation. Radiographics 1994;14(4):807–26 [quiz: 827–8].

44. Mahajan H, Kim EE, Wallace S, et al. Magnetic resonance imaging of malignant fibrous histiocytoma. Magn Reson Imaging 1989;7(3):283–8.

45. Miller TT, Hermann G, Abdelwahab IF, et al. MRI of malignant fibrous histiocytoma of soft tissue: analysis of 13 cases with pathologic correlation. Skeletal Radiol 1994;23(4):271–5.

46. Panicek DM, Casper ES, Brennan MF, et al. Hemorrhage simulating tumor growth in malignant fibrous histiocytoma at MR imaging. Radiology 1991;181(2):398–400.

47. Stacy GS, Nair L. Magnetic resonance imaging features of extremity sarcomas of uncertain differentiation. Clin Radiol 2007;62(10):950–8.

48. Simmons M, Tucker AK. The radiology of bone changes in rhabdomyosarcoma. Clin Radiol 1978;29(1):47–52.

49. deSchepper AM, Vanhoenacker FM, Gielen LM, et al. Imaging of soft tissue tumors. 3rd edition. Berlin (Germany): Springer-Verlag; 2006.

50. Kindblom LG, Angervall L, Svendsen P. Liposarcoma a clinicopathologic, radiographic and prognostic study. Acta Pathol Microbiol Scand Suppl 1975;(253):1–71.

51. Murphey MD, Arcara LK, Fanburg-Smith J. From the archives of the AFIP: imaging of musculoskeletal liposarcoma with radiologic-pathologic correlation. Radiographics 2005;25(5):1371–95.

52. Mentzel T, Fletcher CD. Lipomatous tumours of soft tissues: an update. Virchows Arch 1995;427(4):353–63.

53. Miettinen M. Diagnostic soft tissue pathology. New York: Churchhill Livingstone; 2003.

54. Peterson JJ, Kransdorf MJ, Bancroft LW, et al. Malignant fatty tumors: classification, clinical course, imaging appearance and treatment. Skeletal Radiol 2003;32(9):493–503.

55. Ohguri T, Aoki T, Hisaoka M, et al. Differential diagnosis of benign peripheral lipoma from well-differentiated liposarcoma on MR imaging: is comparison of margins and internal characteristics useful? AJR Am J Roentgenol 2003;180(6):1689–94.

56. Hosono M, Kobayashi H, Fujimoto R, et al. Septum-like structures in lipoma and liposarcoma: MR imaging and pathologic correlation. Skeletal Radiol 1997;26(3):150–4.

57. Arkun R, Memis A, Akalin T, et al. Liposarcoma of soft tissue: MRI findings with pathologic correlation. Skeletal Radiol 1997;26(3):167–72.

58. Kransdorf MJ, Bancroft LW, Peterson JJ, et al. Imaging of fatty tumors: distinction of lipoma and well-differentiated liposarcoma. Radiology 2002;224(1):99–104.

59. Weiss SW, Goldblum JR, Enzinger FM. Liposarcoma. In: Weiss SW, Goldblum JR, editors. Enzinger and Weiss' soft tissue tumors. 5th edition. Philadelphia: Mosby Elsevier; 2008. p. 477–516.

60. Kilpatrick SE, Doyon J, Choong PF, et al. The clinicopathologic spectrum of myxoid and round cell liposarcoma. A study of 95 cases. Cancer 1996;77(8):1450–8.

61. Smith TA, Easley KA, Goldblum JR. Myxoid/round cell liposarcoma of the extremities. A clinicopathologic study of 29 cases with particular attention to extent of round cell liposarcoma. Am J Surg Pathol 1996;20(2):171–80.

62. Allen PW. Myxoid tumors of soft tissues. Pathol Annu 1980;15(Pt 1):133–92.

63. Pearlstone DB, Pisters PW, Bold RJ, et al. Patterns of recurrence in extremity liposarcoma: implications for staging and follow-up. Cancer 1999;85(1):85–92.

64. Jelinek JS, Kransdorf MJ, Shmookler BM, et al. Liposarcoma of the extremities: MR and CT findings in the histologic subtypes. Radiology 1993;186(2):455–9.

65. Sung MS, Kang HS, Suh JS, et al. Myxoid liposarcoma: appearance at MR imaging with histologic correlation. Radiographics 2000;20(4):1007–19.

66. Tateishi U, Hasegawa T, Beppu Y, et al. Prognostic significance of MRI findings in patients with myxoid-round cell liposarcoma. AJR Am J Roentgenol 2004;182(3):725–31.

67. Weiss SW, Goldblum JR, Enzinger FM. Enzinger and Weiss's soft tissue tumors. 4th edition. St Louis (MO): Mosby; 2001.

68. Israels SJ, Chan HS, Daneman A, et al. Synovial sarcoma in childhood. AJR Am J Roentgenol 1984;142(4):803–6.

69. Ishida T, Iijima T, Moriyama S, et al. Intra-articular calcifying synovial sarcoma mimicking synovial chondromatosis. Skeletal Radiol 1996;25(8):766–9.

70. Fletcher C, Unni K, Mertens F. World Health Organization Pathology and Genetics of tumors of soft tissue and bone. Lyon (France): IARC Press; 2002.

71. Cadman NL, Soule EH, Kelly PJ. Synovial sarcoma; an analysis of 34 tumors. Cancer 1965;18:613–27.

72. Murphey MD, Gibson MS, Jennings BT, et al. From the archives of the AFIP: imaging of synovial sarcoma with radiologic-pathologic correlation. Radiographics 2006;26(5):1543–65.

73. Ryan JR, Baker LH, Benjamin RS. The natural history of metastatic synovial sarcoma: experience of the Southwest Oncology group. Clin Orthop Relat Res 1982;(164):257–60.

74. Paulino AC. Synovial sarcoma prognostic factors and patterns of failure. Am J Clin Oncol 2004;27(2):122–7.

75. Wright PH, Sim FH, Soule EH, et al. Synovial sarcoma. J Bone Joint Surg Am 1982;64(1):112–22.

76. Horowitz AL, Resnick D, Watson RC. The roentgen features of synovial sarcomas. Clin Radiol 1973;24(4):481–4.

77. Jones BC, Sundaram M, Kransdorf MJ. Synovial sarcoma: MR imaging findings in 34 patients. AJR Am J Roentgenol 1993;161(4):827–30.

78. Weiss SW, Goldblum JR, Enzinger FM. Malignant tumors of the peripheral nerves. In: Weiss SW, Goldblum JR, editors. Enzinger and Weiss' soft

tissue tumors. 5th edition. Philadelphia: Mosby Elsevier; 2008. p. 903–44.

79. Ducatman BS, Scheithauer BW, Piepgras DG, et al. Malignant peripheral nerve sheath tumors. A clinicopathologic study of 120 cases. Cancer 1986;57(10): 2006–21.

80. Mann FA, Murphy WA, Totty WG, et al. Magnetic resonance imaging of peripheral nerve sheath tumors. Assessment by numerical visual fuzzy cluster analysis. Invest Radiol 1990;25(11):1238–45.

81. Bredella MA, Torriani M, Hornicek F, et al. Value of PET in the assessment of patients with neurofibromatosis type 1. AJR Am J Roentgenol 2007;189(4): 928–35.

82. Cardona S, Schwarzbach M, Hinz U, et al. Evaluation of F18-deoxyglucose positron emission tomography (FDG-PET) to assess the nature of neurogenic tumours. Eur J Surg Oncol 2003;29(6):536–41.

83. Ferner RE, Golding JF, Smith M, et al. [18F]2-fluoro-2-deoxy-D-glucose positron emission tomography (FDG PET) as a diagnostic tool for neurofibromatosis 1 (NF1) associated malignant peripheral nerve sheath tumours (MPNSTs): a long-term clinical study. Ann Oncol 2008;19(2):390–4.

84. Brenner W, Friedrich RE, Gawad KA, et al. Prognostic relevance of FDG PET in patients with neurofibromatosis type-1 and malignant peripheral nerve sheath tumours. Eur J Nucl Med Mol Imaging 2006;33(4):428–32.

85. Enzinger FM. Clear-cell sarcoma of tendons and aponeuroses. An analysis of 21 cases. Cancer 1965;18:1163–74.

86. Chung EB, Enzinger FM. Malignant melanoma of soft parts. A reassessment of clear cell sarcoma. Am J Surg Pathol 1983;7(5):405–13.

87. De Beuckeleer LH, De Schepper AM, Vandevenne JE, et al. MR imaging of clear cell sarcoma (malignant melanoma of the soft parts): a multicenter correlative MRI-pathology study of 21 cases and literature review. Skeletal Radiol 2000;29(4):187–95.

88. Miettinen M. Hemangioendotheliomas, angiosarcomas, and Kaposi's sarcoma. Modern soft tissue pathology: tumors and non-neoplastic conditions. Cambridge (NY): Cambridge University Press; 2010. p. 617–59.

89. Weiss SW, Goldblum JR, Enzinger FM. Hemangioendothelioma, vascular tumors of intermediate malignancy. In: Weiss SW, Goldblum JR, editors. Enzinger and Weiss' soft tissue tumors. 5th edition. Philadelphia: Mosby Elsevier; 2008. p. 681–732.

90. Murphey MD, Fairbairn KJ, Parman LM, et al. From the archives of the AFIP. Musculoskeletal angiomatous lesions: radiologic-pathologic correlation. Radiographics 1995;15(4):893–917.

91. Enjoji M, Hashimoto H. Diagnosis of soft tissue sarcomas. Pathol Res Pract 1984;178(3):215–26.

92. Brenton GE, Johnson DE, Eady JL. Leiomyosarcoma of the hand and wrist. Report of two cases. J Bone Joint Surg Am 1986;68(1):139–42.

93. Shmookler BM, Lauer DH. Retroperitoneal leiomyosarcoma. A clinicopathologic analysis of 36 cases. Am J Surg Pathol 1983;7(3):269–80.

94. Wile AG, Evans HL, Romsdahl MM. Leiomyosarcoma of soft tissue: a clinicopathologic study. Cancer 1981;48(4):1022–32.

95. Hartman DS, Hayes WS, Choyke PL, et al. From the archives of the AFIP. Leiomyosarcoma of the retroperitoneum and inferior vena cava: radiologic-pathologic correlation. Radiographics 1992;12(6): 1203–20.

96. Kevorkian J, Cento DP. Leiomyosarcoma of large arteries and veins. Surgery 1973;73(3):390–400.

97. Berlin O, Stener B, Kindblom LG, et al. Leiomyosarcomas of venous origin in the extremities. A correlated clinical, roentgenologic, and morphologic study with diagnostic and surgical implications. Cancer 1984;54(10):2147–59.

98. Bush CH, Reith JD, Spanier SS. Mineralization in musculoskeletal leiomyosarcoma: radiologic-pathologic correlation. AJR Am J Roentgenol 2003;180(1):109–13.

99. Rouhani P, Fletcher CD, Devesa SS, et al. Cutaneous soft tissue sarcoma incidence patterns in the U.S.: an analysis of 12,114 cases. Cancer 2008;113(3): 616–27.

Soft Tissue Masses in Children

Oscar M. Navarro, MD[a,b,*]

KEYWORDS

• Soft tissue masses • Ultrasound • MRI • Children

There is a large number and wide spectrum of pathologic entities that may present as a soft tissue mass in the pediatric age. Although in many instances a diagnosis can be established based solely on the clinical findings, a significant number of cases requires further imaging evaluation. This article reviews and illustrates the most common causes of soft tissue masses that require imaging in children.

CLINICAL EVALUATION AND IMAGING APPROACH

Attempting to make the diagnosis of a soft tissue mass in a child in the absence of any clinical information is often futile because there is extensive overlapping of the imaging appearances of many of these conditions. Clinical information often adds significant clues that may narrow the differential diagnosis. Crucial clinical information includes age of the child, presence of pre-existing conditions that may be associated with specific tumors, location of the mass, duration of the presence of the mass (especially if congenital), pattern of growth of the lesion, overlying skin abnormalities (in particular discoloration), tumor consistency, changes in the appearance of the mass, and associated systemic symptoms.

Further evaluation with imaging studies is usually required when the clinical findings are not completely contributory for a final diagnosis, to determine extent and relation of the mass to adjacent anatomic structures, when there is uncertainty as to whether the mass is arising from the soft tissues or underlying bones, and when the presence of the mass is not entirely clear on the physical examination. In most cases, the initial imaging evaluation of choice is with ultrasonography (US), which is particularly useful for small and superficial lesions. US has the advantages of being a modality that is highly available, easy to perform, does not require sedation or general anesthesia, lacks ionizing radiation exposure, is of relatively low cost, and practically does not have contraindications. For these reasons, US is ideally suited for the pediatric population. US should be performed with linear-array transducers of the highest frequency available, although in some cases complementary use of convex-array lower-frequency probes may be needed, particularly to assess larger and deeper lesions. In addition to gray-scale imaging, spectral and color Doppler US should be routinely done because information about the absence or presence of intralesional flow and the degree of vascularization is useful. Even in those cases when US is not diagnostic, it can provide useful information especially regarding the differentiation of cystic from solid lesions and can also help planning further imaging.

MR imaging is the diagnostic modality of choice for most large and deep lesions and for some of those for which US has not been diagnostic. MR imaging offers high tissue contrast and multiplanar capability. In contrast to US, MR imaging is often less available, requires sedation or general anesthesia in younger children, and is more expensive. A combination of T1-weighted and T2-weighted images forms the basis of the MR imaging

The author has nothing to disclose.

[a] Department of Medical Imaging, University of Toronto, Toronto, ON, Canada

[b] Department of Diagnostic Imaging, The Hospital for Sick Children, 555 University Avenue, Toronto, ON M5G 1X8, Canada

* Department of Diagnostic Imaging, The Hospital for Sick Children, 555 University Avenue, Toronto, ON M5G 1X8, Canada.

E-mail address: oscar.navarro@sickkids.ca

Radiol Clin N Am 49 (2011) 1235–1259

doi:10.1016/j.rcl.2011.07.008

examination. Fat suppression should be added to the T2-weighted pulse sequence because this is particularly useful when evaluating lesions that involve the subcutaneous fat tissues. In some instances, a T1-weighted fat suppressed sequence may also be added, especially to evaluate lesions that are at least partly hyperintense on the T1-weighted images, such as fat-containing masses. A gradient-echo sequence may also be helpful in the detection of hemosiderin and high-flow vessels. The administration of intravenous gadolinium chelates is used frequently to help in the differentiation between cystic and solid tumors, in the differentiation between venous and lymphatic malformations and in the evaluation of viable tumor.[1]

It has to be emphasized that MR imaging even when correlated with the clinical findings may not only have limitations in providing a specific diagnosis but may also be limited in the differentiation of benign from malignant masses. Fortunately, most pediatric soft tissue masses are benign. It has been estimated that after excluding small benign cutaneous and subcutaneous lesions, approximately 75% of the soft tissue masses requiring imaging are still benign.[2] Furthermore, MR imaging is helpful for making diagnosis of the most common benign masses, including hemangioma, lymphatic and venous malformations, lipoma, periarticular cysts, hematoma, giant cell tumor of the tendon sheath, neurofibroma, and fat necrosis.[3] Even in those cases that MR imaging is not diagnostic, it remains useful for the assessment of tumor extent, involvement of adjacent structures, response to therapy, and recurrence.

The role of other imaging modalities is more limited. Plain radiographs may be useful to exclude or confirm the osseous origin of a presumed soft tissue mass or to assess bone involvement by a soft tissue mass. CT is rarely used due to radiation exposure and less tissue contrast compared with MR imaging. Its main indication is in the evaluation of myositis ossificans although occasionally it may be used in younger children in whom sedation or anesthesia may not be indicated and thus cannot have an MR imaging examination.

The interpretation of the imaging findings also requires the use of appropriate nomenclature. The tumors should be referred to by terms that are not ambiguous and are correctly recognized by all physicians. In that regard, for most entities it is recommended to use the classification proposed by the World Health Organization, which was last revised in 2002.[4] The exception to this are the vascular tumors, for which the most accepted terminology is that included in the classification proposed by Mulliken and Glowacki[5] that has been subsequently adopted by the International Society for the Study of Vascular Anomalies.

PSEUDOTUMORS

This section discusses lesions that are neither neoplastic nor vascular in origin.

Fat Necrosis

Fat necrosis is often a traumatic soft tissue injury associated with nonlacerating compressive force.[6] There is commonly a prolonged time between the trauma and the recognition of a soft tissue mass and in many instances the traumatic event is not recalled by the patient. Other causes of fat necrosis apart from trauma have also been described, including cold exposure, iatrogenic injections, autoimmune disorders, vasculitis, and sickle cell disease.[7] Although fat necrosis can occur at any age, a special affected group is represented by neonates, in whom causes seem to mainly include hypoxia, hypothermia, and obstetric injury. In the author's experience, neonates are the age group in which imaging is most often required for diagnosis of subcutaneous fat necrosis.

Most patients present with a firm, nontender lump, typically in areas of bone prominence that are more prone to trauma, especially shoulders, back, buttocks, thighs, and cheek.[6] The nodule resolves spontaneously in weeks or up to 6 months leaving sometimes atrophy of the subcutaneous tissues resulting in a local depression.

US is often sufficient for diagnosis, particularly when fat necrosis shows a characteristic appearance of a hyperechoic nodule in the subcutaneous tissues with fuzzy margins and little vascularity on color Doppler interrogation (**Fig. 1**).[8] Fat necrosis presenting with a hypoechoic appearance or with a hypoechoic halo surrounding a hyperechoic nodule, however, has also been documented.[7] The variability in appearance likely reflects the stage of evolution and the severity of associated hemorrhage, particularly in posttraumatic cases.

MR imaging of fat necrosis demonstrates abnormal linear signal intensity in the subcutaneous tissues, which is often hypointense on T1-weighted images and mixed hyperintense and hypointense on T2-weighted images.[6] No discrete mass is identified.

Subcutaneous Granuloma Annulare

The subcutaneous form is 1 of 4 types of granuloma annulare, an idiopathic, benign self-limited, inflammatory process included in the category of necrobiotic granulomatous dermatoses.[9] It is

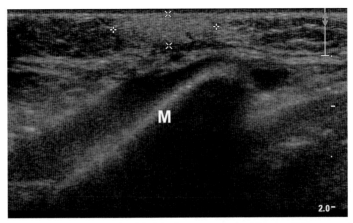

Fig. 1. Subcutaneous fat necrosis in a 4-week-old girl who presented with a small firm, nontender nodule in the right mandibular region. There was history of vaginal delivery that required the use of forceps. Longitudinal US image shows a hyperechoic area with fuzzy margins in the subcutaneous tissues (between cursors), superficial to the angle of the right mandible (M). The lesion gradually disappeared over a few weeks.

usually seen between the ages of 2 and 5 years and presents more frequently as a rapidly growing, nontender subcutaneous mass in the pretibial region and in the scalp, especially in the occiput.[9]

The few cases described on US in the literature have shown subcutaneous granuloma annulare as an ill-defined hypoechoic mass, confined to the subcutaneous tissues and in intimate relation to the superficial fascia of the underlying muscles (Fig. 2).[9,10] On MR imaging, the mass is also ill defined, always extending to but not traversing the underlying fascia, hypointense on T1-weighted images, and hyperintense on T2-weighted images (Fig. 3), with variable enhancement after gadolinium administration.[8,9]

Axillary Breast Tissue

Failure of regression of the embryologic milk streak may lead to formation of ectopic breast tissue, most commonly in the axilla. This often becomes only evident in peripubertal age due to response to hormonal influence. The accessory or ectopic breast tissue presents as a slowly growing mass, tender to palpation.[11]

US findings have been considered nonspecific although US can demonstrate the increased echogenicity of normal breast tissue.[11] On MR imaging, axillary breast tissue appears as an ill-defined subcutaneous mass with signal characteristics similar to the normal orthotopic breast tissue (Fig. 4) and may only differ in the amount of interspersed fat.[11]

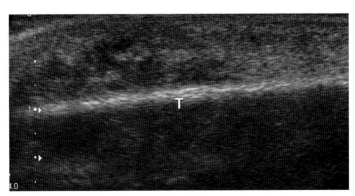

Fig. 2. Subcutaneous granuloma annulare in 3-year-old girl who presented with a rapidly growing, painless mass in the right pretibial region. Longitudinal US image shows an ill-defined hypoechoic area in the subcutaneous tissues that extends superficial to the tibia (T) but without cortical disruption. The adjacent subcutaneous tissues are heterogeneous and hyperechoic. The final diagnosis was made on biopsy.

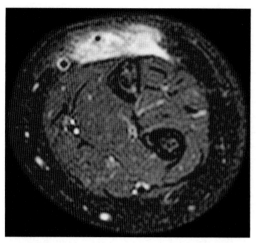

Fig. 3. Subcutaneous granuloma annulare in a 4-year-old girl who presented with a 3-month history of progressively growing nontender mass in the right forearm. Axial fat-suppressed T2-weighted MR image of the right forearm reveals a hyperintense mass with irregular margins in the subcutaneous tissues that abuts the superficial fascial planes but without extending into the underlying muscle planes or bone. The final diagnosis was confirmed on histology.

VASCULAR LESIONS

This category, vascular lesions, represents the most common cause of soft tissue masses in children, encompassing 2 distinct types of lesions: hemangiomas (vascular tumors) and vascular malformations. Although the biology, clinical evolution, and management of each of these lesions can be different, the term, *hemangioma*, is often indiscriminately used to designate almost any type of vascular lesions, including vascular malformations, creating confusion not only to patients and their families but also among physicians, and this may lead to errors in treatment. The use of appropriate nomenclature is imperative to facilitate diagnosis and management of these patients and to improve communication with referring physicians and other specialists.

From an imaging point of view, vascular lesions can also be classified into 2 groups according to the type of flow present within the lesion: high-flow lesions, which include hemangioma, arteriovenous malformation and arteriovenous fistula, and low-flow lesions, which include capillary malformations, venous malformations, and lymphatic malformations.

Hemangiomas

Hemangiomas are neoplastic lesions characterized by hyperplasia of endothelial cells. Several specific entities are now included in the group of hemangiomas, of which the most common in children requiring imaging include hemangioma of infancy, congenital hemangiomas (rapidly involuting and noninvoluting forms), and kaposiform hemangioendothelioma (KH). Tufted angioma and pyogenic granuloma (lobular capillary hemangioma) are also included in the category of hemangiomas; however, these superficial tumors are usually diagnosed clinically and are not referred for imaging. Many lesions diagnosed as "intramuscular hemangiomas" are probably better designated as "venous malformations" (discussed later); however, some investigators think that true intramuscular hemangiomas do occur in older children and adults (see the article "Magnetic Resonance Imaging of Benign Soft Tissue Neoplasms in the Adult" by Walker and colleagues elsewhere in this issue). It is possible that some of these intramuscular hemangiomas represent noninvoluting congenital hemangiomas diagnosed later in life.

Hemangioma of infancy

Hemangioma of infancy or infantile hemangioma is the most common vascular tumor in infants, occurring in up to 5% to 10% of all white infants by 1 year of age, affecting female infants 3 times as often as male infants.[12] Immunohistochemical stains have shown that hemangioma of infancy has a vascular phenotype that resembles placental microvasculature as it is positive for glucose transporter 1 (GLUT1); this is an important diagnostic marker as congenital hemangiomas

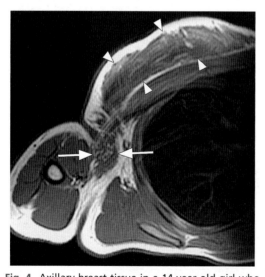

Fig. 4. Axillary breast tissue in a 14-year-old girl who presented with an enlarging axillary mass. Axial T1-weighted MR image shows an irregular mass in the right axilla (*arrows*), which is predominantly isointense to muscle with central hyperintense foci compatible with fatty tissue. The appearance is similar to the orthotopic right breast tissue (*arrowheads*).

and all other vascular tumors as well as the vascular malformations are negative for GLUT1.

Hemangioma of infancy is usually a solitary lesion but can be multiple in up to 15% of cases. It can occur in any area of the body, most frequently in the face and neck (60%) and less frequently in the trunk (25%) and extremities (15%).[12] The superficial lesion has a bright red lobulated appearance (strawberry mark) whereas in a deeper lesion the skin surface may be normal or have a bluish color. Hemangiomas of infancy exhibit a characteristic natural history given by 2 distinct phases: proliferation and involution. In some instances, there may be an inconspicuous precursor lesion noted at or just after birth but the stage of proliferation is often only clinically evident in the first weeks or months of life, in which the lesion shows initial rapid growth. The lesion continues to grow up to approximately 9 to 12 months of life. At approximately 1 year of age, the involution starts to become evident, although at a much slower pace compared with the prolifer-ative phase, proceeding over many years so that 90% of hemangiomas of infancy have reached maximal involution by age 9 years.[12] The lesion may completely disappear or leave a small re-sidue. At histology, the phase of involution is char-acterized by fibrofatty proliferation and the lesion becomes softer and more compressible clinically.

In most cases, the diagnosis of hemangioma of infancy can be made clinically. Imaging is often required, however, in atypical presentations, in deep lesions, and before therapy. US with Doppler interrogation is usually the initial diagnostic mo-dality of choice. Hemangioma of infancy appears on US as a well-defined solid lesion, more often hypoechoic although hyperechoic and occasion-ally heterogeneous appearances have been described (**Fig. 5**).[13] Intralesional vessels and calcifications are not commonly seen on gray-scale US. Color Doppler interrogation typically shows high vessel density, which is defined by the presence of more than 5 vessels per cm^2 in the area of greatest vascularization within the lesion (see **Fig. 5**).[13] Spectral Doppler analysis of the intralesional arteries often reveals a maximum systolic Doppler shift greater than 2 kHz,[13] although some investigators have not corrobo-rated the validity of this latter finding.[14] Dubois and colleagues[13] found that using these 2 Doppler criteria the diagnosis of hemangioma can be made in 84% of such lesions with a specificity of 98%. High vascular density has also been reported in arteriovenous malformation, KH, and congenital hemangiomas; however, there are other gray-scale US and clinical findings that can help in the differentiation of these entities from hemangiomas of infancy (discussed later). As the hemangioma of

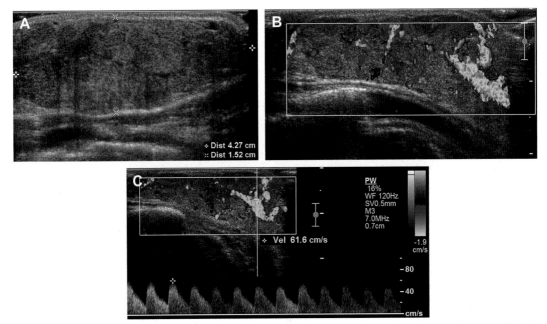

Fig. 5. Hemangioma of infancy in an 11-week-old girl who presented with an enlarging strawberry mark in the left chest wall. (*A*) Transverse US image shows a well-defined, slightly hyperechoic, solid mass confined to the subcutaneous tissues. (*B*) Color Doppler US shows high vascular density of the mass. (*C*) Spectral Doppler analysis reveals arterial flow with relatively high peak systolic velocities. These US features in the appropriate clinical setting are diagnostic of hemangioma of infancy.

infancy enters the phase of involution or undergoes treatment, the intralesional vascularization progressively decreases.[13,14]

The MR imaging appearances of hemangiomas of infancy also depend on their evolutionary phase. Proliferative hemangiomas appear as well-defined, homogeneous, lobulated masses that are isointense to muscle on T1-weighted images and hyperintense on T2-weighted images (**Fig. 6**).[15] The prominent intralesional high-flow vessels, which tend to be more peripheral in distribution, appear as foci of signal void on spin-echo sequences (see **Fig. 6**) and as high–signal intensity foci on gradient-echo sequences. The enhancement after gadolinium administration is usually homogeneous (see **Fig. 6**). As hemangiomas of infancy undergo involution, the lesions become hyperintense on T1-weighted images due to fatty replacement and show less prominent enhancement.

Congenital hemangiomas

Congenital hemangiomas were traditionally considered part of the spectrum of hemangiomas of infancy. In view of their different pathology and postnatal evolution, however, they are now included in a separate category.[16] Two subtypes of congenital hemangiomas are recognized: rapidly involuting congenital hemangioma (RICH) and non-involuting congenital hemangioma (NICH). In contrast to hemangiomas of infancy, congenital hemangiomas have in common a prenatal growth phase, lack of female predominance and negative GLUT1 stain.

RICHs are hemangiomas that are already at their maximum growth at birth and undergo a rapid spontaneous involution that is completed before the age of 14 months.[16] They are more often seen in extremities close to a joint and in the face, although sparing the centrofacial area, and appear at birth as large bulging tumors.

NICHs are also hemangiomas that are already fully grown at birth but that do not exhibit involution. Some NICHs may even show growth that is commensurate with the child mimicking venous malformations clinically. NICHs tend to be smaller than RICHs and often flat, occurring in the head and neck (43%), limbs (38%), and trunk (19%).[17]

Congenital hemangiomas appear more frequently on US as heterogeneous lesions, with visible prominent intralesional vessels on grayscale imaging in contrast to hemangiomas of infancy (**Fig. 7**). Both RICHs and NICHs also exhibit high vascular density on color Doppler interrogation (see **Fig. 7**). Although not a common feature, calcifications are more frequently seen in congenital hemangiomas and only rarely present in hemangiomas of infancy.[16] MR imaging appearances of congenital hemangiomas are similar to hemangiomas of infancy (see **Fig. 7**).

Kaposiform hemangioendothelioma

KH is a type of hemangioma that has a characteristic histology including lymphatic abnormalities, lack of spontaneous involution, and common association with the Kasabach-Merritt phenomenon.[18] Kasabach-Merritt phenomenon is a consumption coagulopathy that is practically only seen with KH and less frequently with the closely related tufted angioma and is characterized by early onset of extremely low blood levels of platelet (<20,000/µL) and fibrinogen, much lower than those documented with coagulopathy associated

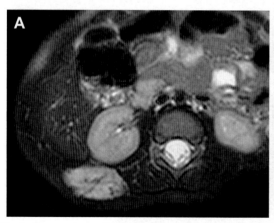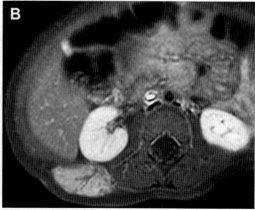

Fig. 6. Hemangioma of infancy in an 11-month-old girl who presented with enlarging mass in the right flank first noticed at 2 weeks of age. (*A*) Axial fat-suppressed T2-weighted MR image shows a well-defined hyperintense mass in the right lumbar region involving the subcutaneous soft tissues and quadratus lumborum muscle and extending into the right perinephric space. Foci of signal void noted within the lesion represent high-flow vessels. (*B*) Axial gadolinium-enhanced fat-suppressed T1-weighted MR image shows avid, diffuse, and relatively homogeneous enhancement of the mass.

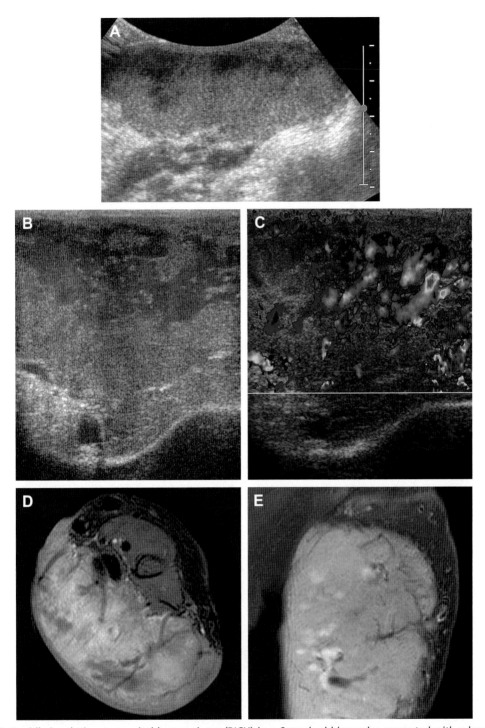

Fig. 7. Rapidly involuting congenital hemangioma (RICH) in a 6-week-old boy who presented with a large left arm mass diagnosed antenatally. (A) Longitudinal US image obtained with curved-array low-frequency transducer shows a well-defined, slightly heterogeneous, mildly hyperechoic mass in the subcutaneous tissues. (B) Longitudinal US image obtained with linear-array high-frequency transducer shows that the heterogeneous appearance is due to distended irregular vascular spaces. (C) Color Doppler US image shows high vascular density of the lesion. (D) Axial fat-suppressed T2-weighted MR image shows an extensive, well-defined hyperintense mass involving and expanding the subcutaneous tissues in the posterior aspect of the left upper arm with prominent intralesional vessels. (E) Coronal gadolinium-enhanced fat-suppressed T1-weighted MR image shows avid and diffuse enhancement of the mass. The clinical evolution with subsequent progressive decrease in size of the mass confirmed the diagnosis.

with large venous malformations or with infantile fibrosarcoma.[12,18]

Most KHs present in the first year of life and not rarely they are congenital, affecting more often an extremity, with variable cutaneous appearance and discoloration that may range from scarlet to purple. They can be aggressive locally with involvement of superficial and deep soft tissues and even adjacent bones.[12]

On US, KHs have poorly defined margins making difficult the differentiation of tumor from normal surrounding soft tissues.[19] The lesion shows variable echogenicity, may contain calcifications, and Doppler interrogation reveals a moderate degree of vascularization, higher than most soft tissue tumors but only rarely to the same degree as hemangiomas of infancy.[19] On MR imaging, KHs are hypointense- or isointense to muscle on T1-weighted images and hyperintense and slightly heterogeneous on T2-weighted and postgadolinium images (**Fig. 8**).[20] The masses are frequently subcutaneous but can also be intramuscular or involve all soft tissue layers. Common findings include presence of signal voids due to prominent vascular channels, cutaneous thickening and subcutaneous stranding as well as hemosiderin deposition (see **Fig. 8**).[20] Biopsy is often required for final diagnosis.

Vascular Malformations

In contrast to hemangiomas, which are neoplastic lesions, vascular malformations are considered errors in vascular development. They occur in approximately 0.3% to 0.5% of the population and have equal gender distribution.[21] Although they are all present at birth, many are not detected until later in life due to slow growth, commensurate with the child's growth. A more rapid growth of these lesions may be caused by trauma, clotting, and hormonal influence at puberty and/or pregnancy.[12]

Arteriovenous malformations

Arteriovenous malformations are high-flow lesions in which there is direct shunting between arteries and veins without intervening arterioles or capillary bed. They are diagnosed at birth in 40% to 60% of cases.[21] Clinically they are divided in 4 stages: (1) dormancy, (2) expansion, (3) destruction, and (4) destruction plus congestive failure. Most lesions during childhood are asymptomatic (stage 1). The progression to stage 2 often occurs in adolescence, in which along with lesion growth, there are skin changes, increase of local temperature, tenderness, thrill, or pulsations. In stage 3, there is skin necrosis, ulceration, or hemorrhage and lytic bone lesions may occur.

On US, similar to hemangiomas of infancy, arteriovenous malformations exhibit high vascular density and high Doppler shift (**Fig. 9**).[13,14] The main differentiating factor is the absence of a solid mass in arteriovenous malformations (see **Fig. 9**). This is also evident on MR imaging, which demonstrates the nidus as a tangle of prominent vessels, with signal void on spin-echo sequences or high

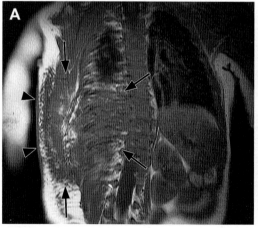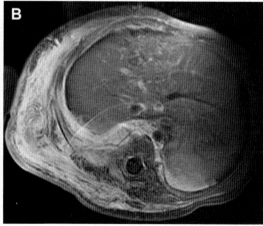

Fig. 8. KH in a 6-month-old boy with 5-month history of enlarging thoracoabdominal wall mass and recent development of Kasabach-Merritt phenomenon. (*A*) Coronal T1-weighted MR image shows a large irregular mass involving the right chest and upper abdominal wall, predominantly isointense to muscle (*arrows*), associated with stranding of the subcutaneous tissues and skin thickening (*arrowheads*). A few signal void foci representing intralesional high flow arteries are also seen. (*B*) Axial gadolinium-enhanced fat-suppressed T1-weighted MR image shows the extensive lesion with avid enhancement and involvement of multiple tissue planes. The combination of imaging findings in association with Kasabach-Merritt phenomenon is compatible with KH.

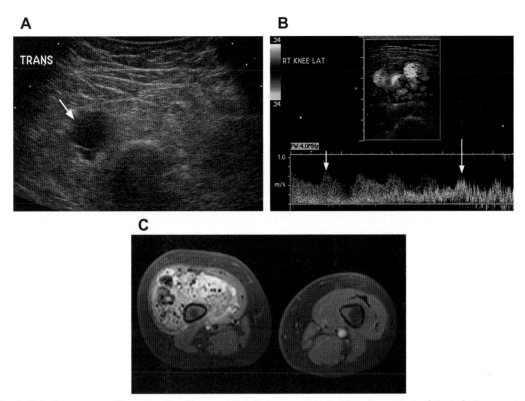

Fig. 9. Arteriovenous malformation in a 7-year-old boy who presented with enlargement of the inferior aspect of the right thigh and audible bruit above the patella. (*A*) Transverse US image of the right thigh shows ill-defined area of increased echogenicity within the quadriceps musculature with at least one rounded hypoechoic structure in the lateral aspect compatible with a large vessel (*arrow*). (*B*) Color Doppler interrogation (*top*) shows the presence of multiple vessels much more than expected from the gray-scale images. Spectral Doppler analysis (*bottom*) reveals prominent arteries, which have a low resistance pattern (*short arrow*) and veins with prominent, turbulent, pulsatile flow (*long arrow*) due to the direct arteriovenous communication. (*C*) Axial gadolinium-enhanced fat-suppressed T1-weighted MR image shows enlargement of the right quadriceps musculature with heterogeneous enhancement due to the increased vascularity in this region; this should not be confused with a solid neoplastic mass. There are multiple signal void foci representing the high flow vessels that are characteristic of this entity.

signal intensity on flow-enhanced gradient-echo sequences due to the high flow (see **Fig. 9**).[15] Perilesional edema with associated increased vascularity, however, is not uncommon and this may appear as an ill-defined area of abnormal signal and enhancement that should not be mistaken for a solid neoplastic mass (see **Fig. 9**).

Venous malformations
Venous malformations are low-flow lesions composed of anomalous ectatic venous channels, which can occur locally or in a segmental distribution, without associated abnormalities or as part of a complex syndrome. Thrombosis of these venous spaces may occur, which may give rise to phleboliths. Although these lesions are designated *cavernous hemangiomas* in some classification systems, the author and most physicians involved in the specialized care of pediatric patients with vascular lesions prefer the term venous malformation to describe these true vascular malformations that are usually present at birth although may not become symptomatic until later in life.

They are found in the head and neck (40%), extremities (40%), and trunk (20%).[1] The superficial variety is often evident at birth appearing as a bluish-colored lesion, soft and compressible on palpation, and increasing in size when the affected area is in a dependent position, with exertion or with crying.[13,21] Deeper lesions are more difficult to diagnose due to lack of cutaneous changes and, therefore, often require imaging.

On US, venous malformations often appear as relatively well-defined sponge-like masses, which are hypoechoic in relation to the adjacent subcutaneous tissue, although isoechoic and hyperechoic appearances have also been described (**Fig. 10**).[14,22] Other appearances include dilated channels

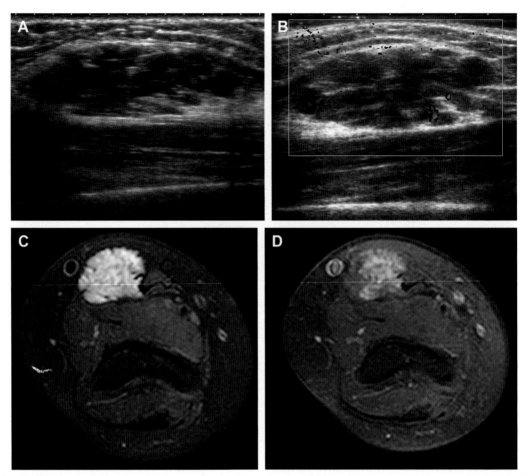

Fig. 10. Venous malformation in a 5-year-old girl who presented with an intermittently tender, soft lump in the right upper arm just proximal to the elbow. (*A*) Longitudinal US image shows the presence of a relatively well-defined mass within the distal aspect of the right biceps muscle, which is partially compressible with the transducer. The mass is hypoechoic and heterogeneous with multiple small irregular anechoic areas giving the appearance of a sponge. (*B*) Color Doppler interrogation reveals little vascularity in the mass. (*C*) Axial fat-suppressed T2-weighted MR image shows a well-demarcated mass within the biceps muscle, which is hyperintense and composed of multiple small locules separated by thin hypointense septa. (*D*) Axial gadolinium-enhanced fat-suppressed T1-weighted MR image shows patchy enhancement of the lesion, which is characteristic of venous malformations.

diffusely involving the subcutaneous tissues and isoechoic thickening of subcutaneous tissues without recognizable channels.[14] The demonstration of phleboliths, appearing as foci of calcification (hyperechoic with posterior shadowing) is helpful and often seals the diagnosis in the appropriate clinical setting (**Fig. 11**). In children, however, phleboliths have been reported to occur only in 9% to 16% of venous malformations.[14,22] Doppler interrogation confirms the low-flow pattern of these lesions, showing low vascular density, mostly venous, and in approximately 16% of cases no flow is detected at all.[22]

On MR imaging, venous malformations may appear as dilated veins or more often as lobulated masses comprised of multiple small locules. They are often hypointense on T1-weighted images and hyperintense on T2-weighted images and may occasionally contain signal voids due to phleboliths or more rarely fluid-fluid levels.[15] After gadolinium administration, there are easily recognizable patchy areas of enhancement (**Fig. 12**).

Lymphatic malformations

Lymphatic malformations are developmental anomalies of the lymphatic system, often referred to as lymphangiomas or cystic hygromas. The localized lymphatic malformations can be classified in 2 groups: microcystic and macrocystic types, although combined microcystic and macrocystic

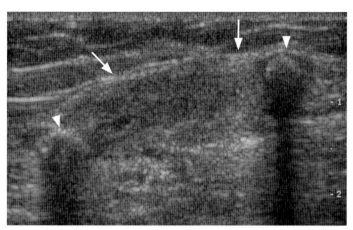

Fig. 11. Venous malformation in an 8-year-old boy who presented with a 3-month history of mass in the right lower thigh. Longitudinal US image shows a deep subcutaneous hypoechoic mass (*arrows*) with two foci of calcifications representing phleboliths (*arrowheads*). The recognition of intralesional calcifications helps to narrow the differential diagnosis. The diagnosis of venous malformation was subsequently confirmed with MR imaging.

lymphatic malformations are common. Lymphatic malformations involve the head and neck in 48% of cases and the trunk and extremities in 42% and can be visceral or internal in location in 10%.[12]

Microcystic lymphatic malformations consist of multiple microscopic cavities and clinically often present as grouped clear or sometimes hemorrhagic vesicles anywhere on the body surface, of variable size, often with a deep component. On US, there are small cysts that measure less than 1 cm or often, due to their small size, the cystic spaces per se are not seen, but the multiple interfaces caused by these tiny cysts result in an ill-defined area of thickening and increased echogenicity (**Fig. 13**).[22] On MR imaging, the microcystic lymphatic malformations have a nonspecific appearance of diffuse areas of low signal intensity on T1-weighted images and high signal intensity on T2-weighted images, with no evident or mild diffuse enhancement after gadolinium administration due to enhancement of the septa that separate the microcysts (**Fig. 14**).[15]

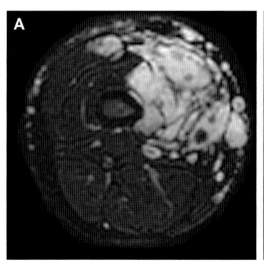
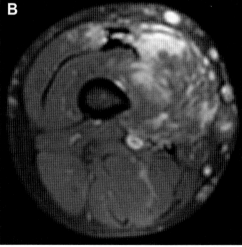

Fig. 12. Venous malformation in a 17-year-old boy. (*A*) Axial fat-suppressed T2-weighted MR image shows a large, irregular hyperintense mass partially involving the musculature and subcutaneous planes in the anteromedial aspect of the right thigh. The mass is composed of multiple locules of varying size representing dilated venous spaces separated by hypointense septa. Some of the intralesional hypointense nodular foci represent phleboliths. There are also dilated superficial veins. (*B*) Axial gadolinium-enhanced fat-suppressed T1-weighted MR image shows patchy enhancement of the lesion, which is characteristic of venous malformations.

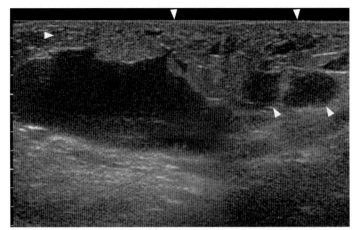

Fig. 13. Combined microcystic and macrocystic lymphatic malformation of the left arm in an 8-month-old boy. Longitudinal US image shows a macrocyst of irregular shape superiorly, whereas anteriorly and inferiorly there is echogenic tissue with small cystic areas (*arrowheads*) representing the microcystic component of the lymphatic malformation.

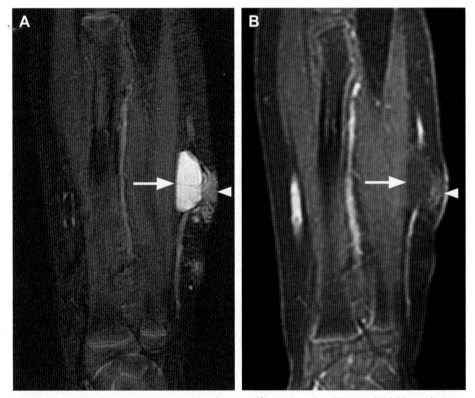

Fig. 14. Combined microcystic and macrocystic lymphatic malformations in a 23-month-old boy who was noted to have two soft tissue lumps in the left forearm at birth, which have grown commensurately with the child. (*A*) Coronal STIR image shows two subcutaneous lesions. The more proximal larger lesion has 2 components: a more superficial slightly hyperintense irregular area (*arrowhead*), which corresponds to the microcystic component, and a deeper hyperintense septated cystic area (*arrow*), which corresponds to the macrocystic component. The smaller distal lesion represents a second microcystic lymphatic malformation. (*B*) Coronal gadolinium-enhanced fat-suppressed T1-weighted MR image shows lack of enhancement of the macrocystic component (*arrow*) with faint enhancement of the microcystic component of the lymphatic malformation (*arrowhead*).

Macrocystic lymphatic malformations often present clinically as cool, soft, smooth, translucent masses without abnormality or with bluish discoloration of the overlying skin.[14] They are often diagnosed before the age of 2 years, although they may present later as a mass of sudden appearance due to superimposed hemorrhage or infection. On US, macrocystic lymphatic malformations appear as large, anechoic cavities, separated by septa (see **Fig. 13**).[22] No flow is demonstrated within the lesion except for the septa that may have arterial and/or venous flow on Doppler interrogation.[14,22] The cysts may contain echoes or fluid-debris levels if complicated by infection or hemorrhage or due to the presence of proteinaceous material. On MR imaging, the lesions appear as well-defined cysts separated by thin septa. The cysts are often of low signal intensity on T1-weighted images and markedly hyperintense on T2-weighted images (see **Fig. 14**; **Fig. 15**).[15] Occasionally, however, the content of the cysts is hyperintense on T1-weighted images due to hemorrhage. After gadolinium administration, there is septal enhancement but no enhancement of the cystic spaces allowing differentiation from venous malformations.

Capillary malformations

Capillary malformations are the most common vascular malformations occurring in approximately 3 of 1000 infants. These include lesions often known as port-wine stains (nevus flameus) and telangiectases. With a variable cutaneous appearance, they are usually diagnosed at birth and may present on any surface of the skin but are more commonly encountered in the head and neck.[21]

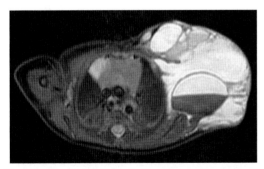

Fig. 15. Macrocystic lymphatic malformation in a 5-day-old boy who presented with a large left chest wall mass diagnosed antenatally. Axial fat-suppressed T2-weighted MR image shows a large macrocystic lymphatic malformation involving the left chest wall and left upper arm. The mass is multiloculated with mostly hyperintense fluid-filled spaces. A fluid-fluid level is noted in one of the largest cysts with low signal intensity of the dependent fluid due to blood products.

The diagnosis is often made clinically without the need of imaging. They may occasionally, however, be associated with congenital hypertrophy of underlying soft tissues and bones, or other vascular or ectodermal anomalies (Sturge-Weber, Klippel-Trénaunay, and Proteus syndromes), for which imaging may be required. The capillary malformations themselves are often not apparent on imaging or sometimes may just show thickening of skin and subcutaneous tissues.[14,15]

Complex Combined Vascular Malformations and Vascular Malformation Syndromes

There is an extensive list of conditions presenting with complex combined vascular malformations and syndromes associated with vascular malformations. This article does not intend to review these entities in detail and for that purpose readers are referred to the excellent review by Lobo-Mueller and colleagues.[23] It is important to emphasize that in these conditions, MR imaging plays a major role because there are often changes in the adjacent soft tissues and skeleton. Of those complex combined vascular malformations and syndromes associated with vascular malformations affecting the extremities most commonly seen in the pediatric age, only 2 include high-flow lesions: Parkes Weber syndrome and Bannayan-Riley-Ruvalcaba syndrome. All the others include exclusively low-flow lesions.

In Parkes Weber syndrome there is usually involvement of an entire limb with hypertrophy of the soft tissues and bone overgrowth. There are arteriovenous fistulas, which cause a red vascular stain of the overlying skin (high-flow pseudocapillary malformation) and dilated cutaneous veins.[23] There may be localized or diffuse lymphedema. In most patients the diagnosis is made clinically.

Bannayan-Riley-Ruvalcaba syndrome includes among its predominant clinical features the presence of capillary or combined vascular malformations.[23] Vascular anomalies most commonly found are high-flow malformations with some degree of arteriovenous shunting. Patients with this syndrome may also present with low flow vascular malformations (capillary, venous, and lymphatic).

Klippel-Trénaunay syndrome is characterized by the clinical triad of capillary malformation of the skin (port-wine stain), venous malformations/varicosities, and hypertrophy of soft tissues/bone.[12,23] It usually affects the lower extremities, more often unilateral, although involvement of both lower extremities is not rare. The most common venous anomaly is the presence in more than half of cases of a persistent embryonic vein known as the lateral marginal vein or vein of

Servelle. There may also be subcutaneous varicosities, intramuscular and intra-articular venous malformations, and an absent or hypoplastic deep venous system. Also common are lymphedema and localized macrocystic and microcystic lymphatic malformations.

Proteus syndrome is another overgrowth disorder that commonly involves bone, connective tissue, and the subcutaneous fat.[23] Some type of vascular anomaly is always present, including capillary malformations, macrocystic lymphatic malformations, varicosities, and complex combined vascular malformations, as in Klippel-Trénaunay syndrome but not as extensive. No high-flow vascular malformation is seen.

Maffucci syndrome is characterized by dyschondroplasia of one or more limbs, multiple enchondromas, and soft tissue venous malformations, the latter coexisting with a reactive vascular tumor, the spindle cell hemangioendothelioma (not to be confused with KH).

Blue rubber bleb nevus syndrome is characterized by the presence of multiple venous malformations anywhere on the skin surface and in the gastrointestinal tract. The cutaneous lesions range in size from 1 mm to 2 mm to several centimeters.

ADIPOCYTIC TUMORS

In contrast to adults, adipocytic tumors are rare in children, representing only 6% of all soft tissue neoplasms in the first 2 decades of life.[24] In addition, in the pediatric age, there are other tumors that may contain fat that are not adipocytic in origin and should be considered in the differential diagnosis according to the clinical context. These include fibroblastic/myofibroblastic tumors, such as fibrous hamartoma of infancy and lipofibromatosis (discussed later), and vascular tumors, in particular hemangioma of infancy during the phase of involution (discussed previously).

Lipoma

Lipomas represent approximately two-thirds of all adipocytic tumors in children.[24] The clinical and MR imaging features do not differ from those seen in adults; therefore, they are discussed in the article "Magnetic Resonance Imaging of Benign Soft Tissue Neoplasms in the Adult" by Walker and colleagues elsewhere in this issue.

Lipoblastoma

Lipoblastoma represents approximately 30% of adipocytic tumors in children, typically diagnosed under the age of 3 years, and only rarely seen over the age of 8 years.[1,24,25] It is a benign tumor composed of an admixture of mature adipocytes and lipoblasts in different stages of development, accompanied by varying degrees of myxoid stromal tissue.[4,25] Two forms are recognized: lipoblastoma proper, which refers to the more common superficial encapsulated lesion, and lipoblastomatosis, which designates a diffuse, nonencapsulated and infiltrative variant more often seen in the deeper adipose tissue with extension into the adjacent muscle planes. Clinically, lipoblastoma presents as a progressively enlarging, nontender mass in the trunk or extremities, often with a more rapid growth pattern compared with lipoma.

On US, lipoblastomas more often appear as homogeneous, hyperechoic masses, although isoechoic and hypoechoic lesions in comparison with muscle as well as lesions of mixed echogenicity or containing small cystic areas have also been described (**Fig. 16**).[25] On MR imaging, the features reflect the relative amounts of mature fat versus lipoblasts and myxoid tissue present within the lesion. Those lipoblastomas composed mainly of mature fat appear predominantly hyperintense on T1-weighted images and hypointense on fat-suppressed sequences. With larger amounts of lipoblasts and myxoid tissue, the mass becomes more heterogeneous, with areas that are hypointense on T1-weighted images and hyperintense on fat-suppressed T2-weighted images and that also may show enhancement after gadolinium administration (**Fig. 17**). The imaging appearance does not allow differentiation from liposarcoma and histology is required for final diagnosis.

Liposarcoma

The most important information about liposarcoma in children is that these are rare tumors and

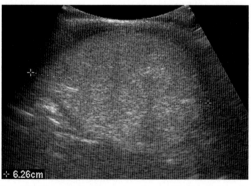

Fig. 16. Lipoblastoma in a 9-month-old boy who presented with an enlarging mass in the left flank. Longitudinal US image shows a large, relatively homogenous, solid, hyperechoic mass involving the left paraspinal muscles. The pattern of echogenicity is suggestive although not specific of a fatty mass.

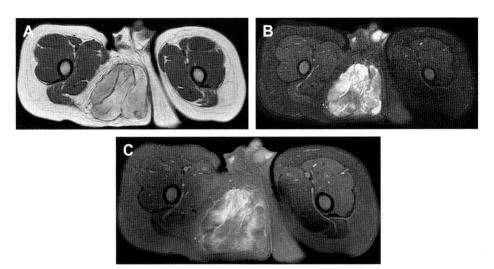

Fig. 17. Lipoblastoma in a 2-year-old boy who presented with a 9-month history of enlarging mass in the right buttock. (*A*) Axial T1-weighted image shows a relatively well-defined mass in the right perineal region that is slightly heterogeneous and predominantly hyperintense, suggestive of fat, although large areas show less signal intensity compared with the subcutaneous fat. (*B*) Axial fat-suppressed T2-weighted MR image shows heterogeneous signal intensity of the mass with both hyperintense and hypointense areas, not characteristic for mature adipocytic tissue. (*C*) Axial gadolinium-enhanced fat-suppressed T1-weighted MR image shows heterogeneous enhancement of the lesion. Although the imaging appearances are compatible with liposarcoma, at this patient's age the most likely diagnosis is lipoblastoma as was confirmed on histology.

most are diagnosed in children older than 10 years of age.[24] The most common liposarcoma in this age group is the myxoid type. The clinical and imaging features of liposarcoma are discussed in the article "Magnetic Resonance Imaging of Malignant Soft Tissue Tumors in the Adult" by Walker and colleagues elsewhere in this issue.

FIBROBLASTIC/MYOFIBROBLASTIC TUMORS

The category, fibroblastic/myofibroblastic tumors, frequent in children, includes a large variety of tumors, most of which have in common the presence of both fibroblastic and myofibroblastic cells. The most common or significant seen in the pediatric age are discussed, with exception of some tumors that are also seen in adults, such as deep fibromatosis, which are discussed in the article "Magnetic Resonance Imaging of Benign Soft Tissue Neoplasms in the Adult" by Walker and colleagues elsewhere in this issue.

Nodular Fasciitis

Nodular fasciitis is a benign fibrous proliferation usually subcutaneous in distribution but sometimes also seen in intramuscular and intermuscular locations. It is more commonly seen in the third or fourth decades, but it has also been described in children, and the cranial form is almost exclusive to children under the age of 2 years.[1] The clinical

and imaging features are described in the article "Magnetic Resonance Imaging of Benign Soft Tissue Neoplasms in the Adult" by Walker and colleagues elsewhere in this issue.

Fibrous Hamartoma of Infancy

Fibrous hamartoma of infancy is an uncommon, usually solitary, benign superficial tumor, most frequently diagnosed in the first 2 years of life with approximately 25% of cases congenital. It is composed of a mixture of well-defined intersecting trabeculae of dense fibrous tissue, primitive mesenchymal cells in a mucoid matrix, and mature fat.[26] It is usually painless, measures less than 5 cm in size, and, although it can arise anywhere in the body, the most common locations are the shoulder girdle, axilla, and upper arm.[26,27]

On US, fibrous hamartoma of infancy has been described as a predominantly hyperechoic subcutaneous mass with a hypoechoic peripheral component and, in the author's experience, also showing hypoechoic internal strands (**Fig. 18**).[27] MR imaging reveals a subcutaneous mass comprised of tightly packed strands of intermediate to low signal intensity on both T1-weighted and T2-weighted images similar to muscle that correspond with the trabeculae of fibrous tissue seen at histology. In-between the strands there is fatty tissue of high signal intensity on T1-weighted images and low signal intensity on fat-suppressed

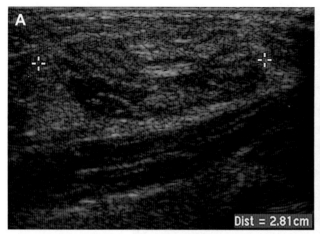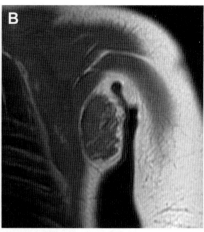

Dist = 2.81 cm

Fig. 18. Fibrous hamartoma of infancy in an 8-month-old boy who presented with a 2-month history of rapidly growing left axillary mass. (*A*) Transverse US image shows a relatively well-defined subcutaneous mass with areas of similar echogenicity to the adjacent subcutaneous fat separated by hypoechoic strands resulting in a multilobulated appearance. (*B*) Coronal T1-weighted MR image shows a well-defined subcutaneous mass that is predominantly isointense to muscle due to fibrous tissue but also containing bands of hyperintense tissue representing fat. This organized pattern of fibrous and adipocytic tissue in a mass is suggestive of fibrous hamartoma of infancy.

images, which blends imperceptibly with the subcutaneous fat.[26]

Myofibroma/Myofibromatosis

Myofibromas/myofibromatosis are common benign tumors that can present as a solitary mass (myofibroma) or as multicentric masses (myofibromatosis). At histology, myofibromas appear as nodules formed by 2 components: one component of plump myofibroblasts arranged in short fascicles or whorls, usually peripheral, and the other component, often central in distribution, of less-differentiated cells usually arranged around hemangiopericytoma-like vessels.[4] It is now thought that the infantile hemangiopericytoma is part of the spectrum of myofibromas, in which the hemangiopericytomatous component predominates over the myofibroblastic component.[4]

Approximately half of the solitary myofibromas are cutaneous/subcutaneous, with most of the other half found in skeletal muscle or aponeurosis, and a minority involving bone, especially the skull.[4] The multicentric myofibromatosis involves both soft tissue and bone and in approximately 15% to 20% of cases there is involvement of deep soft tissues and viscera.[4] Myofibromatosis with visceral involvement has a poor prognosis with mortality rates up to 75%.[28]

Myofibromas can be seen at any age but it has been reported that approximately 88% of cases occur in children under the age of 2 years and approximately 60% are diagnosed at birth.[1,28]

Tumor size is variable, up to 8 cm,[29] and when superficial they appear clinically as a firm, reddish-purple nodule in the skin.[28] The nodules may increase in size and number until approximately 1 year of age. This is followed by a slow spontaneous regression that may take a few years.

On US, the appearances are variable but myofibromas often manifest as well demarcated nodules with an anechoic center and a thick hypoechoic wall (target sign), likely due to central necrosis.[28,29] Others may appear as solid hypoechoic nodules with or without central calcification[10,19,28] (**Fig. 19**) or as isoechoic nodules.[19] They are poorly vascularized on color Doppler interrogation.[13,19] On MR imaging, myofibromas appear hypointense on T1-weighted images and often hyperintense on T2-weighted images, although in some cases with a hypointense center that may reflect calcification (see **Fig. 19**).[28] The enhancement pattern of the lesion after gadolinium administration can be either diffuse or limited to the periphery (target sign) due to central necrosis.[28,29]

Lipofibromatosis

Lipofibromatosis is a rare fibrofatty tumor only recently recognized as a separate entity that often presents as an ill-defined mass involving the subcutaneous or deep soft tissues.[30] It occurs exclusively in the pediatric age, from 11 days to 12 years with a median age of 1 year.[30] The tumor is composed of abundant adipose tissue traversed by bundles of fibroblast-like cells. It can present in

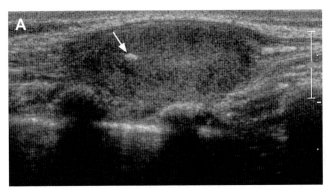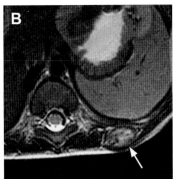

Fig. 19. Myofibroma in a 4-month-old boy who presented with a firm nodule on the back since birth, not growing. (A) Longitudinal US image shows a well-defined intramuscular mass that is predominantly hypoechoic although with a slightly more echogenic center and a small well-defined hyperechoic focus compatible with calcification (arrow). (B) Axial T2-weighted image shows a well-defined slightly heterogeneous nodule (arrow), which is predominantly hyperintense but with hypointense foci due in part to calcifications. The final diagnosis was made at histology.

the extremities, trunk, face, and neck but has a predilection for the hands and feet.[30] Most lipofibromatoses are usually slow growing, nontender lesions, ranging in size from 1 cm to 12 cm.[30,31]

Based on few case reports available in the literature, lipofibromatosis appears on US as a somewhat heterogeneous, predominantly hyperechoic mass with a small amount of internal flow on color Doppler interrogation (**Fig. 20**).[32] On MR imaging, the features reflect the presence of intralesional fat, appearing hyperintense on T1-weighted images and hypointense on fat-suppressed sequences (**Fig. 21**). Within the intralesional fat, there are hypointense strands due to interspersed muscle and fibrous bands.[33] There may be some enhancement of the fibrous component after gadolinium administration (see **Fig. 21**).[33]

Infantile Fibrosarcoma

Also known as congenital fibrosarcoma, the infantile fibrosarcoma represents 13% of the fibroblastic/myofibroblastic tumors in children and 12% of soft tissue malignancies in infants.[4] It is the most common soft tissue sarcoma in children under 1 year of age and approximately one-third of cases are congenital.[34] This should be differentiated from the adult fibrosarcoma, which can also be seen in children but most commonly between the ages of 10 and 15 years. These two tumors are identical on histology and the differentiation should be made on the basis of the patient's age, clinical characteristics, and cytogenetic analysis.[35] This differentiation is important due to the relatively worse prognosis of the adult fibrosarcoma (survival rate

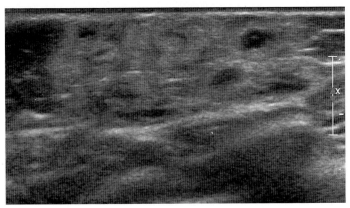

Fig. 20. Lipofibromatosis in a 9-month-old boy who presented with a 3-month history of slowly growing mass in the left lateral chest wall. Longitudinal US image shows a predominantly hyperechoic mass due to mature adipose tissue with scattered hypoechoic nodules and strands due to fascicles of fibrous tissue.

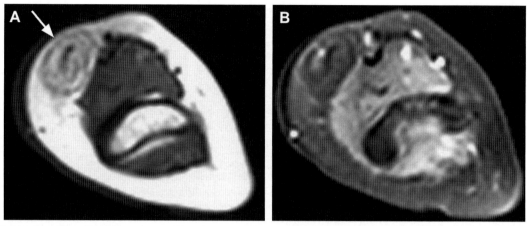

Fig. 21. Lipofibromatosis in a 4-year-old girl who presented with a slowly growing mass in the distal right upper arm since age 6 months. (*A*) Axial T1-weighted image reveals a heterogeneous subcutaneous mass (*arrow*) that has a hyperintense component suggestive of adipose tissue and also hypointense curved bands due to fibrous tissue. The mass is abutting the superficial fascial planes but there is no extension into the underlying muscles. (*B*) Axial gadolinium-enhanced fat-suppressed T1-weighted MR image shows minimal enhancement limited to the anterior aspect of the mass. The diagnosis was confirmed at histology.

(<60%) in comparison with the infantile type (survival rate >80%). The adult fibrosarcoma is discussed in the article "Magnetic Resonance Imaging of Malignant Soft Tissue Tumors in the Adult" by Walker and colleagues elsewhere in this issue.

Infantile fibrosarcoma often presents as a painless, large-size (up to 30 cm), dome-shaped mass, initially with rapid growth, most commonly in the extremities but also seen in the head and neck and in the trunk. It may involve adjacent bone causing erosions. The skin overlying the mass may appear red, tense, and ulcerated and with ectatic superficial veins. Furthermore, it may be associated with disseminated intravascular coagulopathy that may be confused with Kasabach-Merritt phenomenon. Therefore, infantile fibrosarcoma may be misinterpreted as a vascular tumor (hemangioma of infancy, congenital hemangioma, KH, or tufted angioma), leading to a delay in diagnosis and appropriate treatment.[35–37]

There is limited information or illustrations of the US appearance of infantile fibrosarcoma in the literature. The tumors have been described as iso-echoic to muscle,[29] predominantly solid,[38] or solid with an eccentric cystic area due to hemorrhage (**Fig. 22**).[36] There are at least two documented

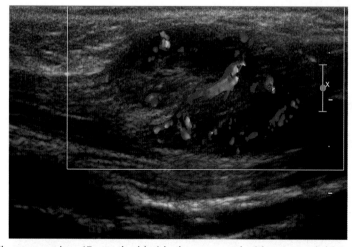

Fig. 22. Infantile fibrosarcoma in a 17-month-old girl who presented with a 4-month history of nontender left cervical mass. Longitudinal color Doppler US image shows a heterogeneous mass with high vascular density expanding the left sternocleidomastoid muscle. Although the appearance may be compatible with fibromatosis colli, the age of presentation is not typical and therefore other neoplastic etiologies must be considered.

cases that have shown increased vascularity on color Doppler interrogation, although there is no information on the degree of vascular density compared with that seen in hemangiomas of infancy.[36,38] On MR imaging, the masses appear isointense to muscle on T1-weighted images and hyperintense on T2-weighted images.[29,34,38] The lesions may appear homogeneous, heterogeneous or with a multiseptated appearance, and after gadolinium administration there is heterogeneous enhancement (**Fig. 23**).[34]

Fibromatosis Colli

Fibromatosis colli is a benign scar-like fibroblastic proliferation specific to the sternocleidomastoid muscle that is thought to be reactive to muscle injury occurring in the last trimester of pregnancy or during delivery.[4] It presents as a firm, rubbery neck mass in a neonate or young infant, more often between 2 and 8 weeks of age, causing torticollis in 14% to 30% of cases.[33] It is usually unilateral and more commonly affects the right side. The mass usually resolves spontaneously or with the aid of physiotherapy.

US is the modality of choice for diagnosis and rarely further imaging or biopsy are needed. On US, fibromatosis colli appears as focal or diffuse enlargement of the sternocleidomastoid muscle, usually fusiform, and predominantly affecting the lower two-thirds of the muscle (**Fig. 24**).[39] The area of abnormality can be hypoechoic, isoechoic, or hyperechoic compared with normal muscle and can be homogenous or heterogeneous.[39] Color Doppler imaging shows increased vascularity either diffuse or focal. MR imaging confirms the fusiform enlargement of the sternocleidomastoid muscle with variable but predominantly increased signal on T2-weighted images.[33,39]

RHABDOMYOSARCOMA

Rhabdomyosarcoma is the most common soft tissue sarcoma in the pediatric age, representing approximately two-thirds of all sarcomas in children and 7% to 8% of all pediatric malignant solid tumors.[40] Although rhabdomyosarcoma is thought to arise from mesenchymal cells committed to skeletal muscle differentiation, it can occur in many different organs, even in those that lack striated muscle.[40] In children, 2 major categories are recognized: embryonal and alveolar. The embryonal is the most common subtype although it is more frequently found in the head and neck and in the genitourinary tract, presenting in the extremities in less than 9% of cases.[4] The alveolar rhabdomyosarcoma is the most common subtype that presents as a soft tissue mass in the extremities. The embryonal subtype is most commonly seen in children less than 5 years of age whereas the alveolar type may present at any age throughout childhood. The alveolar rhabdomyosarcoma subtype has a poorer prognosis than the embryonal subtype, and location in extremities or trunk is considered an unfavorable anatomic site.

Although most cases of rhabdomyosarcoma are sporadic, they occur with a higher frequency in certain predisposing conditions, including neurofibromatosis type 1, Beckwith-Wiedemann syndrome, and Li-Fraumeni syndrome.[2] Clinically, they present as a nontender mass, sometimes quite small but that may be associated with metastatic lymphadenopathy.[40]

On US, rhabdomyosarcoma has been described as a well-defined, slightly hypoechoic heterogeneous mass (**Fig. 25**) that can show significantly increased vascularity on color Doppler

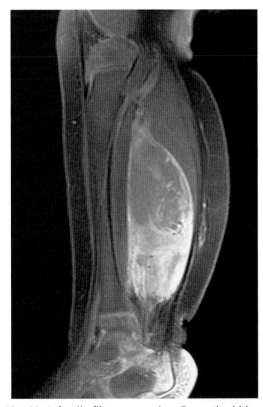

Fig. 23. Infantile fibrosarcoma in a 7-month-old boy who presented with a nontender mass in the right lower leg. Sagittal gadolinium-enhanced fat-suppressed T1-weighted MR image shows a well-defined heterogeneous mass involving the musculature in the right calf. The mass shows enhancing areas as well as areas that do not enhance due to cystic degeneration and necrosis. The diagnosis was confirmed at histology.

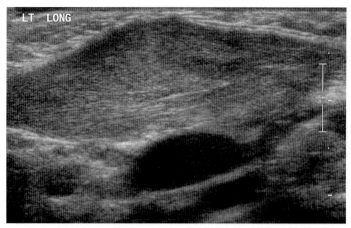

Fig. 24. Fibromatosis colli in a 4-week-old girl who presented with a 1-week history of enlarging left cervical mass. There was history of vaginal delivery that required the use of forceps. Longitudinal US image shows fusiform enlargement of the left sternocleidomastoid muscle with loss of the normal fibrillar pattern centrally and anteriorly. In the appropriate clinical setting, particularly in a patient of this age, this US appearance is diagnostic of fibromatosis colli.

interrogation[41] although cases with low vascular density have also been documented.[14] On MR imaging, rhabdomyosarcomas may appear isointense or slightly hyperintense to muscle on T1-weighted images, of intermediate to high signal intensity on T2-weighted images, and with strong enhancement after administration of gadolinium (see **Fig. 25**).[3,41] Occasionally, they may have

a predominantly cystic appearance.[41] The final diagnosis requires biopsy.

TUMORS OF UNCERTAIN DIFFERENTIATION
Angiomatoid Fibrous Histiocytoma

Angiomatoid fibrous histiocytoma used to be considered a subtype of malignant fibrous histiocytoma.

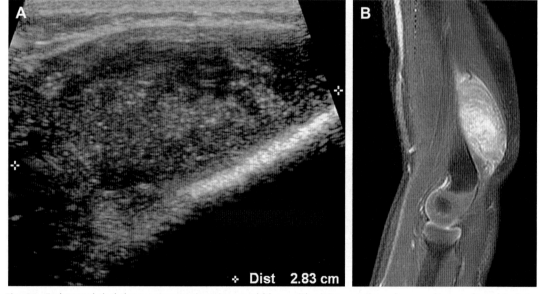

Fig. 25. Embryonal rhabdomyosarcoma in a 3-year-old boy with Li-Fraumeni syndrome who was found to have a mass in the right arm during routine medical check-up. (*A*) Longitudinal US image shows a solid mass of mixed echogenicity within the triceps muscle. (*B*) Sagittal gadolinium-enhanced fat-suppressed T1-weighted MR image shows a well-defined heterogeneous mass involving the triceps muscle. The imaging appearances are nonspecific and the final diagnosis was made at histology.

In view of its distinct morphology and clinical features (earlier age of presentation, more superficial location, and lower metastatic potential and better prognosis), however, it is now considered a different entity.[42] The precise cellular line of differentiation of this tumor remains unknown. At histology there are 4 key diagnostic features that tend to show some correlation with the imaging findings: (1) multinodular cellular proliferation, (2) pseudoangiomatoid spaces, (3) thick fibrous pseudocapsule, and (4) pericapsular lymphoplasmacytic infiltrate.[4]

Angiomatoid fibrous histiocytoma can occur throughout childhood, even at birth.[4] It usually presents as a slow-growing, nontender subcutaneous mass, most frequently in one extremity, although they have also been described in the trunk, head, and neck.[42] Associated systemic symptoms can also be noted, including anemia, weight loss, and fever. It may recur locally after excision in 11% to 16% of cases but distant metastasis are uncommon, occurring in approximately 1% to 5% of cases, accounting for its categorization as an intermediate-grade tumor.[42]

There are no descriptions of the US appearance of angiomatoid fibrous histiocytoma. In the author's experience they may present as heterogeneous hypoechoic masses with posterior acoustic enhancement or as complex, predominantly cystic masses, composed of compartments filled with echogenic fluid or fluid-debris levels that represent the blood-filled pseudoangiomatoid spaces. Doppler interrogation reveals peripheral vascularity. MR imaging shows a well-defined mass that is predominantly hypointense or isointense to muscle on T1-weighted images and predominantly hyperintense on T2-weighted images, although often heterogeneous due to intralesional cystic spaces with hemorrhage and fluid-fluid levels (**Fig. 26**).[42] The recognition of these fluid-fluid levels is useful for narrowing the differential

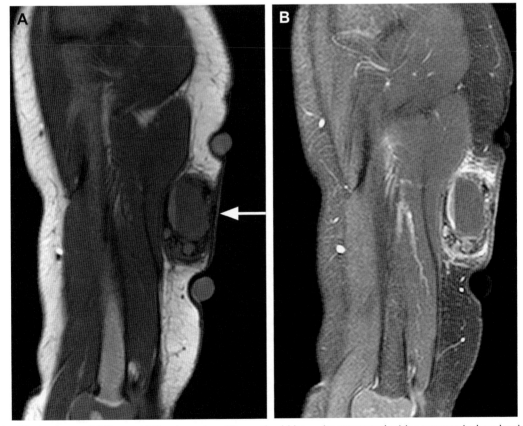

Fig. 26. Angiomatoid fibrous histiocytoma in a 15-month-old boy who presented with a progressively enlarging mass in the left arm. (*A*) Sagittal T1-weighted MR image shows a well demarcated, multiloculated, subcutaneous mass. There is a fluid-fluid level in the larger cystic component with dependent hyperintense fluid due to blood products (*arrow*). (*B*) Sagittal gadolinium-enhanced fat-suppressed T1-weighted MR image reveals peripheral enhancement. Note the presence of low signal areas in the periphery of the lesion due to hemosiderin deposition. The identification of fluid-fluid levels is helpful in narrowing the differential diagnosis. Final diagnosis was made at histology.

diagnosis, although fluid-fluid levels can also be noted in other soft tissue masses in children, particularly in lymphatic and venous malformations but also in synovial sarcoma.[43] The pseudocapsule appears as a hypointense rim on both T1-weighted and T2-weighted images. After gadolinium administration there is marked enhancement of the solid components and of the pseudocapsule.[42]

Synovial Sarcoma

Synovial sarcoma is the second most common soft tissue sarcoma in children after rhabdomyosarcoma.[43] Although it has been reported in a child as young as 2 years of age, in children, it is more frequently seen in the second decade. It is not uncommon in adults and for that reason the clinical and imaging features are discussed in the article "Magnetic Resonance Imaging of Malignant Soft Tissue Tumors in the Adult" by Walker and colleagues elsewhere in this issue.

Ewing Sarcoma/Primitive Neuroectodermal Tumor

Ewing sarcoma and primitive neuroectodermal tumor are round cell sarcomas that have the same molecular genetic abnormality and share immunophenotypic similarities, indicating that they are tumors at different stages in the same line of neuroectodermal tumor differentiation.[44] This is more commonly a skeletal tumor, with extraskeletal presentations being rare although well documented in the paravertebral regions, thoracic wall (formerly known as Askin tumor), retroperitoneum, lower extremities, and other parts of the body.[45,46] Patients present with a soft tissue mass, which may be painful.[45]

On US, extraskeletal Ewing sarcoma/primitive neuroectodermal tumor has been reported to present as a well-circumscribed mass, predominantly hypoechoic, but also with anechoic components and a mixed echogenicity pattern.[45] MR imaging also reveals a well-defined mass of intermediate signal intensity (isointense or hyperintense to muscle) on T1-weighted images, heterogeneous hyperintensity on T2-weighted images, and with variable enhancement after gadolinium administration **(Fig. 27)**.[44,47]

PILOMATRICOMA

Pilomatricoma, also known by the old term, calcifying epithelioma of Malherbe, or by the etymologically incorrect, pilomatrixoma, is a benign subcutaneous tumor that arises from the hair cortex cells. Although this entity is not known by many radiologists, it represents the third most commonly

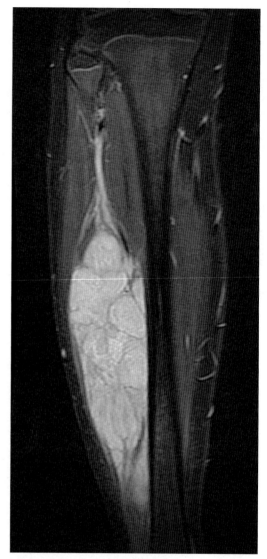

Fig. 27. Primitive neuroectodermal tumor in a 13-year-old boy who presented with a 6-month history of progressively growing mass in the right lower leg that had become painful over the last month. Coronal STIR MR image shows a large, well-defined, hyperintense, intramuscular mass composed of multiple lobules separated by thin hypointense septa. There was no involvement of the adjacent bones. Final diagnosis was made at histology.

resected superficial tumor in children after dermoid/epidermoid cysts and lymph nodes.[48,49]

Pilomatricomas can occur practically at any age but are more common in children and adolescents. They can appear in any area of hair-bearing skin and are most frequently seen in the head (particularly the periauricular region), neck, and upper extremity.[48,49] Most of them grow slowly over months or years and tend to be small in size, on

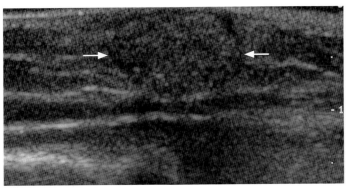

Fig. 28. Pilomatricoma in a 12-year-old girl who presented with a firm, nontender lump in the distal aspect of the right upper arm. Longitudinal US image shows a well-defined subcutaneous nodule with heterogeneous echogenicity and a hypoechoic rim (*arrows*). Within the nodule there are scattered hyperechoic punctate foci that represent small calcifications. There is subtle perilesional increased echogenicity reflecting chronic inflammation due to foreign body reaction. The US appearance is highly suggestive of pilomatricoma, which was confirmed at histology.

average less than 2 cm in diameter, although lesions as big as 18 cm have been reported.[48] They present as a nontender, freely movable, hard nodule of irregular surface, sometimes with bluish discoloration of the overlying skin.

On US, most pilomatricomas have a characteristic appearance allowing a correct preoperative diagnosis in 76% of cases.[48] The lesion presents as a well-defined hyperechoic or isoechoic nodule with a hypoechoic rim and variable number of internal hyperechoic punctate foci due to calcification (**Fig. 28**). In some instances the nodule is markedly hyperechoic with posterior shadowing due to extensive calcification.[48] Color Doppler interrogation reveals the presence of some flow, mainly peripheral (70% of cases) or peripheral and central (10%) in distribution.[48] Rarely, there may be intralesional cystic degeneration.[49] In approximately half of the cases, there is slight increased peritumoral echogenicity representing chronic inflammation due to foreign body reaction.[49]

On MR imaging, pilomatricoma appears as a well-demarcated nodule of intermediate signal intensity on T1-weighted images and heterogeneous signal intensity on T2-weighted images. After gadolinium administration, there is peripheral enhancement, which may be associated with an internal patchy and reticulate pattern of enhancement.[49] The peritumoral inflammatory changes due to chronic inflammation are evident in 60% of cases appearing as stranding of the adjacent subcutaneous tissues and dermis.[49]

SUMMARY

Imaging plays a significant role in the evaluation of soft tissue masses in children. US is in most instances the primary imaging modality and is particularly useful in the diagnosis of vascular lesions, the most common cause of a pediatric soft tissue mass. US also aids in the diagnosis of fibromatosis colli, some pseudotumors, periarticular cysts, and pilomatricoma. MR imaging is also useful, especially in larger and deeper lesions. The interpretation of imaging findings, however, requires correlation with clinical findings. Histology is still needed in many cases for a final diagnosis.

REFERENCES

1. Navarro OM, Laffan EE, Ngan BY. Pediatric soft tissue tumors and pseudotumors: MR Imaging with pathologic correlation. Part 1. Imaging approach, pseudotumors, vascular lesions and adipocytic tumors. Radiographics 2009;29:887–906.

2. Brisse H, Orbach D, Klijanienko J, et al. Imaging and diagnostic strategy of soft tissue tumors in children. Eur Radiol 2006;16:1147–64.

3. Stein-Wexler R. MR imaging of soft tissue masses in children. Magn Reson Imaging Clin N Am 2009;17: 489–507.

4. Fletcher CD, Unni KK, Mertens F, editors. World Health Organization classification of tumours. Pathology and genetics of tumours of soft tissue and bone. Lyon (France): IARC Press; 2002.

5. Mulliken JB, Glowacki J. Hemangiomas and vascular malformations in infants and children: a classification based on endothelial characteristics. Plast Reconstr Surg 1982;69:412–22.

6. Tsai TS, Evans HA, Donnelly LF, et al. Fat necrosis after trauma: a benign cause of palpable lumps in children. AJR Am J Roentgenol 1997;169:1623–6.

7. Walsh M, Jacobson JA, Kim SM, et al. Sonography of fat necrosis involving the extremity and torso

with magnetic resonance imaging and histologic correlation. J Ultrasound Med 2008;27:1751–7.

8. Navarro OM. Imaging of benign pediatric soft tissue tumors. Semin Musculoskelet Radiol 2009;13:196–209.

9. Vandevenne JE, Colpaert CG, De Schepper AM. Subcutaneous granuloma annulare: MR imaging and literature review. Eur Radiol 1998;8:1363–5.

10. Navarro OM, Parra DA. Pediatric musculoskeletal ultrasound. Ultrasound Clin 2009;4:457–70.

11. Laor T, Collins MH, Emery KH, et al. MRI appearance of accessory breast tissue: a diagnostic consideration for an axillary mass in a peripubertal or pubertal girl. AJR Am J Roentgenol 2004;183:1779–81.

12. Frieden I, Enjolras O, Esterly N. Vascular birthmarks and other abnormalities of blood vessels and lymphatics. In: Schachner LA, Hansen RC, editors. Pediatric dermatology. 3rd edition. New York: Mosby; 2003. p. 833–62.

13. Dubois J, Patriquin H, Garel L, et al. Soft-tissue hemangiomas in infants and children: diagnosis using Doppler sonography. AJR Am J Roentgenol 1998;171:247–52.

14. Paltiel HJ, Burrows PE, Kozakewich HP, et al. Soft-tissue vascular anomalies: utility of US for diagnosis. Radiology 2000;214:747–54.

15. Konez O, Burrows PE. Magnetic resonance of vascular anomalies. Magn Reson Imaging Clin N Am 2002;10:363–88.

16. Gorincour G, Kokta V, Rypens F, et al. Imaging characteristics of two subtypes of congenital hemangiomas: rapidly involuting congenital hemangiomas and non-involuting congenital hemangiomas. Pediatr Radiol 2005;35:1178–85.

17. Enjolras O, Soupre V, Picard A. Uncommon benign infantile vascular tumors. Adv Dermatol 2008;24:105–24.

18. Lyons LL, North PE, Lai FM, et al. Kaposiform hemangioendothelioma. A study of 33 cases emphasizing its pathologic, immunophenotypic, and biologic uniqueness from juvenile hemangioma. Am J Surg Pathol 2004;28:559–68.

19. Dubois J, Garel L, David M, et al. Vascular soft tissue tumors in infancy: distinguishing features on Doppler sonography. AJR Am J Roentgenol 2002;178:1541–5.

20. Gruman A, Liang MG, Mulliken JB, et al. Kaposiform hemangioendothelioma without Kasabach-Merritt phenomenon. J Am Acad Dermatol 2005;52:616–22.

21. Garzon MC, Huang JT, Enjolras O, et al. Vascular malformations. Part 1. J Am Acad Dermatol 2007;56:353–70.

22. Trop I, Dubois J, Guibaud L, et al. Soft-tissue venous malformations in pediatric and young adult patients: diagnosis with Doppler US. Radiology 1999;212:841–5.

23. Lobo-Mueller E, Amaral JG, Babyn PS, et al. Complex combined vascular malformations and vascular malformation syndromes affecting the extremities in children. Semin Musculoskelet Radiol 2009;13:255–76.

24. Miller GG, Yanchar NL, Magee JF, et al. Lipoblastoma and liposarcoma in children: an analysis of 9 cases and a review of the literature. Can J Surg 1998;41:455–8.

25. Moholkar S, Sebire NJ, Roebuck DJ. Radiological-pathological correlation in lipoblastoma and lipoblastomatosis. Pediatr Radiol 2006;36:851–6.

26. Loyer EM, Shabb NS, Mahon TG, et al. Fibrous hamartoma of infancy: MR-pathologic correlation. J Comput Assist Tomogr 1992;16:311–3.

27. Arioni C, Bellini C, Oddone M, et al. Congenital fibrous hamartoma of the knee. Pediatr Radiol 2006;36:453–5.

28. Koujok K, Ruiz RE, Hernandez RJ. Myofibromatosis: imaging characteristics. Pediatr Radiol 2005;35:374–80.

29. Eich GF, Hoeffel JC, Tschäppeler H, et al. Fibrous tumours in children: imaging features of a heterogeneous group of disorders. Pediatr Radiol 1998;28:500–9.

30. Fetsch JF, Miettinen M, Laskin WB, et al. A clinicopathologic study of 45 pediatric soft tissue tumors with an admixture of adipose tissue and fibroblastic elements, and a proposal for classification as lipofibromatosis. Am J Surg Pathol 2000;24:1491–500.

31. Canto C, Zapata S, Wise S, et al. Lipofibroma of the neck in children: an unusual diagnosis with special surgical implications. Otolaryngol Head Neck Surg 2007;137:976–8.

32. Walton JR, Green BA, Donaldson MM, et al. Imaging characteristics of lipofibromatosis presenting as a shoulder mass in a 16-month-old girl. Pediatr Radiol 2010;40(Suppl 1):S43–6.

33. Murphey MD, Ruble CM, Tyszko SM, et al. Musculoskeletal fibromatoses: radiologic-pathologic correlation. Radiographics 2009;29:2143–76.

34. Canale S, Vanel D, Couanet D, et al. Infantile fibrosarcoma: magnetic resonance imaging findings in six cases. Eur J Radiol 2009;72:30–7.

35. Cecchetto G, Carli M, Alaggio R, et al. Fibrosarcoma in pediatric patients: results of the Italian Cooperative Group studies (1979–1995). J Surg Oncol 2001;78:225–31.

36. Boon LM, Fishman SJ, Lund DP, et al. Congenital fibrosarcoma masquerading as congenital hemangioma: report of two cases. J Pediatr Surg 1995;30:1378–81.

37. Yan AC, Chamlin SL, Liang MG, et al. Congenital infantile fibrosarcoma: a masquerader of ulcerated hemangioma. Pediatr Dermatol 2006;23:330–4.

38. Lee MJ, Cairns RA, Munk PL, et al. Congenital-infantile fibrosarcoma: magnetic resonance imaging findings. Can Assoc Radiol J 1996;47:121–5.

39. Ablin DS, Jain K, Howell L, et al. Ultrasound and MR imaging of fibromatosis colli (sternomastoid tumor of infancy). Pediatr Radiol 1998;28:230–3.

40. McDowell HP. Update on childhood rhabdomyosarcoma. Arch Dis Child 2003;88:354–7.

41. Van Rijn RR, Wilde JC, Bras J, et al. Imaging findings in noncraniofacial childhood rhabdomyosarcoma. Pediatr Radiol 2008;38:617–34.

42. Ajlan AM, Sayegh K, Powell T, et al. Angiomatoid fibrous histiocytoma: magnetic resonance imaging appearance in 2 cases. J Comput Assist Tomogr 2010;34:791–4.

43. McCarville MB, Spunt SL, Skapek SX, et al. Synovial sarcoma in pediatric patients. AJR Am J Roentgenol 2002;179:797–801.

44. Laffan EE, Ngan BY, Navarro OM. Pediatric soft-tissue tumors and pseudotumors: MR imaging features with pathologic correlation: part 2. Tumors of fibroblastic/myofibroblastic, so-called fibrohistiocytic, muscular, lymphomatous, neurogenic, hair matrix, and uncertain origin. Radiographics 2009;29:e36.

45. O'Keefe F, Lorigan JG, Wallace S. Radiological features of extraskeletal Ewing sarcoma. Br J Radiol 1990;63:456–60.

46. Chow E, Merchant TE, Pappo A, et al. Cutaneous and subcutaneous Ewing's sarcoma: an indolent disease. Int J Radiat Oncol Biol Phys 2000;46:433–8.

47. Dick EA, McHugh K, Kimber C, et al. Imaging of non-central nervous system primitive neuroectodermal tumors: diagnostic features and correlation with outcome. Clin Radiol 2001;56:206–15.

48. Hwang JY, Lee SW, Lee SM. The common ultrasonographic features of pilomatricoma. J Ultrasound Med 2005;24:1397–402.

49. Lim HW, Im SA, Lim GY, et al. Pilomatricomas in children: imaging characteristics with pathologic correlation. Pediatr Radiol 2007;37:549–55.

Mimics of Bone and Soft Tissue Neoplasms

G. Scott Stacy, MD*, Avnit Kapur, MD

KEYWORDS

- Bone tumor • Soft tissue tumor • Pseudotumor
- Mimic • Imaging • Radiology

Many benign nonneoplastic entities can mimic bone and soft tissue tumors on imaging examinations. Distinguishing between neoplastic and nonneoplastic entities depends on history and physical examination findings as well as imaging findings, and is an important early step in the patient's overall workup and treatment plan. This article describes some of the pseudotumors seen on imaging studies of patients who have been referred to our orthopedic oncology clinic, as well as mimics of bone and soft tissue neoplasms described in the medical literature. Tumor mimics resulting from anatomic and developmental variants, trauma, infection and inflammation, osteonecrosis and myonecrosis, articular and juxta-articular conditions, and miscellaneous causes are discussed. For simplicity, the word tumor is used synonymously with neoplasm throughout this article, representing both benign and malignant entities.

NORMAL IMAGING FEATURES AND DEVELOPMENTAL VARIANTS THAT MIMIC TUMORS

Sites of Muscle/Tendon Attachment and Metaphyseal Cortical Irregularities

Tug lesions refer to cortical irregularities that occur at sites of tendon and muscle attachment. Some appear as small spurlike entities (eg, along the distal femur at the adductor magnus tendon insertion[1] or the fibular neck at the soleus attachment[2]). These lesions may persist into adulthood, mimicking a small exostosis, but do not require a workup. However, a different type of tug lesion has a more sinister radiographic appearance, resulting in irregular cortical ossification that can mimic an aggressive bone tumor, particularly in adolescents. The best known example is the so-called cortical desmoid (also known as metaphyseal cortical irregularity or avulsive cortical irregularity) arising along the medial supracondylar femur (**Fig. 1**).[3,4] The lesion is not a desmoid in the traditional sense of the word; instead, it is self-limiting and considered by some to be a normal developmental variant and by others to result from repetitive traction of the medial head of the gastrocnemius or the aponeurosis of the adductor magnus. It is typically discovered incidentally on knee radiographs in adolescent boys. In most cases, it does not correspond to the site of the patient's knee pain, although mild pain is occasionally localized to the region of the irregularity.[3] On radiographs, the lesion may manifest either as a lucency or a proliferative abnormality[5] with aggressive-appearing features (eg, periosteal reaction and spicules) that mimic osteosarcoma. This variant is generally smaller than most osteosarcomas, does not result in a soft tissue mass, and in most cases, the typical location and appearance of the lesion allow for proper diagnosis and avoidance of workup; however, for equivocal cases, additional imaging may be warranted. Radiographs of the contralateral knee could be considered, because this lesion is bilateral in one-third of cases. Magnetic resonance (MR) imaging excludes a soft tissue mass and medullary invasion, arguing against an aggressive neoplasm. The lesion may be inconspicuous on MR imaging, but typically presents as cortically based low signal intensity on T1-weighted (T1W) images and intermediate to high, sometimes cystic signal intensity on T2-weighted (T2W) images,

Department of Radiology, University of Chicago Medical Center, 5841 South Maryland Avenue, MC2026, Chicago, IL 60637, USA
* Corresponding author.
E-mail address: sstacy@radiology.bsd.uchicago.edu

Radiol Clin N Am 49 (2011) 1261–1286
doi:10.1016/j.rcl.2011.07.009

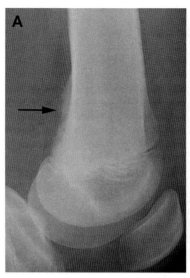
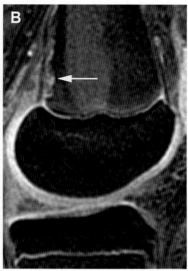

Fig. 1. 12-year-old boy referred with mild knee pain. (*A*) Lateral radiograph of the left knee shows a bony proliferative abnormality (*arrow*) along the posterior aspect of the distal femoral metaphysis. (*B*) Sagittal gradient-echo MR image shows corresponding irregularity of the posterior margin of the femur (*arrow*), but no associated soft tissue mass, confirming cortical desmoid.

with an underlying low signal intensity rim. Enhancement is noted after intravenous gadolinium chelate injection,[6] and adjacent marrow and soft tissue edema may be noted after trauma.[4] Computed tomography (CT) shows small areas of cortical erosion associated with cortical thickening. Lesions may show no activity or slightly increased activity on skeletal scintigraphy; activity may be more pronounced on 2-(fluorine-18)-fluoro-2-deoxy-D-glucose positron emission tomography (PET).[7]

Keats and Joyce[8] along with other investigators[9,10] have described a variety of notchlike metaphyseal cortical irregularities in children. Included in this group of irregularities is the cortical desmoid. The investigators suggest that these lesions may represent variations of normal growth rather than by-products of stress or avulsion, citing fenestrations in the metaphyseal cortex in neonatal pathology specimens that could persist beyond the neonatal period. However, other cortical irregularities seem to be associated with chronic forces at sites of musculotendinous attachment, such as those described in asymptomatic gymnasts along the anterior aspect of the proximal humerus at the pectoralis major insertion.[11,12] A spectrum of bone irregularities mimicking malignancy has also been described at the insertions of the deltoid muscle (pseudotumor deltoideus)[13,14] and the latissimus dorsi muscle on the humerus,[15] at the origins of the sartorius and rectus femoris muscles on the ilium, along the ischium at the hamstring origin,[16] and at the insertion of the biceps tendon on the radius.[17] These pseudotumors may result in increased activity on skeletal scintigraphy[18] as

well as mild cortical irregularity and eccentric marrow abnormality on MR imaging and CT. The absence of a soft tissue mass combined with the recognition of the site of abnormality as the location of tendon attachment can help to exclude malignancy.

Foramina, Fossae, and Other Radiolucent Tumor Mimics

A foramen is a naturally occurring passageway through or into a bone. Occasionally an anomalous foramen develops in a bone and mimics a lucent lesion. For example, an anomalous foramen in the central portion of the inferior half of the body of the sternum[19] may simulate a small lytic tumor on imaging studies; however, it is often associated with an adjacent thin vertically oriented sclerotic band and, in our experience, is at least partially filled with fat: features that can help distinguish it from tumor. Anomalous foramina also occur in a variety of locations within the scapula, including the neck, superior fossa, and body.[20,21] On radiographs, the resultant lucencies usually have sclerotic margins, which can assist with differentiation from metastasis and myeloma. Normal vascular foramina within the scapula may become particularly prominent at the site of transition between the scapular neck and body, and at the root of the scapular spine.

A fossa represents a depression of a bone. When a fossa becomes unusually prominent, it too may mimic a destructive lesion; such fossae are often at sites of ligamentous attachment. For example, irregularity and concavity of the cortex along the undersurface of the medial clavicle at the attachment of the costoclavicular (rhomboid) ligament may mimic neoplasm when pronounced (**Fig. 2**). This rhomboid fossa is often more prominent on the side of the patient's handedness.[17,22] Another fossa in the anterior end of the first rib may enlarge and mimic a lesion; although the abnormality may be unilateral, it is consistent in location, and should not be confused with true bone destruction.[23] CT shows these fossae as benign entities.

The femoral neck herniation pit and dorsal defect of the patella result in small round lesions that can be confused with osteoid osteoma or other neoplastic entities. Classically the former is believed to represent a normal variant related to herniation of synovium through the anterior cortex of the proximal superior quadrant of the femoral neck,[24] although investigators have also suggested that it may arise because of acquired degenerative changes from chronic abrasive effects[25]; an association with femoroacetabular impingement is controversial.[26,27] The pit is recognized on radiographs and CT as a small round radiolucency surrounded by a thin sclerotic margin.[24] It is well-marginated on MR imaging, extending to the anterior cortex, with variable signal intensity centrally surrounded by a low signal intensity rim.[25] Its characteristic appearance and location should allow confident differentiation from osteoid osteoma, which is typically associated with reactive new bone formation and marrow edema. The dorsal defect of the patella is an uncommon lesion of unknown cause[28] usually discovered in adolescents and young adults.[29] On radiographs, it creates a 1-cm to 2-cm round lucency with a sclerotic margin in the superolateral aspect of the patella. MR imaging shows a well-defined but often heterogeneous area of abnormal signal intensity along the posterior margin of the patella[30]; there may be ingrowth of cartilage into

the defect[28] with interruption of the dorsal cortex, which is an unusual presentation for an intramedullary tumor. The lesion can be symptomatic and associated with increased activity on skeletal scintigraphy. Its characteristic location in the superolateral aspect of the patella allows for a confident diagnosis in most cases.

Schmorl nodes represent herniation of disc material through the vertebral endplate into the vertebral body.[31] They can be confused with malignancy and lead to a request for biopsy. On radiographs, they result in a lucent defect in the vertebral body that borders on the disk and is surrounded by sclerosis.[32] Although the nodes may become unusually large or show surrounding marrow edema on MR imaging, reformatted cross-sectional imaging typically shows a well-delineated lesion in the vertebral body connected to a degenerative disk[33] via an endplate defect, allowing for proper diagnosis. Cystic varieties have also been described. Although Schmorl nodes may arise as idiopathic developmental variants, they also can result from processes that weaken the cartilaginous surface or subchondral bone of the vertebral body, including underlying malignancy.

Another common normal variant that results in referrals to our orthopedic oncology clinic based on imaging findings is the asymmetric ischiopubic synchondrosis. The ischiopubic synchondroses enlarge bilaterally in early childhood as a normal phenomenon of growth.[34] However, in older children this enlargement is commonly seen unilaterally, particularly on the side of the nondominant limb. This enlargement manifests on radiographs as radiolucent expansion caused by delayed fusion, and mimics a lucent lesion on CT (**Fig. 3**). On MR imaging, fusiform edema along the synchondrosis with signal alteration and contrast enhancement of marrow and adjacent soft tissues may also resemble tumor. A smooth hypointense band in the center of the edema representing

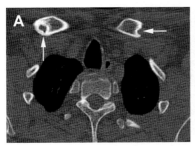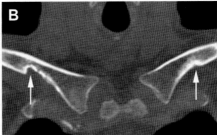

Fig. 2. 42-year-old man referred to rule out clavicular tumor. (*A*) Transverse CT image shows bilateral rhomboid fossae (*arrows*), the one on the right mimicking a lucent lesion with sclerotic margins; (*B*) CT scan reformatted in the coronal plane shows rhomboid fossae (*arrows*) to better advantage.

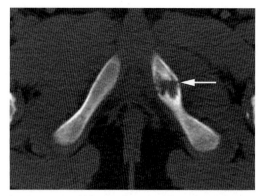

Fig. 3. 7-year-old boy referred with suspected tumor of left obturator ring. CT scan shows irregular lucency and expansile remodeling of the left ischiopubic junction, compatible with delayed fusion. Follow-up radiographs (not shown) revealed complete resolution of abnormality.

fibrous bridging across the synchondrosis can help distinguish this variant[35] from neoplasm.

Physiologic radiolucencies occur when a normal paucity of trabeculae creates the appearance of a lucent lesion. Such pseudotumors have been described in the glenoid,[23] the greater tuberosity of the humeral head,[36] the proximal end of the ulna,[15] the femoral neck (Ward triangle),[17] the fibular head,[1] and the junction of the neck and body of the calcaneus.[37,38] Although lack of aggressive features such as periosteal reaction and cortical destruction, combined with the characteristic location of these pseudotumors, should lead to the correct diagnosis, cross-sectional imaging may be performed in difficult cases to confirm the presence of normal marrow.

Accessory Muscles

Numerous accessory muscles have been described in the literature[39] that clinically can present as masses. Diagnosis of an accessory muscle on cross-sectional imaging is generally straightforward, because the accessory muscle has characteristics similar to the normal musculature, including points of origin and insertion. On occasion, accessory muscles may be mistaken for tumor[40,41]; for example, an accessory muscle may be injured, and the resultant edema can create a confusing picture, resulting in an erroneous diagnosis of neoplasm (**Fig. 4**).

Hematopoietic Marrow

Bone marrow contains both fat and hematopoietic cells. When the fatty element predominates the marrow is described as yellow; the marrow is described as red when the hematopoietic element predominates. In adults, hematopoietic marrow persists in the axial skeleton and often in the metaphyses of the proximal femora and humeri[42]; islands of residual red marrow may persist elsewhere in the skeleton as well (eg, the distal femur of adolescents or women of menstruating age). The signal intensity of yellow marrow on MR imaging is similar to that of normal subcutaneous fat, with interspersed reticular low signal intensity trabeculae. On fat-suppressed T2W images, hematopoietic marrow has an intermediate signal intensity higher than that of the suppressed yellow marrow, similar to that of skeletal muscle. Such red marrow can be mistaken for a neoplastic process when presenting focally in the medullary space amidst a background of normal fatty

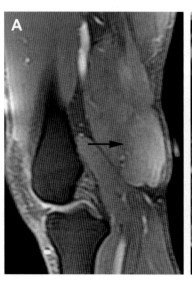
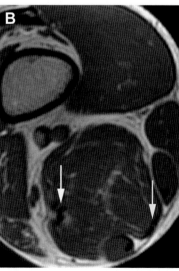

Fig. 4. 25-year-old man referred with a posterior thigh mass. (A) Fat-suppressed T1W sagittal MR image of the lower thigh after intravenous administration of gadolinium chelate shows an enhancing posterior soft tissue mass (arrow). (B) T1W transverse image through the mass shows a large, anomalous semimembranosus muscle with 2 tendons (arrows). T2W images (not shown) revealed mild feathery edema consistent with strain of the anomalous muscle.

marrow. However, on T1W images, normal red marrow, which contains an admixture of fatty elements and hematopoietic elements, typically has a signal intensity lower than that of fatty marrow but higher than that of skeletal muscle; neoplastic infiltration is generally, although not consistently, isointense or hypointense to skeletal muscle on T1W images.[42] Furthermore, tumor deposits tend to be rounded and sharply defined, whereas the margins of red marrow islands are typically poorly defined and interdigitate with yellow marrow. In clinical settings of increased hematopoietic demand, fatty marrow may revert back to red marrow. In chronically ill patients with advanced marrow reconversion, as well as in patients with myeloproliferative disorders, the signal intensity of red marrow may appear isointense or even hypointense to that of skeletal muscle on T1W images, and the margins of the marrow may become more sharply defined.[42] Distinguishing normal from pathologic marrow in these patients may be difficult. Opposed-phase gradient-echo MR imaging and diffusion-weighted imaging show some promise for distinguishing red marrow from pathologic marrow.[42-44]

TRAUMA
Stress Injuries of Bone

Stress fractures are overuse injuries, and occur when normal bone is exposed to abnormal repetitive stress (fatigue fractures) or when osteoporotic bone is exposed to normal stress (insufficiency fractures).[45] Most fatigue fractures occur in the lower extremities, particularly in the tibia and metatarsals, but upper extremity fatigue fractures can be seen in certain athletes. The pelvis, proximal femur and vertebral bodies are common sites for insufficiency fractures. In most cases, clinical features are highly suggestive of the diagnosis of a stress fracture, particularly when a specific activity leads to pain in an area prone to such an injury. Radiographic manifestations vary in accordance with the site and stage of the injury, and are often normal in the early stages. Subsequent findings range from subtle periosteal reaction and endosteal sclerosis to exuberant callus formation, cortical thickening, and a lucent fracture line.[46] Bone along the fracture may undergo resorption; expansile remodeling of the bone may also occur. Although the radiographic features are usually diagnostic or strongly suggestive of a stress fracture, difficulty with diagnosis may arise if the fracture is in an atypical location or presents with exaggerated radiographic findings; in such cases a bone tumor may be erroneously included in the differential diagnosis.[47,48] The imaging features of stress fracture may mimic osteoid osteoma in particular; however, the lucent nidus of osteoid osteoma is typically rounded, whereas a stress fracture is more commonly linear in configuration.

MR imaging can detect marrow edema of stress injuries before emergence of radiographic findings. This edema may be mistaken for neoplastic infiltration. A discrete hypointense fracture line within the area of edema allows a proper diagnosis (**Fig. 5**). Increased signal intensity in the adjacent cortex may also be visible, particularly in the long bones.[49] However, marrow and periosteal edema may be evident before development of a discrete fracture line. Furthermore, adjacent soft tissue edema and

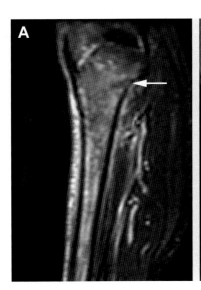 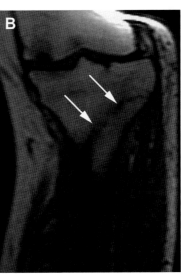

Fig. 5. 54-year-old man referred with painful tibial lesion. (*A*) Fat-suppressed T2W sagittal MR image of the tibia shows edema throughout the visualized marrow, as well as in the adjacent soft tissues. Note the horizontally oriented low signal intensity band in proximal tibia (*arrow*) representing the fracture. (*B*) T1W coronal image the shows the fracture line to better advantage (*arrows*). Note that the remainder of the marrow appears relatively normal on the T1W image. The patient had a history of multiple previous stress fractures as well.

enhancement can be extensive and, in combination with marrow edema, mimic soft tissue extension of an intramedullary neoplasm. In difficult cases such as these, the radiologist must rely on typical clinical manifestations and locations of stress fractures to offer a correct diagnosis. In our experience, marrow edema associated with stress injuries is frequently more pronounced on fat-suppressed T2W images than on T1W images and is often ill-defined; in contrast, neoplasms typically present as well-defined hypointense lesions on T1W images. In some instances, CT may be necessary to provide the specificity needed to diagnose a stress fracture, particularly in the sacrum.[50] Fottner and colleagues[47] retrospectively reviewed 22 cases of stress fractures that presented as bone tumors, and noted that CT was required as the key to diagnosis in 15 of the patients. It is important for radiologists to remember that pathologic fractures can occur in bone tumors; as with nonfractured tumors, tumors with pathologic fractures typically exhibit well-defined T1 marrow alterations, and may be associated with endosteal scalloping and an adjacent soft tissue mass. The use of in-phase and out-of-phase MR sequences may help differentiate benign stress fractures from pathologic fracture.[51]

Other Posttraumatic Pseudotumors of Bone

Posttraumatic cortical lucencies are uncommon entities after fractures in children (Fig. 6). Most of these pseudotumors have been described in the distal radius, although distal tibial and femoral posttraumatic lesions have also been reported.[52] Often they appear after minor greenstick fractures.

The pathogenesis of these lesions is unclear. They may arise because of entrapment of intramedullary fat in a subperiosteal hematoma at the fracture site; this is supported by the fact that the lesions are of fat density/signal intensity based on the reports of some investigators.[53] The lesions can mimic tumor or infection, but the clinical history, and, if necessary, cross-sectional imaging characteristics, should allow for a confident diagnosis. Focal bone lesions may also result from chronic impingement/abutment of skeletal structures and mimic epiphyseal tumors on imaging studies. Patients with cystic changes in the posterior aspect of the humeral head on MR imaging associated with internal impingement of the shoulder have been referred to our orthopedic oncology clinic with a diagnosis of chondroblastoma. Accompanying posterosuperior labral disease and undersurface tears of the supraspinatus and infraspinatus tendons in overhead throwing athletes are clues to the correct diagnosis.[54] Throwing athletes may also develop osteochondral lesions in the elbow. Those lesions occurring in the capitellum are familiar to most radiologists as part of the constellation of findings seen with little league elbow; however, osteochondral lesions occurring in the humeral trochlea are encountered less commonly, and may be mistaken for an epiphyseal tumor such as chondroblastoma.[55] A variety of surgical procedures, including tendon transfers, bone graft harvesting, and bone biopsy, may produce lucent defects that mimic small metastatic or myelomatous foci. Knowledge of such procedures and their characteristic imaging manifestations is crucial for accurate diagnosis.

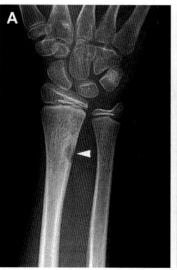 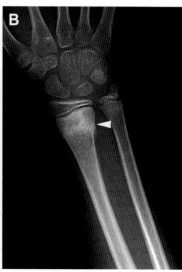

Fig. 6. Young girl referred with distal radius lesion. (A) Anteroposterior radiograph of the distal forearm shows a cortically based lucency in the distal metadiaphysis (arrowhead). (B) Radiograph obtained 5 months earlier shows the original fracture (arrowhead) before the development of the lucency. The lucency remained stable on follow-up radiographs, and is presumed to be posttraumatic in cause.

Soft Tissue Injuries

Hematomas may manifest as soft tissue masses that mimic neoplasms in patients with or without a clear history of trauma; however, in most patients, the clinical history and imaging pattern of the mass usually allow a proper diagnosis of hematoma.[56] Sonography can be used for initial evaluation, particularly in children, showing the hematoma as an ill-defined hyperechoic mass in the acute phase that gradually becomes better defined and hypoechoic.[57,58] Hematoma can have a variety of appearances on MR imaging that depend on changes in the structure of the hemoglobin molecule related to the age of the blood.[59] Increased signal intensity within the mass on unenhanced T1W images, particularly when fat-suppressed, is suggestive of methemoglobin and a subacute hematoma (**Fig. 7**); this high signal intensity is often most noticeable in the periphery of the hematoma.[57] Edema surrounding the hematoma is common, diminishing with time. Areas of relatively low signal intensity within or along the periphery of the mass on T2W images caused by intracellular deoxyhemoglobin or hemosiderin deposition also support the diagnosis of hematoma, as does blooming on gradient-echo sequences. Lack of central enhancement after intravenous gadolinium administration is typical; however, fibrovascular tissue within a hematoma may show some enhancement, and delayed imaging after gadolinium administration may allow diffusion of the contrast into the hematoma, with resultant enhancement mimicking that of a tumor.[60] It may be difficult to distinguish a simple hematoma from a hemorrhagic neoplasm at imaging. Nodular or masslike enhancement after intravenous gadolinium administration is suggestive of a neoplasm. The absence of subcutaneous ecchymosis and lack of trauma history or anticoagulation should also arouse suspicion for underlying tumor.[61] If a hematoma is observed, it should be followed until it resolves or decreases in size; otherwise biopsy should be considered if an underlying soft tissue neoplasm is suspected. Open biopsy may be necessary.[62] High signal intensity within a mass on T1W images can also represent fat, such as that which may be seen with a benign or malignant lipomatous tumor; fat-suppressed sequences can help differentiate subacute blood products from adipose tissue.[57]

Hematomas may accompany myotendinous strains and tendon avulsions.[63] A first-degree (mild) myotendinous strain results in edema without architectural distortion, and is usually not confused with neoplasm. Second-degree and third-degree strains, representing partial-thickness and complete-thickness macroscopic tears, respectively,[60] are often accompanied by hematoma formation, and hence are more likely to be misinterpreted as neoplasms (see **Fig. 7**). Complete avulsion of a tendon can likewise mimic a soft tissue neoplasm if associated with a hematoma, or if retraction of the tendon and muscle form a masslike pseudotumor (**Fig. 8**); such pseudotumors may be confirmed by careful evaluation of images in multiple anatomic planes to locate the torn end of the retracted tendon. Partial-thickness tendon tears and tendinosis can result in calcification as well as altered signal intensity and enhancement of the adjacent soft tissues, causing a pseudotumor.[64] The abnormality may extend into the bone, resulting in periosteal edema, cortical defects, and abnormal eccentric marrow signal.[14] Awareness of these findings occurring at the sites of tendon origins and insertions can allow for proper diagnosis. In children, a fragment of bone may be avulsed by tendon because of incompletely fused apophyses, and subsequent healing of the avulsion fracture may result in prominent bone formation that mimics an aggressive neoplasm such as osteosarcoma on radiographs (**Fig. 9**).[65] MR imaging may also result

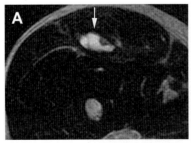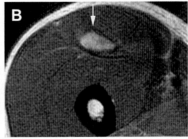

Fig. 7. 20-year-old man with a recent muscle strain referred with a soft tissue mass. (*A*) T2W transverse MR image of the thigh shows a mass of high signal intensity (*arrow*) in the rectus femoris. (*B*) T1W transverse MR image shows the high signal intensity mass (*arrow*) adjacent to the distal tendon of the rectus femoris muscle, compatible with a subacute hematoma from a myotendinous strain injury. The low signal intensity rim that partially surrounds the hematoma represents hemosiderin deposition.

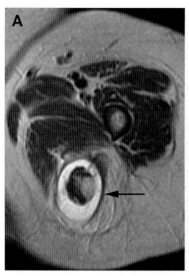

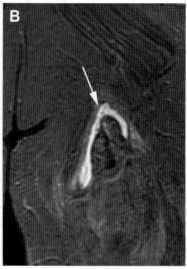

Fig. 8. Middle-aged woman referred with suspected soft tissue tumor. (*A*) T2W transverse MR image of the proximal thigh shows a mass with a target appearance (*arrow*) in the posterior soft tissues that was initially misinterpreted as a nerve sheath tumor. Note the absence of the normal hamstring musculature. (*B*) Fat-suppressed T2W coronal MR image shows that the mass represents torn and retracted hamstring musculature surrounded by fluid (*arrow*).

in confusion if the reactive bone formation produces a mass associated with marrow edema in the underlying bone. CT can usually secure the correct diagnosis by revealing the donor site of the fracture and the benign nature of the ossification.

Posttraumatic myositis ossificans represents a self-limiting, localized reparative lesion consisting of reactive hypercellular fibrous tissue and bone.[66] Soft tissue injury is the initiating event in most cases, although patients may not provide a history of trauma. The anterior musculature of the thigh and arm are most frequently involved. In the early stages, primitive mesenchymal cells with prominent mitotic activity can mimic sarcoma

on biopsy.[67] Myositis ossificans may produce features on imaging studies that also mimic a neoplasm; this is particularly true on MR imaging examinations. As with hematoma, the appearance of myositis ossificans on MR imaging is variable and depends on the maturity of the lesion.[68] During the late or chronic phase of myositis ossificans, lesions typically have an appearance comparable with that of bone, with peripheral low signal intensity and central high signal intensity (marrow fat) on T1W images. However, earlier stages are more likely to mimic a soft tissue neoplasm, with heterogeneous low signal intensity on T1W images, heterogeneous high signal intensity on T2W images, and enhancement after

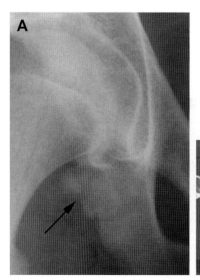

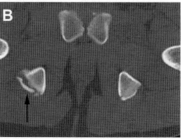

Fig. 9. 15-year-old athlete referred with possible pelvic osteosarcoma. (*A*) Anteroposterior radiograph of the hip shows lobulated ossification (*arrow*) along the proximal ischium. (*B*) Transverse CT image through the pelvis shows a discrete avulsion fracture (*arrow*) arising from the right ischium at the hamstring origin; no tumor was evident.

intravenous gadolinium administration. Soft tissue edema surrounding myositis ossificans during the early or acute phase tends to be more pronounced than that surrounding neoplasms.[59] During the subacute or intermediate phase, a low signal intensity rim, corresponding to peripheral ossification, can suggest the diagnosis of myositis ossificans. Radiographs or CT are often necessary to better characterize the mass, specifically to evaluate the pattern of mineralization. Although initially radiographs and CT may show only soft tissue edema, calcifications become evident 2 to 6 weeks after the onset of symptoms.[66] Unlike soft tissue malignancies, the mineralization of myositis ossificans is most mature at the periphery of the mass, and this is particularly well shown with CT (Fig. 10). Sonography may also be able to detect calcifications at an early point, and, when hematoma is shown, can provide evidence of previous trauma.[67] Parosteal osteosarcoma can mimic myositis ossificans; however, parosteal osteosarcoma arises from the surface of bone, and the ossified portion of the tumor is typically surrounded by a soft tissue component, unlike myositis ossificans. If mineralization of the mass is difficult to characterize but myositis ossificans is suspected clinically, follow-up CT in 4 weeks may be necessary,[60] at which time the calcification may have a more typical appearance. The mass of myositis ossificans tends to decrease in size over time until stabilizing at maturity, and in some cases completely disappears.

Morel-Lavallée lesions (MLLs) represent closed degloving injuries of the soft tissues that develop as a result of a blunt tangential force that separates the hypodermis from the underlying fascia.[69] The sheared hemolymphatic supply of the tissue subsequently fills the space between the subcutaneous fat and underlying fascia. The hemolymphatic collection becomes surrounded by granulation tissue that may be organized into a fibrous pseudocapsule, preventing reabsorption of fluid.[70] MLLs have been described along the knee, lateral thigh, buttock, and lower back. Although a history of trauma is helpful in directing the clinician to the appropriate diagnosis, patients may sometimes not recall any specific event, and the diagnosis of MLL may initially be missed and the lesion mistaken for a tumor. The imaging appearance of the MLL depends on the age and amount of blood, fat, and lymph tissue within it. Mild enhancement of the fibrous pseudocapsule as well as internal contents of MLLs has been described and is believed to be related to the presence of residual capillaries in the space filled by the lesion.[71] The variable enhancement occasionally seen in these lesions may lead the radiologist to the diagnosis of a soft tissue tumor. The acute angle margin from the peeling back of subcutaneous fat from fascia, history of trauma, and characteristic locations help to distinguish MLLs from neoplasm.[70]

A foreign object in the soft tissues may occasionally produce a pseudotumor as a result of the body's reaction to the object. On MR imaging examinations, high signal intensity surrounding the object on T2W images can represent fluid and granulation tissue. Low signal intensity may result if fibrosis predominates.[72] In many cases, the geometric or angular nature of the central foreign object allows for a correct diagnosis.

INFECTION AND INFLAMMATION
Osteomyelitis

Distinguishing bone infection from bone neoplasm can be difficult, and multiple reports of osteomyelitis resembling tumor, as well as tumor masquerading as infection, are found in the medical literature.[73,74] Osteomyelitis can be caused by direct invasion of bone or hematogenous spread of an infecting agent.[75–77] Most cases in children are hematogenous, typically involving the subphyseal metaphysis of rapidly growing bones. Adults, with their relatively competent immune system, are less

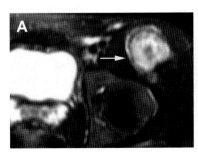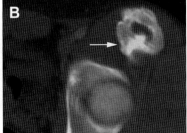

Fig. 10. 15-year-old boy with an anterior proximal thigh mass. (A) T2W transverse MR image of the left hip shows a mass of heterogeneously high signal intensity (arrow) in the soft tissues anterior to the femoral head. (B) Transverse CT image reveals peripheral ossification of the mass typical of myositis ossificans traumatica (arrow).

prone to hematogenous osteomyelitis, and therefore most cases of osteomyelitis in adults are caused by direct penetration of bone at sites of skin ulceration; however, hematogenous spread of infection is still encountered in certain adult patient groups (eg, intravenous drug abusers). Infection of bone can also be subdivided based on the clinical course into acute, subacute, and chronic osteomyelitis. All stages have the potential to mimic neoplasm on imaging studies. Radiographs may not show appreciable findings in the bone for several days or even weeks after the onset of infection.[75] Trabecular destruction and localized osteopenia represent early manifestations. Osteomyelitis may result in geographic, moth-eaten, or permeative lucencies. Lamellated periosteal reaction is frequently encountered, and may be detected before osteolysis. A Codman triangle may occur, although this is more commonly seen with bone malignancies than with osteomyelitis. On MR imaging, areas of infected marrow can be detected before radiographic changes are apparent, showing high signal intensity on fat-suppressed T2W images and low signal intensity on T1W images. Although highly sensitive for acute osteomyelitis, these findings are nonspecific, and can be seen with tumors. However, as a general rule, infected areas of marrow are large and irregularly outlined, with juxtaosseous edema consistently present. The formation of early intraosseous abscesses, with peripheral but not central contrast enhancement, can also support the diagnosis of osteomyelitis. Cortical permeation can be detected on MR imaging and can be used to support a diagnosis of osteomyelitis if an adjacent soft tissue abscess is present.[76]

When the defense mechanisms of the body contain an infection to a localized area within the medullary space, an acute infection of bone may proceed to subacute osteomyelitis, characterized radiographically by a mixture of bone destruction and reactive sclerosis.[75,76] In this setting, a Brodie abscess can form (Fig. 11). This lesion is more common in children, and can be confused with bone tumor. The abscess is characterized on radiographs by a well-defined lytic lesion, typically 1 to 5 cm in size, surrounded by thick reactive sclerosis. Mild periosteal reaction may be present. When small and eccentrically located in the bone, a Brodie abscess can mimic an osteoid osteoma. On MR imaging, a Brodie abscess is generally of high signal intensity on fat-suppressed T2W images. It usually lacks central contrast enhancement, although granulation tissue within the defect may enhance. In long bones, a target appearance is characteristic, created by (1) central nonenhancing pus of low signal intensity on T1W images and high signal intensity on T2W images surrounded by (2) an inner ring of high signal intensity on T1W and T2W images and (3) an outer ring of low signal intensity. This ring in turn is surrounded by (4) a halo of edema.[78] The hyperintense inner ring on T1W images reflecting vascularized granulation tissue has been termed the penumbra sign; its sensitivity for osteomyelitis lies between 20%

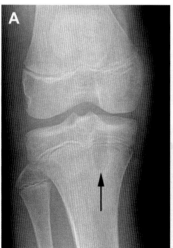 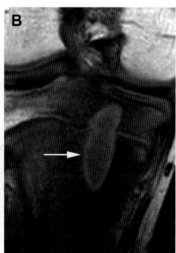 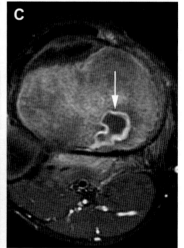

Fig. 11. 13-year-old boy referred with a proximal tibial lesion. (A) Anteroposterior radiograph of the knee shows an ovoid metaepiphyseal lesion with sclerotic margins (*arrow*) crossing the proximal tibial physis. (B) T1W coronal MR image shows the penumbra of high signal intensity (*arrow*), typical of infection, between the central pus and surrounding edema. (C) Fat-suppressed T1W transverse MR image after intravenous administration of gadolinium chelate shows nonenhancing pus centrally surrounded by an enhancing rim (*arrow*), confirming Brodie abscess.

and 75%, depending on the investigator, but its specificity seems to be greater than 90%.[79–81]

There is no clear-cut distinction between subacute osteomyelitis and chronic osteomyelitis. The term chronic osteomyelitis itself is vague, encompassing hypovirulent forms of Brodie abscesses, recurrent exacerbations of exogenous osteomyelitis, as well as granulomatous (fungal and mycobacterial) and other nonbacterial inflammatory bone lesions.[75] However, as a general rule, chronic osteomyelitis is characterized by irregular sclerosis and hyperostosis caused by solid periosteal reaction. The sclerotic region may contain lytic areas representing sites of active infection or granulation tissue. A sequestrum, involucrum, and cloaca may form.[76] The cloaca, representing a direct communication between the infected medullary cavity and the surrounding soft tissue, can be detected readily on cross-sectional imaging studies, and helps to confirm osteomyelitis. Sequestra, pieces of dead bone within infected bone, are important to identify because they must be removed to cure the infection. CT is generally considered to be the best technique for identification of sequestra. Sequestra can be seen with a variety of tumors, including fibrosarcoma, malignant fibrous histiocytoma, lymphoma, desmoplastic fibroma, and eosinophilic granuloma.[82]

Chronic recurrent multifocal osteomyelitis (CRMO) is a poorly understood entity encompassing a variety of chronic/subacute episodes of osteomyelitis affecting children and young adults. As the term suggests, CRMO frequently involves multiple sites, sometimes symmetrically.[75] Although CRMO is generally considered to be a form of low-grade chronic infection, abscesses, cloacae, and sequestra typically do not form, and a causative organism is not usually identified. The metaphyses of long bones and the medial clavicles are typically involved, although the vertebral bodies, pelvis, ribs and mandible may also be affected.[83] The radiographic appearance is that of a lytic lesion that develops progressive sclerosis and hyperostosis over time. CRMO is a diagnosis of exclusion, and the differential diagnosis includes bone malignancies. The combination of features that support the diagnosis of CRMO include multifocality and symmetry, involvement of typical sites such as the medial clavicle, sclerosis, and hyperostosis, and a prolonged clinical course, with most patients being healthy between recurrent episodes (**Fig. 12**). CRMO shares many features with (and may be the same entity as) sclerosing osteomyelitis of Garré, and also has an association with SAPHO syndrome (synovitis, acne, pustulosis, hyperostosis, osteitis), which tends to present at a slightly later age.

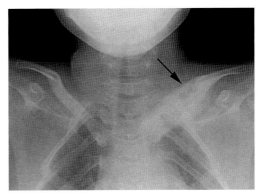

Fig. 12. 12-year-old girl referred with a clavicle lesion. Anteroposterior radiograph of the clavicles shows hyperostosis of the left clavicle (*arrow*) typical of CRMO. Follow-up radiographs (*not shown*) revealed little change.

Soft Tissue Inflammation and Infection

Patients with soft tissue infection usually present with fever, pain, and increased white blood cell count, which prompts the correct diagnosis rather than a misdiagnosis of tumor.[59] In the appropriate clinical context, diagnosis of a soft tissue abscess on MR imaging is generally straightforward if the examination shows a collection of uniform or slightly heterogeneous high signal intensity on fluid-sensitive sequences, with peripheral enhancement on sequences after gadolinium administration.[84] However, the signal intensity of the contents of the abscess cavity can be variable because of blood or proteinaceous material on both T1W and T2W images.[58] Ill-defined edema in the surrounding soft tissues tends to be more pronounced with abscesses than tumors in our experience, although edema may be less marked in immunosuppressed patients.[72] A penumbra sign of high signal intensity surrounding the soft tissue abscess cavity on T1W images has been described, similar to that seen with subacute infection of bone.[80] CT likewise shows a rim-enhancing collection, with typically low internal density that can be influenced by the amount of proteinaceous fluid and cellular debris. Foci of gas may be seen within the collection, which, in the absence of recent penetrating trauma, strongly suggests abscess. Sonography is useful for detection of abscess, which manifests as a heterogeneously hypoechoic fluid collection surrounded by a thick hyperechoic and hyperemic wall. Because an abscess containing thick fluid and debris may appear solid on sonography, compression can help to show the mobility of the contents.[84] Furthermore, the contents should not show vascularity. Although necrotic soft tissue tumors may mimic abscesses, the degree of internal enhancement with tumors, including nodular or masslike components, is usually more than that seen with pus. However, occasionally a soft tissue tumor shows only peripheral enhancement, or an abscess enhances heterogeneously, necessitating aspiration/biopsy.[85] Diffusion-weighted MR imaging may play a role in distinguishing abscess from necrotic tumor of the musculoskeletal system.[86]

Myositis, be it infectious or noninfectious, tends to result in muscle edema and enlargement rather than a discrete mass, and is therefore usually distinguished from sarcoma without difficulty. However, a masslike appearance mimicking sarcoma may occasionally manifest at MR imaging,[87–89] particularly in cases of infectious myositis. What seems to be a mass in 1 imaging plane (eg, the transverse plane), may be more confidently diagnosed as an inflamed muscle in another plane (eg, longitudinal) if the muscle maintains its normal fusiform contour (**Fig. 13**). Persistence of the normal feathery pattern of muscle architecture also argues against tumor. Prominent perilesional inflammatory changes are more in keeping with infection than tumor, but may not be so robust in patients with granulomatous infection or patients who are immunocompromised.[57] Adjacent cellulitis, although not always present, favors a diagnosis of pyomyositis over neoplasm. Also, the margins of soft tissue tumors are typically better defined than those of infected muscle.[89] Needle aspiration/biopsy can provide confirmation in confusing cases. Other causes of abnormal muscle signal intensity (eg, autoimmune myositis, subacute muscle denervation, radiation therapy, compartment syndrome) can usually be distinguished from neoplasm based on the morphology, location and extent of the abnormality, as well as the clinical history. One caveat is that skeletal muscle lymphoma may present as abnormal muscle signal intensity oriented along muscle fascicles rather than as a discrete mass[90]; however, this is a rare occurrence.

Regional lymphadenitis can have features on imaging studies that mimic those of neoplasm.[91] Cat-scratch disease, a bacterial infection caused by *Bartonella henselae*, usually affects young patients and results in lymphadenopathy in an upper extremity. A patient who develops a nodular mass in the medial epitrochlear region of the elbow after being scratched or bitten by a cat is typical. The enlarged nodes associated with cat-scratch disease usually show peripheral enhancement after intravenous gadolinium administration, with central necrosis (**Fig. 14**); this would be an unusual appearance for lymphoma or metastasis before therapy. Furthermore, the nodes of cat-scratch disease may be associated with extensive surrounding edema, which is also unusual with neoplasm. Systemic infection by *B henselae* may also result in bacillary angiomatosis, which can manifest as masslike soft tissue infection and painful osteolytic bone lesions in patients infected with the human immunodeficiency virus.[92] Such bone lesions can progress to extensive cortical destruction, medullary permeation, and aggressive periosteal reaction.

OSTEONECROSIS AND MYONECROSIS
Osteonecrosis

Osteonecrosis is a general term that refers to death of the cellular elements of bone marrow as a result of ischemia.[93] There are many causes,

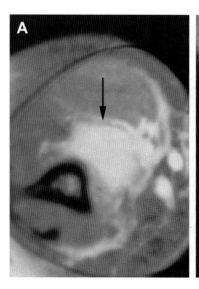
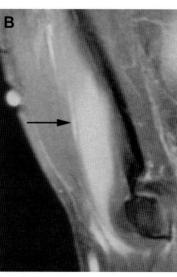

Fig. 13. 39-year-old man with painful swelling of his arm. (*A*) Fat-suppressed T1W transverse MR image of the arm obtained after intravenous administration of gadolinium chelate shows enhancement of the brachialis muscle (*arrow*) mimicking a mass. (*B*) Fat-suppressed T1W sagittal MR image shows diffuse enhancement of the distal brachialis (*arrow*); however, the muscle maintains its normal fusiform contour, compatible with inflammatory myopathy.

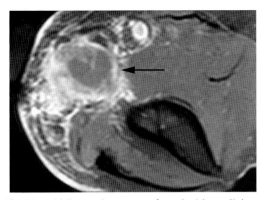

Fig. 14. Middle-aged woman referred with medial epitrochlear arm mass. Fat-suppressed T1W transverse MR image shows a mass (*arrow*) in the medial epicondylar region of the elbow with central necrosis and surrounding inflammation compatible with lymphadenitis. Cat-scratch disease was presumed based on the patient's admission that she was frequently bitten and scratched by her cat. The mass did not enlarge on subsequent imaging studies.

including trauma, hemoglobinopathies, vasculidities, and steroid therapy. Avascular necrosis, which refers to osteonecrosis that occurs in a subarticular location such as the femoral head, has received a great deal of attention in the medical literature and is easily recognized by radiologists. Osteonecrosis occurring in metadiaphyseal locations is termed bone infarction; bone infarction has received little attention in the radiology literature and hence can be a source of uncertainty for radiologists, accounting for a large number of patient referrals to our orthopedic oncology clinic. On radiographs, the typical pattern of bone

infarction is that of a serpentine ringlike band of sclerosis separating a central necrotic area of variable radiolucency from the surrounding normal bone. This pattern, although characteristic, is a late manifestation. Earlier in the disease course, bone infarction may mimic a lytic neoplastic process by presenting as a poorly defined area of lucency within the medullary space (**Fig. 15**).[94,95] Osteonecrosis may also result in periosteal reaction. In questionable cases, bone infarction may be correctly diagnosed with the aid of MR imaging. On T1W MR images, infarction typically manifests as a well-defined serpentine rim of low signal intensity. On T2W MR images, the rim may be of low signal intensity or high signal intensity; when the rim consists of parallel bands of low and high signal intensity, the double line sign is formed, a nearly pathognomonic feature of osteonecrosis. Inside the rim, the necrotic marrow is usually the same signal intensity as that of fat; however, it may be heterogeneously hypointense on T1W images because of fibrosis or calcification.[96] Earlier in the course of disease, osteonecrosis may present on MR imaging as nonspecific marrow edema,[97] and in the acute setting may be associated with edema of the periosteum and adjacent soft tissues. If osteonecrosis is suspected clinically, and the marrow edema is not associated with a definable adjacent lesion, follow-up MR imaging may be warranted to visualize regression of the edema or progression to a pattern more typical of osteonecrosis. Sarcomatous degeneration is a well-known albeit uncommon complication of bone infarction, and should be suspected from imaging if cortical destruction or a soft tissue mass is associated with the infarct.

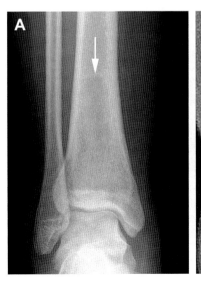

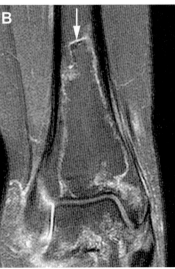

Fig. 15. 15-year-old girl on steroid therapy after liver transplantation referred with a distal tibial lesion. (*A*) Anteroposterior radiograph of the ankle shows a poorly defined lucency (*arrow*) in the distal tibial diaphysis. (*B*) Fat-suppressed proton-density-weighted MR image shows a high signal intensity curvilinear band surrounding bone with signal intensity similar to that of suppressed fat. Note the double line sign (*arrow*), virtually pathognomonic of osteonecrosis. T1W images (*not shown*) also revealed central necrotic bone of fat signal intensity. Osteonecrosis of the talus is evident as well.

Myonecrosis

Infarction of skeletal muscle is uncommon; however, when the normally rich collateral blood flow of muscle is compromised because of trauma, vasculitis, or infection, myonecrosis may occur. Muscle infarction results in enlargement and edema of the affected muscle(s), with heterogeneous high signal intensity on T2W images. However, heterogeneous masslike enhancement can be observed after intravenous gadolinium administration, which can be mistaken for tumor. Streaks of linear, serpentine, nonenhancing signal separated by enhancing linear signal have been described as diagnostic of myonecrosis.[98] The presentation of the patient is also important. For example, if the radiologist encounters an irregular rim of enhancement within edematous musculature without a focal fluid collection, then he or she can suggest the diagnosis of diabetic myonecrosis if the patient has long-standing and poorly controlled diabetes and abrupt onset of painful swelling of the lower extremity without signs of overlying infection. Sonography may also assist in differentiating myonecrosis from necrotic tumor or abscess by revealing a predominantly hypoechoic lesion with visualization of linear muscle fibers, but lack of a dominant anechoic region or swirling fluid.[99]

Calcific myonecrosis represents a late complication of compartment syndrome and trauma, characterized by the replacement of muscle with a calcified mass (Fig. 16). Because of the long delay (often several decades) between injury and presentation with a soft tissue mass, trauma is often not considered as the cause, and the condition is mistaken for a soft tissue neoplasm both clinically and radiologically.[100] Furthermore, the mass may result in pressure erosion along the cortex of the adjacent bone, eventually destroying a segment of the bone.[101] The key to diagnosis is recognizing the calcified mass as fusiform and replacing leg musculature, typically involving the anterior compartment of the leg. MR imaging also shows a fusiform mass with an outer rim of low signal intensity reflecting calcification and fibrosis. This pattern of calcification helps to distinguish this entity from calcifying soft tissue sarcomas, in which the mineralization tends to be distributed centrally as well. Furthermore, unlike soft tissue tumors, calcific myonecrosis does not enhance after intravenous gadolinium administration.

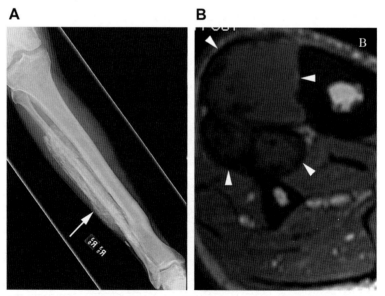

Fig. 16. 62-year-old woman referred with a leg mass. (A) Anteroposterior radiograph of the leg shows an elongated calcified mass (arrow) overlying the fibula. Note deformity of the distal tibia and fibula, indicating healed fractures. (B) T1W transverse MR image of the leg after intravenous administration of gadolinium chelate shows the mass (arrowheads) in cross-section anterior to the fibula and lateral to the tibia, essentially replacing the anterior compartment musculature. The mass does not enhance, and is surrounded by a low signal intensity rim corresponding to calcification. The imaging findings are compatible with calcific myonecrosis; follow-up imaging (not shown) revealed no progression.

ARTICULAR AND JUXTA-ARTICULAR CONDITIONS
Arthritis and Rheumatologic Conditions

Although the diagnosis of a rheumatologic condition on imaging studies is not difficult in most cases, occasionally the process can result in articular, juxta-articular, or subchondral imaging findings that mimic tumor. Osteoarthritis is the most common form of arthritis. Subchondral cysts are common in patients with osteoarthritis. Usually, these cysts are small, multiple, and located on both sides of the joint. However, occasionally a cyst can become large, prompting the radiologist to consider tumor in the differential diagnosis. Patients with large degenerative cysts of the acetabulum and glenoid are not uncommonly referred to our orthopedic oncology clinic. These cysts are usually associated with other features of osteoarthritis (eg, nonuniform cartilage loss/narrowing of the joint, osteophyte formation, and subchondral sclerosis),[102] and the patient is subsequently reassured that the lesion is not neoplastic. However, if the cyst results in destruction of the cortical margins, has a calcified matrix, or is associated with a soft tissue component, biopsy is often performed. Occasionally, biopsy of these cysts may also be warranted to exclude metastasis if the patient is scheduled to undergo joint replacement at the site of the cyst and has a history of a primary tumor elsewhere. Other features of degenerative joint disease can also occasionally mimic tumor. Although osteophyte formation at joints usually does not cause a diagnostic dilemma on radiographs, bone proliferation at the sternoclavicular joint can result in a masslike appearance on MR imaging, as well as a palpable abnormality at physical examination. CT can help with the diagnosis in questionable cases. Likewise, subchondral sclerosis of osteoarthritis rarely mimics tumor; however, premature arthritis as a result of mechanical strain across the sacroiliac joint can produce a robust sclerosis along the auricular portion of the ilium (osteitis condensans ilii) that can occasionally simulate a sclerotic bone tumor or metastasis. Osteitis condensans ilii typically affects women before the fourth decade, often after pregnancy. The characteristic site and well-defined triangular morphology of the sclerosis, along with lack of bone destruction, help to distinguish this entity from malignancy.[103] Neuropathic arthropathy can present in patients with diabetes, syringomyelia, amyloidosis, syphilis, leprosy, and a variety of other conditions.[104] The hypertrophic form results in increased bone density, osseous debris, and marked degenerative changes[105]; this is commonly seen in the feet of diabetic patients, and tumor does not usually enter the differential diagnosis. However, the atrophic form of neuropathic arthropathy can result in aggressive bone erosion that can mimic destruction by a bone tumor, the classic example occurring in the proximal humerus in a patient with syringomyelia. Often there is an associated large joint effusion with bone debris, which can occasionally create a confusing appearance on CT or MR imaging examinations.

Inflammatory arthritides can produce erosions, which, like degenerative subchondral cysts, may become large and occasionally mimic a tumor.[106] On MR imaging, these erosions may be surrounded by marrow edema that can further contribute to the erroneous impression of an aggressive neoplastic process. As with degenerative arthritis, the diagnosis of inflammatory arthritis is based on recognizing the disease process as being joint based, with findings affecting both sides of the joint, multiple joint involvement, and often involvement of nearby tendon sheaths and bursae. If only a single affected joint is imaged, then the diagnosis may become more confusing, and radiologists who are unfamiliar with the MR imaging appearance of a thickened enhancing pannus of inflammatory arthritis may mistake it for an intra-articular tumor, particularly if nodular in morphology. Benign rheumatoid nodules, which typically develop in healthy children but occasionally affect adults, may mimic a soft tissue sarcoma.[107] These lesions are confined to the subcutaneous tissues, mainly distributed along the anterior legs, feet, scalp, forearms, and hands, extending up to but never deep into the underlying fascia. They are usually less than 5 cm in size, may be solid or cystic, and can be of low signal intensity on T2W MR images. Biopsy is usually necessary to confirm the diagnosis.

Gout is characterized by deposition of monosodium urate or urate acid crystals in joints and soft tissues.[108] Radiologists are familiar with the classic radiographic features of calcified tophi and erosion of adjacent bone with overhanging spicules that affect the peripheral joints. However, tophaceous gout can result in masses and bone destruction that mimic malignancy when occurring in unusual locations or isolated and robust. For example, spinal gout, a rare manifestation of the disease, can form paraspinal masses and lytic lesions that at first glance have the appearance of malignancy (Fig. 17). Gout is typically evident elsewhere in such patients, and therefore physical examination should include assessment of the peripheral joints.[108,109] Gouty tophi can also present as masses on MR imaging. Intermediate signal intensity on T1W images is the norm.[110]

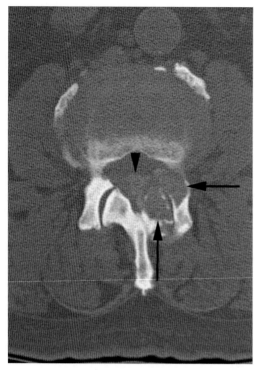

Fig. 17. 71-year-old man with colon cancer referred with spinal lesions. Transverse CT image of the lumbar spine shows lucent lesions (*arrows*) along the facet joint eroding the lamina and pedicle. Note faint calcification of adjacent tophus (*arrowhead*) in spinal canal compatible with gout. Multiple joint-based gouty erosions and tophi were present at other spinal levels (*not shown*), but no vertebral body lesions were evident to suggest metastases.

Although the signal intensity of gouty masses on T2W images is variable, low signal intensity is a characteristic feature that likely corresponds to calcifications. Most tophi enhance homogeneously after intravenous administration of contrast. Intraosseous tophi can manifest as lytic lesions of bone.[111] Such lesions may be accompanied by a soft tissue mass with calcifications.[112] If the lesion is of low signal intensity on T2W MR images or shows internal calcification on CT, then the diagnosis of gout may be entertained in the proper clinical setting.[111]

Other depositional arthritic diseases are less likely to produce findings that are mistaken for tumor. Calcium pyrophosphate dihydrate crystal deposition disease can occasionally result in tophaceous pseudogout, which, like gout, may result in a mass that mimics a soft tissue malignancy.[113] Hydroxyapatite deposition can result in calcific pseudotumors in tendons and bursae that erode into bone, mimicking a destructive neoplasm.[64] Amyloid deposition may also result

in juxta-articular or peritendinous soft tissue masses, as well as a destructive arthropathy that is typically bilateral and most frequently affects the shoulders, hips, knees, and wrists.[106] Amyloid deposits, like tophi, are characterized by low to intermediate signal intensity on MR imaging that may enhance with contrast.

Two additional joint-based entities that deserve a brief mention despite appropriate referral to our orthopedic oncology clinic are pigmented villonodular synovitis (PVNS) and synovial osteochondromatosis. PVNS is a benign, typically monoarticular proliferative disorder of synovium that can manifest as either a masslike diffuse process or focal form within a joint.[106] The intra-articular nature of the disease, combined with characteristic low signal intensity on T2W MR images as a result of hemosiderin deposition, usually allows for a proper diagnosis (**Fig. 18**). Synovial osteochondromatosis is another benign monoarticular disorder of uncertain cause characterized by metaplastic transformation of the synovium with formation of multiple intrasynovial and intra-articular cartilaginous nodules.[106] When the nodules become calcified or ossified,

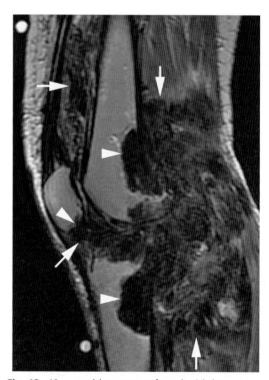

Fig. 18. 40-year-old woman referred with knee mass. Sagittal T2W MR image of the knee shows extensive low signal intensity material within the knee joint and extending into the surrounding soft tissues, compatible with PVNS (*arrows*). Note erosions of the femur, tibia, and patella (*arrowheads*).

the radiographic picture of multiple intra-articular bodies of uniform size is virtually pathognomonic. On MR imaging, the process has a variable appearance, ranging from a noncalcified intra-articular conglomerate mass that is isointense to skeletal muscle on T1W images and hyperintense on T2W images, to clusters of nodules containing hypointense calcification or mature bone with fatty marrow (**Fig. 19**).

Bursae, Recesses, Ganglia, and Cysts

A bursa is generally defined as a synovium-lined compartment separate from a joint, whereas a synovial recess is a synovium-lined extension of the joint cavity. However, this distinction is not always clear-cut, because what constitutes a bursa embryologically may appear at later imaging studies as a synovial recess and vice versa[114] Some investigators use the term synovial cyst to encompass both synovial recess and bursa. Distension of a bursa or synovial recess can result in a mass at physical examination. Proper diagnosis of a distended bursa or recess on imaging studies requires the radiologist to be familiar with bursal/recess anatomy and extent. For example, the diagnosis of a Baker cyst, representing distension of the gastrocnemius-semimembranosus bursa/recess, can be confidently made if one sees a fluid collection in the posteromedial knee with extension toward the joint between the distal tendon of the semimembranosus and the proximal tendon of the medial head of the gastrocnemius muscle. In our experience, distension of less commonly encountered bursa, such as the bicipitoradial bursa of the

elbow and the obturator externus bursa of the hip, is more likely to result in erroneous diagnosis of neoplasm (**Fig. 20**). Another synovial-lined mass that is not uncommonly mistaken for tumor is the acromioclavicular joint cyst, which results in a prominent bump on the superior aspect of the shoulder; usually communication with the acromioclavicular joint is evident on imaging studies,[115] and an association with extensive rotator cuff tearing is typical. When bursae and recesses are distended with homogeneous fluid, a correct diagnosis can be confidently made on cross-sectional imaging studies, including sonography. Peripheral enhancement is noted after intravenous injection of contrast agents; thickened enhancing synovial lining is not uncommon in inflammatory conditions. Loose bodies, blood products, rice bodies, or other material (eg, resulting from chronic synovitis or infection) filling the bursa/recess may produce a more heterogeneous appearance that can lead to an incorrect diagnosis of neoplasm, particularly if associated with pressure erosion of adjacent bone. Radiography or ultrasonography can help confirm the presence of calcified or ossified loose bodies in certain circumstances and allow for a proper diagnosis.

Ganglia are masses of uncertain pathogenesis containing myxoid material surrounded by connective tissue.[116] Although they typically occur near joints, they are not lined by synovium. Juxta-articular ganglia are most commonly found in the hands and feet, often adjacent to tendons. On imaging studies, ganglia typically appear as fluid-filled cystlike masses, although often multilobulated with thin septations (**Fig. 21**). On occasion, ganglia may show intermediate or even high signal

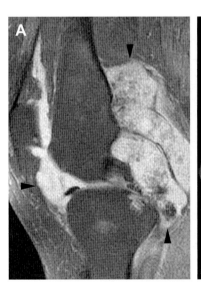
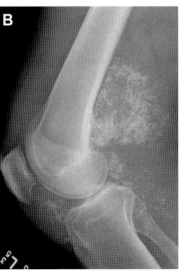

Fig. 19. Young man referred with knee mass. (*A*) Sagittal T2W MR image of the knee with fat suppression shows a hyperintense joint-based conglomerate mass (*arrowheads*). (*B*) Lateral radiograph of the knee shows innumerable joint-based calcifications compatible with synovial chondromatosis.

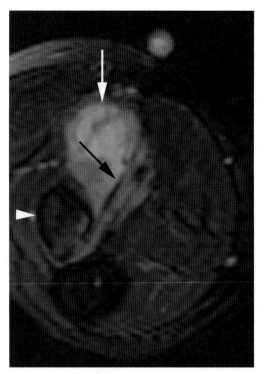

Fig. 20. 27-year-old woman with rheumatoid arthritis referred with anterior elbow mass. Fat-suppressed transverse T2W MR image shows a collection of heterogeneous high signal intensity (*white arrow*) surrounding the distal biceps tendon (*black arrow*) and extending between the tendon and the cortex of the proximal radius (*white arrowhead*), compatible with distension of the bicipitoradial bursa. T1W images obtained after intravenous administration of gadolinium chelate (*not shown*) revealed peripheral enhancement of the collection supporting the diagnosis of bicipitoradial bursitis. No progression was noted on follow-up imaging.

intensity on T1W MR images, and internal echoes on sonography are not uncommon.[58] Thin peripheral and septal enhancement may be noted after contrast administration. Most ganglia are small, but they may extend into muscle or cause pressure erosion of adjacent bone. Ganglia may also occur within joints (eg, adjacent to or within the cruciate ligaments of the knee). Parameniscal and paralabral cysts have similar appearances to ganglia, but are typically associated with meniscal and labral tears, respectively.[58,117,118]

Intraosseous ganglia typically form subchondral lucent lesions with sclerotic margins on radiographs of adult patients with little evidence of arthritis. They may be primarily intraosseous or may arise by penetration of soft tissue ganglia into the underlying bone.[119] They most frequently

involve the medial malleolus, the proximal tibia, the proximal femur, and the carpal bones. Chondroblastomas may have a similar appearance, but typically arise in children, are associated with adjacent marrow edema on MR imaging, and may contain internal calcifications. Giant cell tumors also extend to the subchondral bone, but typically are larger and usually do not form sclerotic margins.

Cystic adventitial disease is characterized by cystic degeneration of a peripheral artery that can present clinically as claudication and pain but also with a soft tissue mass that can be mistaken for sarcoma.[120] The popliteal artery is most commonly affected. Imaging studies typically show multiple cystlike lesions in the arterial wall that may be associated with compromise of the lumen.

The keys to diagnosing benign ganglia, cysts, bursae, and recesses are knowing their common locations and recognizing the typically homogeneous fluidlike nature on cross-sectional imaging studies. Enhancement should be minimal or restricted to a thin rim of peripheral and occasionally septal enhancement. Certain soft tissue malignancies, such as myxoid liposarcoma and synovial sarcoma, can be mistaken for benign cystlike lesions on unenhanced studies; however, they tend to show more heterogeneous or nodular/solid contrast enhancement than do recesses, bursae, and cysts.

OTHER MIMICS OF NEOPLASM
Osteoporosis

Osteoporosis refers to loss of bone mass and is characterized on radiographs by increased radiolucency of bone, cortical thinning, altered trabecular pattern, and ultimately fractures and deformity.[121] Benign vertebral compression fractures of osteoporosis may be difficult to distinguish from compression fractures caused by malignancy. Findings suggesting malignant collapse include location in the upper thoracic region, pedicle or neural arch involvement, and involvement of multiple discontinuous vertebrae. Malignant collapse may be associated with a focal lytic or sclerotic lesion and a paravertebral mass. A bulging posterior border with smooth contours is also an indicator of malignant collapse, whereas collapse as a result of osteoporosis typically results in a posterior border that is concave or has sharp angular margins. MR imaging can assist in distinguishing benign from malignant collapse. For example, compression fractures caused by malignancy often are associated with complete loss of normal marrow signal in the involved vertebra. Chronic benign osteoporotic

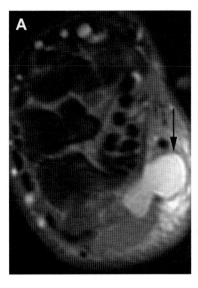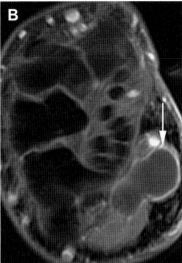

Fig. 21. 38-year-old man referred with wrist mass. (*A*) Transverse T2W MR image of the wrist shows a lobulated homogeneous mass (*arrow*) of fluid signal intensity volar to the hook of the hamate bone. (*B*) Fat-suppressed transverse T1W MR image after intravenous administration of gadolinium chelate shows peripheral enhancement of the mass (*arrow*). The findings are compatible with a ganglion of the Guyon canal.

fractures typically show normal marrow signal intensity, and with acute osteoporotic fractures, low signal intensity on T1W images is usually restricted to the bandlike area of the fracture line. Diffusion-weighted imaging has been successfully used by some investigators for the differentiation of benign and malignant vertebral compression fractures.[122]

Regional osteoporosis may either be the result of disuse of an extremity or a family of conditions that may be grouped under the term bone marrow edema syndrome. With disuse osteoporosis, spotty demineralization of bone resulting from formation of large intertrabecular spaces can simulate the permeative destructive process of neoplastic involvement.[123] However, the extent of bone involvement tends to be better marginated with neoplasm than with disuse osteoporosis. In confusing cases, MR imaging can easily distinguish between osteoporosis, with its fatty marrow, and tumor. Bone marrow edema syndrome includes conditions such as regional migratory osteoporosis, transient osteoporosis of the hip, and reflex sympathetic dystrophy (complex regional pain syndrome).[124] The pathogenesis of these conditions is not clear. On radiographs, they share an eventual onset of periarticular bone demineralization that occurs 3 to 6 weeks after symptoms arise. MR imaging shows edema before osteoporosis seen on radiographs or CT. Marrow edema may or may not be present with reflex sympathetic dystrophy; when present, the process often involves multiple bones in a juxta-articular distribution. Transient osteoporosis (edema) of the hip and regional migratory osteoporosis

(edema) are probably related entities. Like neoplasms, these conditions result in bone marrow edema; however, a discrete tumor focus is not evident on MR imaging.

Hyperparathyroidism and Renal Osteodystrophy

Primary hyperparathyroidism is most often caused by a parathyroid adenoma, and less commonly by parathyroid hyperplasia or carcinoma. Generalized skeletal demineralization is a common finding that, when profound, can mimic diffuse skeletal metastases or multiple myeloma.[125] Brown tumors may be encountered in patients with long-standing hyperparathyroidism,[126] commonly affecting the pelvis, ribs, femur, and mandible. The lesions are radiolucent and may result in expansile remodeling of the bone (**Fig. 22**). Multiple Brown tumors can mimic metastases, multiple myeloma, histiocytoses, leukemia, and other polyostotic processes. However, with Brown tumors, other features of hyperparathyroidism, including acro-osteolysis and subperiosteal resorption, almost invariably affect the skeleton. Serum biochemistry also aids in the diagnosis.

Renal osteodystrophy refers to the skeletal manifestations of chronic renal failure and encompasses not only hyperparathyroidism (secondary) but also osteomalacia, osteoporosis, and soft tissue calcification.[127] Brown tumors can occur with renal osteodystrophy, and although classically associated with primary hyperparathyroidism, may be encountered more frequently with secondary hyperparathyroidism because of the

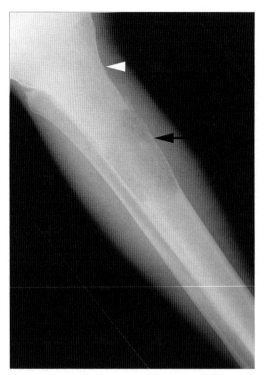

Fig. 22. 33-year-old man with hyperparathyroidism complaining of leg pain after trauma. Anteroposterior radiograph of the leg reveals a lucent lesion (*arrow*) in the proximal tibial diaphysis with a pathologic fracture. Note subperiosteal resorption along the medial aspect of proximal tibial metaphysis (*arrowhead*), indicating hyperparathyroidism. The lesion was presumed to represent a Brown tumor, and additional Brown tumors were noted elsewhere in the patient's skeleton on other radiographs (*not shown*).

larger number of patients with renal failure than with primary parathyroid disease. Lytic bone lesions may also result from amyloid deposition in patients on long-term hemodialysis[128]; unlike metastases or myeloma, amyloidomas typically occur in a juxta-articular distribution. Discovertebral amyloid deposits can result in a destructive spondyloarthropathy that may be more difficult to distinguish from neoplasm if the history of long-term dialysis is not provided. Periosteal new bone formation (periosteal neostosis) occurs in some patients with renal osteodystrophy, and when robust can mimic a neoplasm; however, it is accompanied by other findings such as subperiosteal resorption and osteosclerosis of the central skeleton, indicating a relationship with renal osteodystrophy.[129] Soft tissue calcification may also be robust, particularly about the joints, where masslike deposition of calcium may occur. Although occasionally lumped into the category of tumoral calcinosis, the argument has been made that the term tumoral calcinosis more precisely refers to a familial condition of phosphate metabolic dysfunction, also characterized by calcified periarticular masses, in patients with normal serum calcium levels but increased serum phosphate levels[130]; however, there are no radiologic differences between the masslike calcinosis of chronic renal failure and that of familial tumoral calcinosis. Calcinosis of chronic renal failure typically appears multilobulated, amorphous, and often cystic with fluid levels as a result of calcium sedimentation, and is located in a periarticular distribution; it may diminish in size after hemodialysis. Although soft tissue sarcomas may calcify as well, usually the calcification involves only a portion of the tumor. Calcinosis of renal failure may also mimic parosteal or soft tissue osteosarcoma; involvement of bone or the presence of a noncalcified component of the mass favors neoplasm.

Paget Disease

The true cause of Paget disease is uncertain, but chronic viral infection of bone has been suggested. Paget disease is rare in individuals less than 40 years of age but affects up to 10% of individuals more than 70 years of age. The disease is characterized by abnormal osteoclast and osteoblast activity, leading to accelerated bone turnover and irregular new bone deposition.[131] Paget disease may be polyostotic or monostotic, and is usually asymptomatic. It is most commonly encountered in the pelvis, but the remainder of the skeleton (particularly the axial skeleton and the proximal femur) is also frequently involved. Paget disease is typically recognized on radiographs based on its imaging features, which in turn depend on the phase of the disease. The active or lytic phase is characterized by osteoporosis circumscripta in the skull, and flame-shaped or blade-of-grass osteolysis in the long bones extending from the epiphysis along the diaphysis. The inactive or sclerotic phase is characterized by cortical thickening, trabecular coarsening, and bone enlargement. In the skull and spine, this situation can create appearances (cotton wool skull, ivory vertebra) that can be mistaken for sclerotic metastases or other bone-forming processes. Not uncommonly, an intermediate or mixed phase is encountered, with both lytic and sclerotic components. Although the radiographic findings are usually diagnostic, radiologists may mistake Paget disease for neoplasm if the patient is unusually young or if the process occurs in an atypical location (**Fig. 23**). Diffuse enlargement of the bone or bowing deformities may aid in the correct

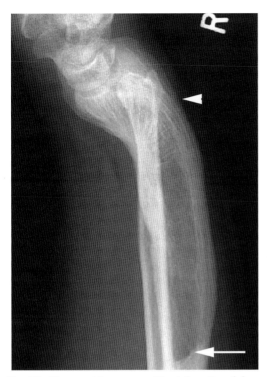

Fig. 23. 64-year-old woman with deformity of forearm and suspicion of tumor. Lateral radiograph of the distal forearm shows the advancing lytic front (*arrow*) typical of the active phase of Paget disease and cortical and trabecular thickening (*arrowhead*) typical of the sclerotic phase, as well as bowing and expansile remodeling of the distal radius.

diagnosis of Paget disease. Increased uptake on isotope bone scans is typical. Clues to the diagnosis include involvement of the whole bone (particularly the pelvis, vertebra, and scapula) and uptake extending from the articular end of a long bone along the diaphysis with a V-shaped leading edge.[132] Paget disease can also result in increased uptake on PET studies.[133] Although CT and MR imaging are usually not necessary for the diagnosis of Paget disease, these modalities may help clarify the diagnosis in confusing cases. The marrow spaces in pagetic bone usually have a density or signal intensity similar to that of fat (or hematopoietic marrow), unlike neoplasm.[134] However, in the active phase, vascular tissue may predominate in the pagetic marrow, resulting in increased signal intensity on fluid-sensitive MR imaging sequences.[135] Elements that are more sclerotic may appear as intermediate signal intensity or low signal intensity areas on T1W images. The presence of small fatty foci supports the diagnosis of Paget disease. Marrow edema in the setting of underlying Paget disease could be

caused by fracture. Sarcoma arising within pagetic bone is a well-recognized but uncommon complication, occurring in less than 1% of patients[136]; radiographic evidence of bone destruction and an associated soft tissue mass are evident in most patients with sarcoma at the time of presentation.

Hemophilic Pseudotumor

Hemophilic pseudotumor represents a slowly expanding mass resulting from recurrent hemorrhage.[137] Intraosseous pseudotumors form osteolytic lesions, typically with well-defined margins and often associated with expansile remodeling of the bone. Subperiosteal pseudotumors result from hemorrhage that has elevated the periosteum and causes pressure necrosis of the underlying bone. Such pseudotumors may extend into the adjacent soft tissue and produce an aggressive-appearing periosteal reaction that can mimic malignancy. Soft tissue pseudotumors are most common in the thigh, gluteal region, and iliopsoas muscle, but may be intramuscular or extramuscular. On MR imaging, fluid-filled lesions with complex signal reflecting recurrent hemorrhage (blood products of various stages of evolution) and clot organization are typical, with low and high signal intensity areas on both T1W and T2W images. Adjacent hemophilic arthropathy can also be a clue to the diagnosis.

Aneurysms

Large aneurysms and pseudoaneurysms can mimic soft tissue neoplasms in the extremities. Clues to the diagnosis include pulsatility, complex signal intensity on T1W and T2W MR images caused by blood products of varying ages often resulting in a laminated appearance,[57] and recognition of continuity with an artery. Sonography is useful in distinguishing aneurysm from tumor.

Melorheostosis

Melorheostosis is an uncommon, benign sclerosing skeletal dysplasia of uncertain cause.[138] The disease may involve 1 bone or multiple bones, usually in a sclerotomal distribution in 1 limb. The characteristic radiographic appearance is that of cortical hyperostosis along 1 side of a long bone resembling melting wax. In later stages, endosteal hyperostosis can obliterate the medullary cavity. The polyostotic form of the disease, with eccentric hyperostosis along a sclerotomal distribution, is usually not a diagnostic dilemma because of its classic radiographic appearance. However, the monostotic form of the disease can have a more variable appearance, and can mimic a bone-forming tumor (**Fig. 24**). Hyperostosis rather than bone destruction is the rule for melorheostosis, which can aid in distinguishing this entity from an osteosarcoma. A potentially confusing variable is associated soft tissue mass formation, particularly near the joints, consisting of osseous, chondroid, vascular, and fibrocartilaginous tissue. These masses may or may not be mineralized, and may or may not be contiguous with the hyperostostic cortex. The MR imaging appearance of these masses is variable, and heterogeneity of signal is the norm. Many show infiltrating margins and enhancement.

Sarcoidosis

Sarcoidosis is a disease of unknown cause, likely caused by an immune response to an unknown antigen. It can involve the skeleton in up to 10% of cases. Usually sarcoidosis affects the small bones of the hands and feet, manifesting radiographically as a lacelike trabecular pattern or granulomatous punched-out lucent lesions. Occasionally, the disease can progress to a highly

destructive form with profound cortical loss mimicking an aggressive tumor, although periosteal reaction is uncommon. Sclerotic lesions are another atypical presentation. Sarcoidosis involving larger bones can resemble metastatic disease and myeloma.[139] Some intramedullary lesions in large bones may also contain central areas corresponding to fat or form a convex margin with marrow fat.[140] In muscles, sarcoidosis can result in nodular masses; a central low signal intensity dark star appearance surrounded by a bright rim has been described on T2W images. Up to 90% of patients with sarcoid involvement of bone have disease elsewhere, particularly in the lungs or mediastinum, which can help secure a more confident diagnosis of the disease.[76]

SUMMARY

Referral of patients with nonneoplastic pseudotumors to the orthopedic oncology clinic is not uncommon.[141,142] The list of entities that can potentially mimic bone and soft tissue tumors is extensive. Radiologists should be aware of these mimics and understand the features that distinguish them from neoplasm. However, in many cases, it is not possible to definitively exclude malignancy. Patients with a suspected bone or soft tissue tumor should be referred to specialists at an orthopedic oncology clinic who are experts in the care of such patients.

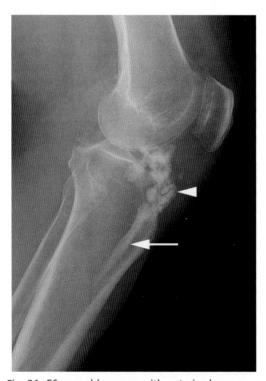

Fig. 24. 56-year-old woman with anterior knee mass. Lateral radiograph of the knee shows lobulated ossification (*arrowhead*) in the fat pad of Hoffa. Bandlike sclerosis in the anterior tibia (*arrow*) extending inferiorly from the soft tissue abnormality is compatible with melorheostosis, which was confirmed with biopsy in this patient.

REFERENCES

1. Keats TE, Anderson MW. The lower extremity. In: Keats TE, Anderson MW, editors. Atlas of normal Roentgen variants that may simulate disease. 8th edition. Philadelphia: Mosby Elsevier; 2007. p. 655–978.
2. Tehranzadeh J. The spectrum of avulsion and avulsion-like injuries of the musculoskeletal system. Radiographics 1987;7:945–74.
3. Kontogeorgakos VA, Xenakis T, Papachristou D, et al. Cortical desmoids and the four clinical scenarios. Arch Orthop Trauma Surg 2009;129:779–85.
4. La Rocca Vieira R, Bencardino JT, Rosenberg ZS, et al. MRI features of cortical desmoids in acute knee trauma. AJR Am J Roentgenol 2011;196:424–8.
5. Resnick D, Greenway G. Distal femoral cortical defects, irregularities, and excavations. Radiology 1982;143:345–54.
6. Suh J, Cho J, Shin K, et al. MR appearance of distal femoral cortical irregularity (cortical desmoid). J Comput Assist Tomogr 1996;20:328–32.
7. Goodin GS, Shulkin BL, Kaufman RA, et al. PET/ CT characterization of fibroosseous defects in

children: 18F-FDG uptake can mimic metastatic disease. AJR Am J Roentgenol 2006;187:1124–8.

8. Keats TE, Joyce JM. Metaphyseal cortical irregularities in children: a new perspective on a multi-focal growth variant. Skeletal Radiol 1984;12:112–8.

9. Ozonoff MB, Ziter FM. The upper humeral notch. Radiology 1974;113:699–701.

10. Ozonoff MB, Ziter FM. The upper femoral notch. Skeletal Radiol 1985;14:198–9.

11. Fulton MN, Albright JP, El-Khoury GY. Cortical desmoid-like lesion of the proximal humerus and its occurrence in gymnasts (ringman's shoulder lesion). Am J Sports Med 1979;7:57–61.

12. Brower A. Cortical defect of the humerus at the insertion of the pectoralis major. AJR Am J Roentgenol 1977;128:677–8.

13. Donnelly LF, Helms CA, Bisset GS. Chronic avulsive injury of the deltoid insertion in adolescents: imaging findings in three cases. Radiology 1999; 211:233–6.

14. Morgan H, Damron T, Cohen H, et al. Pseudotumor deltoideus: a previously undescribed anatomic variant at the deltoid insertion site. Skeletal Radiol 2001;30:512–8.

15. Keats TE, Anderson MW. The upper extremity. In: Keats TE, Anderson MW, editors. Atlas of normal Roentgen variants that may simulate disease. 8th edition. Philadelphia: Mosby Elsevier; 2007. p. 507–654.

16. Keats TE, Anderson MW. The pelvic girdle. In: Keats TE, Anderson MW, editors. Atlas of normal Roentgen variants that may simulate disease. 8th edition. Philadelphia: Mosby Elsevier; 2007. p. 373–414.

17. De Wilde V, De Maeseneer M, Lenchik L, et al. Normal osseous variants presenting as cystic or lucent areas on radiography and CT imaging: a pictorial overview. Eur J Radiol 2004;51:77–84.

18. Fink-Bennett D, Vicuna-Rios J. The deltoid tuberosity–a potential pitfall (the "delta sign") in bone scan interpretation. J Nucl Med 1980;21:211–2.

19. Yekeler E, Tunaci M, Tunaci A, et al. Frequency of sternal variations and anomalies evaluated by MDCT. AJR Am J Roentgenol 2006;186:956–60.

20. Pate D, Kursunoglu S, Resnick D, et al. Scapular foramina. Skeletal Radiol 1985;14:270–5.

21. Cigtay OS, Mascatello VJ. Scapular defects: a normal variation. AJR Am J Roentgenol 1979;132:239–41.

22. Paraskevas G, Natsis K, Spanidou S, et al. Excavated-type of rhomboid fossa of the clavicle: a radiological study. Folia Morphol (Warsz) 2009; 68:163–6.

23. Keats TE, Anderson MW. The shoulder girdle and thoracic cage. In: Keats TE, Anderson MW, editors. Atlas of normal Roentgen variants that may simulate disease. 8th edition. Philadelphia: Mosby Elsevier; 2007. p. 415–506.

24. Pitt MJ, Graham AR, Shipman JH, et al. Herniation pit of the femoral neck. AJR Am J Roentgenol 1982; 138:1115–21.

25. Nokes SR, Vogler JB, Spritzer CE, et al. Herniation pits of the femoral neck: appearance at MR imaging. Radiology 1989;172:231–4.

26. Kim JA, Park JS, Jin W, et al. Herniation pits in the femoral neck: a radiographic indicator of femoroacetabular impingement? Skeletal Radiol 2011;40: 167–72.

27. Tannast M, Siebenrock KA, Anderson SE. Femoroacetabular impingement: radiographic diagnosis–what the radiologist should know. AJR Am J Roentgenol 2007;188:1540–52.

28. Monu JU, De Smet AA. Case report 789. Skeletal Radiol 1993;22:528–31.

29. Haswell DM, Berne AS, Graham CB. The dorsal defect of the patella. Pediatr Radiol 1976;4:238–42.

30. Ho VB, Kransdorf MJ, Jelinek JS, et al. Dorsal defect of the patella: MR features. J Comput Assist Tomogr 1991;15:474–6.

31. Wu HT, Morrison WB, Schweitzer ME. Edematous Schmorl's nodes on thoracolumbar MR imaging: characteristic patterns and changes over time. Skeletal Radiol 2006;35:212–9.

32. Resnick D, Niwayama G. Intravertebral disk herniations: cartilaginous (Schmorl's) nodes. Radiology 1978;126:57–65.

33. Hauger O, Cotton A, Chateil JF. Giant cystic Schmorl's nodes: imaging findings in six patients. AJR Am J Roentgenol 2001;176:969–72.

34. Herneth AM, Philipp MO, Pretterklieber ML, et al. Asymmetric closure of ischiopubic synchondrosis in pediatric patients: correlation with foot dominance. AJR Am J Roentgenol 2004;182:361–5.

35. Herneth AM, Trattnig S, Bader TR, et al. MR imaging of the ischiopubic synchondrosis. Magn Reson Imaging 2000;18:519–24.

36. Helms CA. Pseudocysts of the humerus. AJR Am J Roentgenol 1978;131:287–8.

37. Diard F, Hauger O, Moinard M, et al. Pseudocysts, lipomas, infarcts and simple cysts of the calcaneus: are there different or related lesions? JBR-BTR 2007;90:315–24.

38. Smith RW, Smith CF. Solitary unicameral bone cyst of the calcaneus. J Bone Joint Surg Am 1974;56: 49–56.

39. Sookur PA, Naraghi AM, Bleakney RR, et al. Accessory muscles: anatomy, symptoms, and radiologic evaluation. Radiographics 2008;28:481–99.

40. Bianchi S, Abdelwahab IF, Oliveri M, et al. Sonographic diagnosis of accessory soleus muscle mimicking a soft tissue tumor. J Ultrasound Med 1995;14:707–9.

41. Paul MA, Imanse J, Golding RP, et al. Accessory soleus muscle mimicking a soft tissue tumor. A report of 2 patients. Acta Orthop Scand 1991;62:609–11.

42. Hwang S, Panicek DM. Magnetic resonance imaging of bone marrow in oncology, part 1. Skeletal Radiol 2007;36:913–20.

43. Lang P, Fritz R, Majumdar S, et al. Hematopoietic bone marrow in the adult knee: spin-echo and opposed-phase gradient echo MR imaging. Skeletal Radiol 1993;22:95–103.

44. Long SS, Yablon CM, Eisenberg RL. Bone marrow signal alteration in the spine and sacrum. AJR Am J Roentgenol 2010;195:W178–200.

45. Krestan C, Hojreh A. Imaging of insufficiency fractures. Eur J Radiol 2009;71:398–405.

46. Fayad LM, Kawamoto S, Kamel I, et al. Distinction of long bone stress fractures from pathologic fractures on cross-sectional imaging: how successful are we? AJR Am J Roentgenol 2005;185:915–24.

47. Fottner A, Baur-Melnyk A, Birkenmaier C, et al. Stress fractures presenting as tumours: a retrospective analysis of 22 cases. Int Orthop 2009;33:489–92.

48. Mulligan ME. The "gray cortex": an early sign of stress fracture. Skeletal Radiol 1995;24:201–3.

49. Gaeta M, Minutoli F, Scribano E, et al. CT and MR imaging findings in athletes with early tibial stress injuries: comparison with bone scintigraphy findings and emphasis on cortical abnormalities. Radiology 2005;235:553–61.

50. Brahme SK, Cervilla V, Vint V, et al. Magnetic resonance appearance of sacral insufficiency fractures. Skeletal Radiol 1990;19:489–93.

51. Disler DG, McCauley TR, Ratner LM, et al. In-phase and out-of-phase MR imaging of bone marrow: prediction of neoplasia based on the detection of coexistent fat and water. AJR Am J Roentgenol 1997;169:1439–47.

52. Houshian S, Pedersen NW, Torfing T, et al. Post-traumatic cortical cysts in paediatric fractures: is it a concern for emergency doctors? A report of three cases. Eur J Emerg Med 2007;14:365–7.

53. Papadimitriou NG, Christophorides J, Beslikas TA, et al. Post-traumatic cystic lesion following fracture of the radius. Skeletal Radiol 2005;34:411–4.

54. Giaroli EL, Major NM, Higgins LD. MRI of internal impingement of the shoulder. AJR Am J Roentgenol 2005;185:925–9.

55. Marshall KW, Marshall DL, Busch MT, et al. Osteochondral lesions of the humeral trochlea in the young athlete. Skeletal Radiol 2009;38:479–91.

56. Bush CH. The magnetic resonance imaging of musculoskeletal hemorrhage. Skeletal Radiol 2000;29:1–9.

57. McKenzie G, Raby N, Ritchie D. Non-neoplastic soft-tissue masses. Br J Radiol 2009;82:775–85.

58. Navarro OM. Imaging of benign pediatric soft tissue tumors. Semin Musculoskelet Radiol 2009;13:196–209.

59. Stein-Wexler R. MR imaging of soft tissues masses in children. Magn Reson Imaging Clin N Am 2009;17:489–507.

60. Boutin RD, Fritz RC, Steinbach LS. Imaging of sports-related muscle injuries. Radiol Clin North Am 2002;40:333–62.

61. Ward WG, Rougraff B, Quinn R, et al. Tumors masquerading as hematomas. Clin Orthop Relat Res 2007;465:232–40.

62. Imaizumi S, Morita T, Ogose A, et al. Soft tissue sarcoma mimicking chronic hematoma: value of magnetic resonance imaging in differential diagnosis. J Orthop Sci 2002;7:33–7.

63. Bencardino JT, Rosenberg ZS, Brown RR, et al. Traumatic musculotendinous injuries of the knee: diagnosis with MR imaging. Radiographics 2000;20:S103–20.

64. Anderson SE, Hertel R, Johnston JO, et al. Latissimus dorsi tendinosis and tear: imaging features of a pseudotumor of the upper limb in five patients. AJR Am J Roentgenol 2005;185:1145–51.

65. Resnick JM, Carrasco CH, Edeiken J, et al. Avulsion fracture of the anterior inferior iliac spine with abundant reactive ossification in the soft tissue. Skeletal Radiol 1996;25:580–4.

66. Rosenberg AE. Myositis ossificans and fibroosseous pseudotumor of digits. In: Fletcher CD, Unni KK, Mertens F, editors. World Health Organization Classification of Tumours. Pathology and genetics of tumours of soft tissue and bone. Lyon (France): IARC Press; 2002. p. 52–4.

67. Gindele A, Schwanborn D, Tsironis K, et al. Myositis ossificans traumatic in young children: report of three cases and review of the literature. Pediatr Radiol 2000;30:451–9.

68. Parikh J, Hyare H, Saifuddin A. The imaging features of post-traumatic myositis ossificans with emphasis on MRI. Clin Radiol 2002;57:1058–66.

69. Mellado JM, Bencardino JT. Morel-Lavallée lesion: review with emphasis on MR imaging. Magn Reson Imaging Clin N Am 2005;13:775–82.

70. Borrero CG, Maxwell N, Kavanagh E. MRI findings of prepatellar Morel-Lavallée effusions. Skeletal Radiol 2008;37:451–5.

71. Mellado JM, del Palomar LP, Diaz L, et al. Long-standing Morel-Lavallée lesions of the trochanteric region and proximal thigh: MRI features in five patients. AJR Am J Roentgenol 2004;182:1289–94.

72. Anderson SE, Johnston JO, Steinbach LS. Pseudotumors of the shoulder invited review. Eur J Radiol 2008;68:147–58.

73. Lazarides S, Roysam SG, DeKiewiet G. Acute bone infection resembling neoplasia. Two unusual cases. Eur J Orthop Surg Traumatol 2005;15:247–50.

74. Mathur K, Nazir AA, Sumathi VP, et al. Ewing's sarcoma masquerading as chronic osteomyelitis: a case report. Eur J Orthop Surg Traumatol 2006;16:175–7.

75. Bohndorf K. Infection of the appendicular skeleton. Eur Radiol 2004;14:E53–63.

76. Reinus WR. Imaging approach to musculoskel-etal infections. In: Bonakdarpour A, Reinus WR, Khurana JS, editors. Diagnostic imaging of muscu-loskeletal diseases: a systematic approach. New York: Springer; 2010. p. 363–405.

77. Blickman JG, van Die CE, de Rooy JWJ. Current imaging concepts in pediatric osteomyelitis. Eur Radiol 2004;14:L55–64.

78. Marti-Bonmati L, Aparisi F, Poyatos C, et al. Brodie abscess: MR imaging appearance in 10 patients. J Magn Reson Imaging 1993;3:543–6.

79. Grey AC, Davies AM, Mangham DC, et al. The 'penumbra sign' on T1-weighted MR imaging in subacute osteomyelitis: frequency, cause and significance. Clin Radiol 1998;53:587–92.

80. McGuinness B, Wilson N, Doyle AJ. The "penumbra sign" on T1-weighted MRI for differenti-ating musculoskeletal infection from tumor. Skeletal Radiol 2007;36:417–21.

81. Shimose S, Sugita T, Kubo T, et al. Differential diag-nosis between osteomyelitis and bone tumor. Acta Radiol 2008;49:928–33.

82. Mulligan ME, Kransdorf MJ. Sequestra in primary lymphoma of bone: prevalence and radiologic features. AJR Am J Roentgenol 1993;160: 1245–8.

83. Khanna G, Sato TS, Ferguson P. Imaging of chronic recurrent multifocal osteomyelitis. Radiographics 2009;29:1159–77.

84. Turecki MB, Taljanovic MS, Stubbs AY, et al. Imaging of musculoskeletal soft tissue infections. Skeletal Radiol 2010;39:957–71.

85. Gaskill T, Payne D, Brigman B. Cryptococcal abscess imitating a soft-tissue sarcoma in an immunocompetent host: a case report. J Bone Joint Surg Am 2010;92:1890–3.

86. Harish S, Chiavaras MM, Kotnis N, et al. MR imaging of skeletal soft tissue infection: utility of diffusion-weighted imaging in detecting abscess formation. Skeletal Radiol 2011;40:285–94.

87. May DA, Disler DG, Jones EA, et al. Abnormal signal intensity in skeletal muscle at MR imaging: patterns, pearls and pitfalls. Radiographics 2000; 20:S295–315.

88. Soler R, Rodriguez E, Aguilera C, et al. Magnetic resonance imaging of pyomyositis in 43 cases. Eur J Radiol 2000;35:59–64.

89. Trusen A, Beissert M, Schultz G, et al. Ultrasound and MRI features of pyomyositis in children. Eur Radiol 2003;13:1050–5.

90. Chun CW, Jee WH, Park HJ, et al. MRI features of skeletal muscle lymphoma. AJR Am J Roentgenol 2010;195:1355–60.

91. Wang CW, Chang WC, Chao TK, et al. Computed tomography and magnetic resonance imaging of cat-scratch disease: a report of two cases. Clin Imaging 2009;33:318–21.

92. Baron AL, Steinbach LS, LeBoit PE, et al. Osteolytic lesions and bacillary angiomatosis in HIV infection: radiologic differentiation from AIDS-related Kaposi sarcoma. Radiology 1990;177:77–81.

93. Jaramillo D. What is the optimal imaging of osteo-necrosis, Perthes, and bone infarcts? Pediatr Ra-diol 2009;39:S216–9.

94. Munk PL, Helms CA, Holt RG. Immature bone infarcts: findings on plain radiographs and MR scans. AJR Am J Roentgenol 1989;152:547–9.

95. Resnick D, Sweet DE, Madewell JE. Osteonecrosis: pathogenesis, diagnostic techniques, specific situ-ations, and complications. In: Resnick D, editor. Diagnosis of bone and joint disorders. 4th edition. Philadelphia: Saunders; 2002. p. 3599–685.

96. Saini A, Saifuddin A. MRI of osteonecrosis. Clin Ra-diol 2004;59:1079–93.

97. Barr MS, Anderson MW. The knee: bone marrow abnormalities. Radiol Clin North Am 2002;40: 1109–20.

98. Kattapuram TM, Suri R, Rosol MS, et al. Idiopathic and diabetic skeletal muscle necrosis: evaluation by magnetic resonance imaging. Skeletal Radiol 2005;34:203–9.

99. Delaney-Sathy LO, Fessel DP, Jacobson JA, et al. Sonography of diabetic muscle infarction with MR imaging, CT, and pathologic correlation. AJR Am J Roentgenol 2000;174:165–9.

100. Dhillon M, Davies AM, Benham J, et al. Calcific myo-necrosis: a report of ten new cases with an emphasis on MR imaging. Eur Radiol 2004;14:1974–9.

101. Zohman GL, Pierce J, Chapman MW, et al. Calcific myonecrosis mimicking an invasive soft-tissue neoplasm. A case report and review of the litera-ture. J Bone Joint Surg Am 1998;80:1193–7.

102. Gupta KB, Duryea J, Weissman BN. Radiographic evaluation of osteoarthritis. Radiol Clin North Am 2004;42:11–41.

103. Mitra R. Osteitis condensans ilii. Rheumatol Int 2010;30:293–6.

104. Shoots IG, Slim FJ, Busch-Westborek TE, et al. Neuro-osteoarthropathy of the foot–radiologist: friend or foe? Semin Musculoskelet Radiol 2010; 14:365–76.

105. Steinbach LS, Anderson S, Panicek D. MR imaging of musculoskeletal tumors in the elbow region. Magn Reson Imaging Clin N Am 1997;5:619–53.

106. Sheldon PF, Forrester DM, Learch TF. Imaging of intra-articular masses. Radiographics 2005;25: 105–19.

107. Osanai T, Tsuchiya T, Hasegawa T, et al. Large benign rheumatoid nodules of the trunk in an elderly patient: radiologic appearance mimicking a soft-tissue sarcoma. Mod Rheumatol 2006;16:312–5.

108. Chan AT, Leung JL, Sy AN, et al. Thoracic spinal gout mimicking metastasis. Hong Kong Med J 2009;15:143–5.

109. Nakajima A, Kato Y, Yamanaka H, et al. Spinal to-phaceous gout mimicking a spinal tumor. J Rheumatol 2004;31:1459–60.

110. Yu JS, Chung C, Recht M, et al. MR imaging of tophaceous gout. AJR Am J Roentgenol 1997;168:523–7.

111. Liu SZ, Yeh L, Chou YJ. Isolated intraosseous gout in hallux sesamoid mimicking a bone tumor in a teenaged patient. Skeletal Radiol 2003;32:647–50.

112. Recht MP, Seragini F, Kramer J, et al. Isolated or dominant lesions of the patella in gout: a report of seven patients. Skeletal Radiol 1994;23:113–6.

113. Havitçioğlu H, Tatari H, Baran O, et al. Calcium pyrophosphate dihydrate crystal deposition disease mimicking malignant soft tissue tumor. Knee Surg Sports Traumatol Arthrosc 2003;11:263–6.

114. Morrison JL, Kaplan PA. Water on the knee: cysts, bursae and recesses. Magn Reson Imaging Clin N Am 2000;8(2):349–70.

115. Tshering Vogel DW, Steinbach LS, Hertel R, et al. Acromioclavicular joint cyst: nine cases of a pseudotumor of the shoulder. Skeletal Radiol 2005;34:260–5.

116. Kransdorf MJ, Murphey MD. Synovial tumors. In: Kransdorf MJ, Murphey MD, editors. Imaging of soft tissue tumors. 2nd edition. Philadelphia: Lippincott Williams & Wilkins; 2006. p. 381–436.

117. Beaman FD, Peterson JJ. MR imaging of cysts, ganglia, and bursae about the knee. Magn Reson Imaging Clin N Am 2007;15:39–52.

118. Tirman PFJ, Feller JF, Janzen DL, et al. Association of glenoid labral cysts with labral tears and glenohumeral instability: radiologic findings and clinical significance. Radiology 1994;190:653–8.

119. Schajowicz F, Sainz MC, Slullitel JA. Juxta-articular bone cysts (intra-osseous ganglia): a clinicopathological study of eighty-eight cases. J Bone Joint Surg Br 1979;61:107–16.

120. Peterson JJ, Kransdorf MJ, Bancroft LW, et al. Imaging characteristics of cystic adventitial disease of the peripheral arteries: presentation as soft-tissue masses. AJR Am J Roentgenol 2003;180:621–5.

121. Gopinathan A, Guglielmi G, Peh WCG. Radiology of osteoporosis. Radiol Clin North Am 2010;48:497–518.

122. Dietrich O, Biffar A, Reiser MF, et al. Diffusion-weighted imaging of bone marrow. Semin Musculoskelet Radiol 2009;13:134–44.

123. Joyce JM, Keats TE. Disuse osteoporosis: mimic of neoplastic disease. Skeletal Radiol 1986;15:129–32.

124. Korompilias AV, Karantanas AH, Lykissas MG, et al. Bone marrow edema syndrome. Skeletal Radiol 2009;38:425–36.

125. Polat P, Kantarci M, Alper F, et al. The spectrum of radiographic findings in primary hyperparathyroidism. Clin Imaging 2002;26:197–205.

126. Scholl RJ, Kellet HM, Neumann DP, et al. Cysts and cystic lesions of the mandible: clinical and radiologic-histopathologic review. Radiographics 1999;19:1107–24.

127. Sundaram M. Renal osteodystrophy. Skeletal Radiol 1989;18:415–26.

128. Ross LV, Ross GJ, Mesgarzadeh M, et al. Hemodialysis-related amyloidomas of bone. Radiology 1991;178:263–5.

129. Meema HE, Oreopoulos DG, Rabinovich S, et al. Periosteal new bone formation (periosteal neostosis) in renal osteodystrophy: relationship to osteosclerosis, osteitis fibrosa, and osteoid excess. Radiology 1974;110:513–22.

130. Olsen KM, Chew FS. Tumoral calcinosis: pearls, polemics, and alternative possibilities. Radiographics 2006;26:871–85.

131. Whitehouse RW. Paget's disease of bone. Semin Musculoskelet Radiol 2002;6:313–22.

132. Hain SF, Fogelman I. Nuclear medicine studies in metabolic bone disease. Semin Musculoskelet Radiol 2002;6:323–9.

133. Mahmood S, Martinez de Llano SR. Paget disease of the humerus mimicking metastatic disease in a patient with metastatic malignant mesothelioma on whole body F-18 FDG PET/CT. Clin Nucl Med 2008;33:510–2.

134. Vande Berg BC, Malghem J, Lecouvet FE, et al. Magnetic resonance appearance of uncomplicated Paget's disease of bone. Semin Musculoskelet Radiol 2001;5:69–77.

135. Roberts MC, Kressel HY, Fallon MD, et al. Paget disease: MR imaging findings. Radiology 1989;173:341–5.

136. Sundaram M, Khanna G, El-Khoury GY. T1-weighted MR imaging for distinguishing large osteolysis of Paget's disease from sarcomatous degeneration. Skeletal Radiol 2001;30:378–83.

137. Park JS, Ryu KN. Hemophilic pseudotumor involving the musculoskeletal system: spectrum of radiologic findings. AJR Am J Roentgenol 2004;183:55–61.

138. Suresh S, Muthukumar T, Saifuddin A. Classical and unusual imaging appearances of melorheostosis. Clin Radiol 2010;65:593–600.

139. Moore SL, Teirstein A, Golimbu C. MRI of sarcoidosis patients with musculoskeletal symptoms. AJR Am J Roentgenol 2005;185:154–9.

140. Moore SL, Teirstein AE. Musculoskeletal sarcoidosis: spectrum of appearances at MR imaging. Radiographics 2003;23:1389–99.

141. Stacy GS, Dixon LB. Pitfalls in MR image interpretation prompting referrals to an orthopedic oncology clinic. Radiographics 2007;27:805–28.

142. Heck RK, O'Malley AM, Kellum EL, et al. Errors in the MRI evaluation of musculoskeletal tumors and tumor-like lesions. Clin Orthop Relat Res 2007;459:28–33.

Musculoskeletal Neoplasms: Biopsy and Intervention

Ambrose J. Huang, MD, Susan V. Kattapuram, MD*

KEYWORDS

- Biopsy • Intervention • Tumor • Infection • Spondylodiscitis
- Sarcoma • Metastasis

There are few musculoskeletal lesions that can be diagnosed confidently based on imaging features alone. Even if a lesion is likely to be a particular entity (eg, metastasis in a patient with innumerable osseous lesions and a known primary malignancy), the implications for treatment are such that a definitive diagnosis is usually required. In these situations, biopsy of the suspicious lesion is warranted. Lesions that clinically and radiologically appear benign do not necessarily demand a biopsy. Some lesions that are benign radiologically appear aggressive or malignant histologically and potentially lead to overtreatment.[1,2]

The most common indications for biopsy of a bone or soft tissue lesion are to evaluate for neoplasm or infection. Knowledge of the tissue type of a neoplasm is used both for pretreatment (neoadjuvant chemotherapy or preoperative radiation) and treatment planning. A biopsy of a lesion in the setting of a known primary malignancy can confirm that it represents a metastasis, or it may be used to identify the primary malignancy if that is unknown. Sites of infection often appear aggressive on imaging and can be difficult to discriminate from malignancy. Differentiating spondylodiscitis from severe degenerative disc disease or other arthropathy can be challenging as well. Clinical and laboratory findings in the setting of suspected infection are often nonspecific.[3] Biopsy can be helpful to distinguish infection from neoplastic or other inflammatory conditions, and identification of the causative organism allows initiation of

an antibiotic regimen to which the organism is sensitive.

Although the mechanical aspects of performing a biopsy are straightforward, factors such as which part of a particular lesion to biopsy and the approach to take to reach the lesion can determine the difference between a successful and an unsuccessful biopsy. The consequences of an unsuccessful biopsy range from a delay in diagnosis to departure from the optimum treatment plan, including unnecessary amputation and worsening of prognosis and survival.[4,5]

BIOPSY METHODS

The 2 main ways of acquiring a tissue diagnosis are open biopsy and percutaneous, typically image-guided, biopsy. Advantages of open biopsy include the possibility of definitive therapy (when used in conjunction with frozen section evaluation), larger sample size, which permits the performance of ancillary studies (eg, flow cytometry, cytogenetics, immunohistochemistry), and lack of exposure of the patient and/or the care team to ionizing radiation (as opposed to fluoroscopic-guided or computed tomography [CT]–guided biopsy).[6] Disadvantages of open biopsy include increased procedure time; risks inherent to any open procedure, such as complications related to wound healing; and increased costs, such as those related to the operating room, hospital stay, and anesthesia.[7] Advantages

The authors have nothing to disclose.

Department of Radiology, Harvard Medical School, Massachusetts General Hospital, 55 Fruit Street, Yawkey 6E, Boston, MA 02114, USA

* Corresponding author.

E-mail address: skattapuram@partners.org

doi:10.1016/j.rcl.2011.07.010

of percutaneous needle biopsy include decreased cost, procedure time, and patient morbidity. In addition, a preoperative diagnosis may permit patient counseling, multidisciplinary collaboration, and initiation of preoperative chemotherapy and/or radiation therapy. The wide range of diagnostic accuracies is the main disadvantage of percutaneous biopsy, with studies reporting accuracies ranging from 74% to 97%.[6–13] Accuracy is generally greatest for metastatic disease and least for primary bone tumors.[14] Even in series in which percutaneous biopsy was highly accurate in distinguishing a benign from a malignant process, determining the exact histologic type and grade of the lesion from a needle sample can remain problematic.[15] Both open and percutaneous biopsies, if poorly planned, are susceptible to complicating the definitive surgical treatment. In both types of biopsies, there are the possibilities of suboptimal selection of the incision site or needle entry site as well iatrogenic spread of malignant cells, either by seeding of the biopsy track in percutaneous cases or spillage of tumor in open cases.[8]

Percutaneous biopsies can be further subdivided into fine-needle aspirations and core needle biopsies. Because the needles used in fine-needle aspirations are of smaller gauge, there is a smaller risk of hemorrhage and damage to soft tissues. However, smaller-gauge needles are more difficult to steer into a lesion, especially if the lesion is deep. Smaller tissue sample size can increase the risk of a nondiagnostic specimen or sampling error, although some experienced centers and groups can achieve a high degree of diagnostic accuracy.[16] Usually, fine-needle aspirates provide adequate tissue for diagnosis of metastatic disease and infection, whereas core needle biopsies are preferred for assessing the lesion's architecture, cell type, and histologic grade, which are needed for diagnosis of a primary bone or soft tissue malignancy.[17]

PREPROCEDURAL STEPS
Imaging

Once a lesion is detected, either clinically or by imaging, workup of the lesion usually begins with cross-sectional imaging for further characterization of the lesion. Magnetic resonance (MR) imaging is helpful for visualizing a soft tissue mass or the soft tissue component of a primarily osseous lesion, especially its relationship to neural and vascular structures and the extent of muscular involvement. CT is helpful for assessing bony integrity or destructive changes and for detecting foci of internal mineralization. For osseous lesions, whole-body technetium 99m methylene diphosphonate skeletal scintigraphy is useful for detecting other lesions that would suggest the diagnosis of metastatic disease and may reveal another lesion that is safer or easier to biopsy than the original lesion.

If more than 1 lesion is a candidate for biopsy, the largest and most superficial lesion is usually the preferred target. Other factors to consider include proximity of the lesion to adjacent structures, such as lung, nerve, or artery, and whether the lesion contains viable tissue. Because bone and soft tissue tumors often have heterogeneous imaging features, the location of the biopsy within the lesion is important. It is possible to obtain a biopsy specimen that does not represent the main disease process, resulting in a diagnosis that is incorrect because of sampling error. Metabolic imaging, such as with ^{18}F-deoxyglucose positron emission tomography, can reveal areas of the lesion that are more likely to yield diagnostic tissue when sampled. Postcontrast imaging can identify enhancing areas or areas that are more vascular. These areas are more likely to yield diagnostic tissue than areas of nonenhancement, which may reflect necrotic or cystic areas. Ultrasound can provide similar information and distinguish solid or vascular areas from cystic areas as well as identify vascular structures to be avoided during the biopsy.

Planning the Biopsy Route

A bone or soft tissue lesion that is one of many similar-appearing lesions throughout the body, or that occurs in a patient with a known primary malignancy, suggests metastatic disease. Surgical resection is usually not indicated in this situation, so a percutaneous biopsy can be performed along the easiest and safest trajectory. However, if a bone or soft tissue lesion is solitary, primary sarcoma is usually a consideration, as is the possibility of surgical resection.[18] The radiologist should collaborate with the orthopedic oncologist to determine a biopsy trajectory that coincides with the potential surgical route so that the biopsy track can be excised along with the tumor, should the lesion turn out to be amenable to limb-sparing surgery.[19]

In the extremities, knowledge of anatomic compartments is important when considering bone and soft tissue sarcomas[20,21] because these tumors tend to enlarge radially or spherically within their compartments of origin until they encounter barriers to such growth. These barriers include muscular attachment sites, muscular fascia or other firm fibrous septa, articular cartilage, and bony cortex. Once a barrier is encountered, the tumor enlarges and elongates along the path of least resistance. Tumors that traverse these barriers and spread into adjacent compartments are more aggressive.

In addition, it is assumed that during a biopsy, cells from the lesion will be deposited along, or seed, the needle track (**Fig. 1**). Therefore, the biopsy route must be selected in collaboration with the treating surgeon to ensure that the track lies within the planned resection bed, so that it can be removed with the same wide margins as the primary lesion. Furthermore, the biopsy route should be selected so that the needle does not traverse an unaffected compartment or

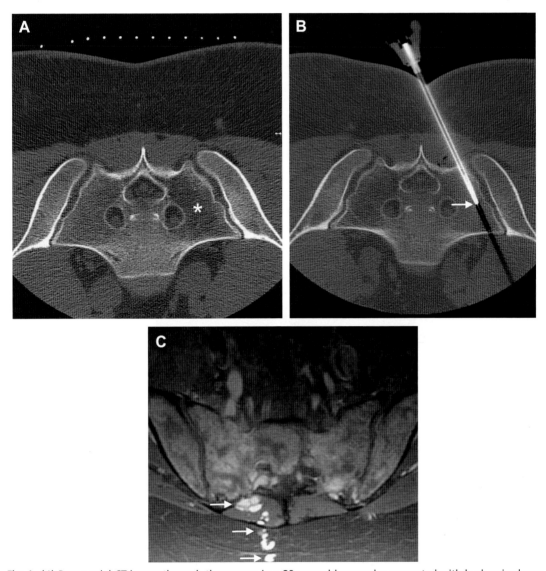

Fig. 1. (A) Prone axial CT image through the sacrum in a 29-year-old man who presented with back pain shows a lytic lesion in the right sacral ala (*asterisk*). Imaging workup at an outside hospital revealed multiple lesions throughout the spine and pelvis. (B) The lesion was biopsied using an 11-gauge diamond-tipped marrow biopsy needle (*arrow*). The final diagnosis was metastatic poorly differentiated round cell and spindle sarcoma from an unknown primary. Subsequently, the patient developed right calf pain. Imaging revealed a large soft tissue mass, which was biopsied and revealed grade 2/3 myxoid and round cell liposarcoma (not shown). Additional staging imaging revealed lung metastases as well. (C) Axial T1-weighted, fat-suppressed, postgadolinium MR image from a follow-up examination 7 months later shows enhancing foci in the soft tissues overlying the right sacrum, along the course of the biopsy needle track, consistent with tumor seeding (*arrows*).

a neurovascular bundle. Contamination of an unaffected compartment or neurovascular bundle requires a more extensive surgical resection or a wider radiation field to combat the greater chance of local recurrence and can result in a greater functional deficit.[22]

This article reviews soft tissue compartmental anatomy in the extremities. The specific approaches for intraosseous lesions that are described and illustrated are general guidelines, applicable in most but not necessarily all cases. Each lesion should be approached on a case-by-case basis, and collaboration with the treating surgeon cannot be overemphasized.

There are 3 soft tissue compartments in the thigh (**Fig. 2**). The anterior compartment includes the quadriceps muscle group, the iliopsoas, sartorius, and tensor fascia lata muscles, and the iliotibial band. The medial compartment includes the adductor muscle group and the gracilis muscle. The posterior compartment includes the hamstring muscle group. The femoral neurovascular bundle is extracompartmental structure in the proximal thigh and becomes the popliteal neurovascular bundle in the posterior compartment after passing through the adductor hiatus of the adductor

magnus. The sciatic nerve is a posterior compartment structure. Generally, it is recommended to biopsy lesions within the femoral diaphysis from a lateral approach, anterior to the lateral femoral intermuscular septum. It is important to avoid traversing the rectus femoris, because its resection results in a substantial functional deficit. Lesions in the distal femoral metaphyseal or epiphyseal areas can usually be approached either medially or laterally, with care taken not to traverse the knee joint capsule. It is recommended to access lesions in the femoral head or neck using a lateral trochanteric approach. The needle should be directed superomedially through the femoral neck into the lesion without entering the hip joint (**Fig. 3**).

There are 4 soft tissue compartments in the lower leg (**Fig. 4**). The anterior compartment includes the tibialis anterior, extensor hallucis longus, and extensor digitorum longus muscles, the anterior tibial artery and vein, and the deep peroneal nerve. The lateral compartment includes the peroneus longus and brevis muscles and the common peroneal nerve, which becomes the superficial peroneal nerve after the takeoff of the deep peroneal nerve. The superficial posterior compartment includes the gastrocnemius, soleus, and plantaris muscles. The deep posterior compartment includes the tibialis posterior, flexor digitorum longus, and flexor hallucis longus muscles, as well as the peroneal and posterior tibial neurovascular bundles. Lesions in the tibia can be accessed anteromedially, with the needle traversing only subcutaneous fat before reaching the tibial surface. Fibula shaft lesions should be approached laterally through the peroneus longus muscle with care taken to avoid the superficial peroneal nerve. For lesions in the proximal and distal tips of the fibula, a lateral approach requires the needle tip to traverse only subcutaneous fat before reaching the fibula surface.

There are 2 soft tissue compartments in the upper arm (**Fig. 5**). The anterior compartment includes the biceps, brachialis, and coracobrachialis muscles. The triceps muscle comprises the posterior compartment. The brachial artery and vein and the median and ulnar nerves are extracompartmental structures in the proximal upper arm. In the distal upper arm, the brachial artery and vein and the median nerve are anterior compartment structures, whereas the ulnar nerve continues in the extracompartmental space. The radial neurovascular bundle is a posterior compartment structure in the proximal upper arm and becomes an anterior compartment structure in the distal upper arm. It is recommended to biopsy lesions within the humeral shaft from an

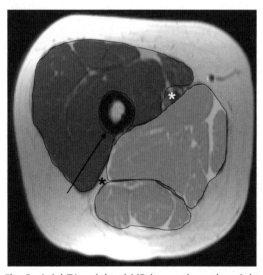

Fig. 2. Axial T1-weighted MR image through a right proximal thigh depicts the anterior (*red shaded area*), medial (*green shaded area*), and posterior (*blue shaded area*) compartments. The femoral neurovascular bundle is extracompartmental in the proximal thigh (*white asterisk*). The arrow denotes the recommended lateral approach, through the anterior compartment, for biopsy of a lesion within the femoral diaphysis. The lateral femoral intermuscular septum (*black asterisk*) separates the anterior from the posterior compartments.

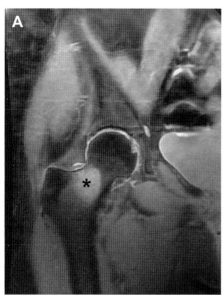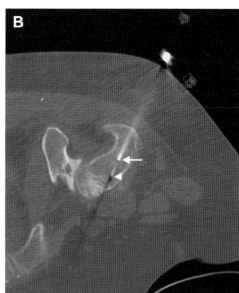

Fig. 3. (*A*) Coronal proton density-weighted, fat-suppressed MR image of the right hip in a 58-year-old woman who presented with hip pain shows a solitary hyperintense lesion (*asterisk*) in the femoral neck with a small extra-osseous soft tissue component. (*B*) Prone axial image from a CT-guided biopsy. A 14-gauge bone penetration set was advanced through the inferior aspect of the greater trochanter of the femur just inside the edge of the lesion (*arrow*), and a 16-gauge trephine-type biopsy needle (*arrowhead*) was advanced coaxially through the introducer to obtain multiple core samples. Because sarcoma remained in the differential diagnosis, the biopsy route was specifically chosen to coincide with the location of the surgical incision that would be made should the lesion turn out to be a primary bone tumor amenable to surgical resection. The final diagnosis was plasmacytoma.

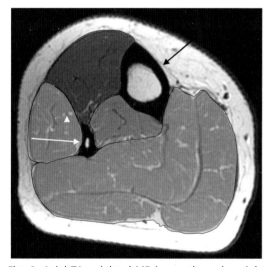

Fig. 4. Axial T1-weighted MR image through a right proximal lower leg depicts the anterior (*red shaded area*), lateral (*green shaded area*), deep posterior (*yellow shaded area*), and superficial posterior (*blue shaded area*) compartments. The black arrow denotes the generally recommended anteromedial approach for biopsy of a lesion within the tibial shaft, which can usually be accomplished by traversing only subcutaneous fat. The white arrow denotes the generally recommended lateral approach, through the peroneus longus muscle, for biopsy of a lesion within the fibula shaft. The trajectory is posterior to the superficial peroneal nerve (*arrowhead*).

anterolateral approach, posterior to the cephalic vein. Lesions within the medial and lateral humeral epicondyles can be approached directly, with the needle traversing only subcutaneous fat.

There are 2 soft tissue compartments in the forearm (**Fig. 6**). The posterior compartment includes the extensors of the wrist and digits, abductor pollicis longus, brachioradialis, and the supinator muscles. The anterior compartment includes the flexors of the wrist and digits, pronator teres, pronator quadratus, and palmaris longus muscles. Three-compartment and 4-compartment descriptions of the forearm exist, but the fascial planes used for the additional subdivisions do not completely separate the muscle groups. The radial and ulnar artery and vein and the median and ulnar nerves are anterior compartment structures. The radial nerve divides into a superficial branch, located in the anterior compartment, and a deep branch, located in the posterior compartment. Lesions in the radius can be approached laterally or posterolaterally, and lesions in the ulna can be approached medially or posteromedially, both using trajectories that traverse minimal muscle and avoid the posterior interosseous neurovascular bundle. Lesions within the olecranon can be approached posteriorly, with the needle traversing only subcutaneous fat.

In the spine, the presence of nearby viscera, blood vessels, and other important structures limits

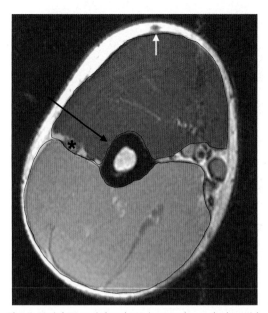

Fig. 5. Axial T1-weighted MR image through the mid-to-distal aspect of a right upper arm depicts the anterior (*red shaded area*) and posterior (*blue shaded area*) compartments. The black arrow denotes the generally recommended anterolateral approach for biopsy of a lesion within the humeral shaft. The trajectory is anterior to the radial neurovascular bundle (*asterisk*), which is an anterior compartment structure in the distal upper arm, and posterior to the cephalic vein (*white arrow*). On the medial side, the brachial vessels and the median and ulnar nerves are extracompartmental structures.

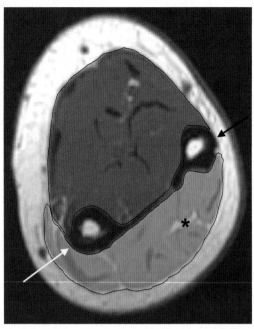

Fig. 6. Axial T1-weighted MR image through the mid-to-distal aspect of a right forearm depicts the anterior (*red shaded area*) and posterior (*blue shaded area*) compartments. The white arrow denotes the generally recommended lateral or posterolateral approach for biopsy of a lesion within the radial shaft. The black arrow denotes the generally recommended medial approach for biopsy of a lesion within the ulnar shaft, which can usually be accomplished by traversing only subcutaneous fat. Both trajectories can avoid the posterior interosseous neurovascular bundle (*asterisk*).

the number of viable paths to the lesion. Preprocedural cross-sectional imaging is helpful in planning biopsies of the spine and paraspinal soft tissues to ensure that the biopsy needle avoids these important structures. In the cervical spine, anterior lesions can usually be accessed via an anterolateral approach (**Fig. 7**). Posterior lesions can usually be accessed using transpedicular or posterolateral approaches. Occasionally, anterior lesions are more easily approached posteriorly (**Fig. 8**). In the thoracic and lumbar spine, almost all lesions are approached posteriorly. Lesions in the pedicles or off-midline aspects of the vertebral bodies can be accessed using a transpedicular approach (**Fig. 9**). Smaller lesions in the midline aspects of the vertebral bodies usually cannot be reached from a transpedicular approach but can usually be accessed from a posterolateral approach,[23] including transforaminodiscal,[24] transcostovertebral, and transcostotransverse approaches. The posterolateral approach can also be used to access the intervertebral disc, especially in the lumbar spine, and the inferior aspects of vertebral

bodies. Thoracic intervertebral discs are accessible using a transcostotransverse approach. Small midline sacral lesions can be accessed using a trans–sacroiliac joint approach (**Fig. 10**).

Pain Control

Many bone and soft tissue biopsies can be performed on an outpatient basis using only 1% lidocaine for local anesthesia. Although there is no general consensus regarding the handling of anticoagulant therapy before percutaneous interventions of the musculoskeletal system, it is common practice to instruct patients to terminate any blood-thinning medications for 5 to 7 days. For simple procedures in healthy patients, laboratory values and an American Society of Anesthesiologists (ASA) assessment are typically unnecessary. For some cases, intravenous conscious sedation (eg, using fentanyl and midazolam) with continuous cardiac monitoring and pulse oximetry administered by dedicated conscious sedation nursing staff is necessary. Cases performed under

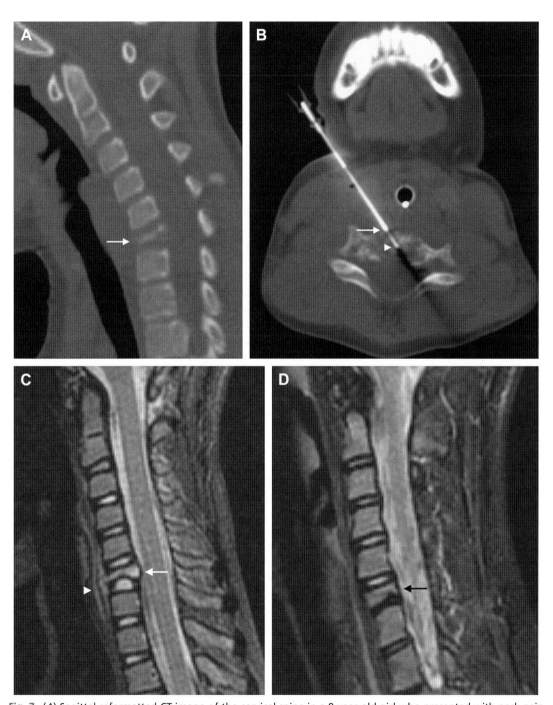

Fig. 7. (A) Sagittal reformatted CT image of the cervical spine in a 9-year-old girl who presented with neck pain reveals vertebra plana at C6 (arrow). (B) Axial image from a CT-guided biopsy with the patient lying supine shows a 19-gauge introducer inserted to the edge of the vertebral body using a right anterolateral approach (arrow). Subsequently, a 22-gauge aspiration needle (arrowhead) was inserted coaxially through the introducer to obtain aspirates for analysis. The final diagnosis was Langerhans cell histiocytosis, and 40 mg of methylprednisolone was injected for treatment. (C) Sagittal short tau inversion recovery (STIR) MR image of the cervical spine before injection shows C6 compression fracture with marrow edema (arrow) and prevertebral soft tissue swelling (arrowhead). (D) Follow-up sagittal STIR MR image of the cervical spine 4 years after injection shows preservation of C6 height (arrow) and resolution of marrow edema and prevertebral soft tissue swelling. To date, the patient remains symptom free.

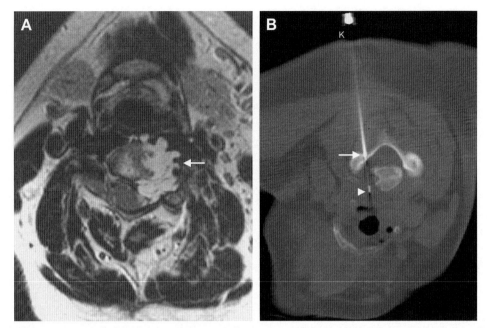

Fig. 8. (*A*) Axial T2-weighted MR image of the cervical spine in a 57-year-old woman reveals a T2-hyperintense mass arising from the left aspect of the C3 vertebral body (*arrow*) that enlarges the left C3 to C4 neural foramen, extends into the spinal canal, and displaces the spinal cord to the right. The mass was detected incidentally on cervical spine CT ordered as part of an emergency department workup when the patient presented after falling and fracturing her radial head. (*B*) Prone axial image from a CT-guided biopsy. A 14-gauge bone penetration set was used to drill through the left C3 lamina using a posterolateral approach (*arrow*). The drill was then exchanged for a 20-gauge, spring-loaded, side-cutting biopsy needle (*arrowhead*), which was inserted coaxially through the introducer into the lesion to obtain multiple core samples. The final diagnosis was chordoma.

conscious sedation are those in which patient pain, discomfort, or anxiety is anticipated to be high or if the patient is otherwise not expected to be able to remain still for the duration of the biopsy. As examples, biopsy of a suspected peripheral nerve sheath tumor or suspected infection is expected to be uncomfortable or painful and hence can be scheduled to be performed under conscious sedation. In these cases, the patient undergoes workup and physical examination by the nursing and physician staff, including ASA assessment. Laboratory samples may be drawn, for example, if the patient is known to take blood-thinning medications that have not been discontinued before the biopsy.

Contraindications

Relative contraindications to percutaneous core needle biopsy include (1) inability of the patient to lie still in the appropriate position on the procedure table or otherwise cooperate for the duration of the biopsy; (2) inability to identify a safe pathway from the skin surface to the lesion, such as when cross-sectional imaging reveals no way to access the lesion from the skin surface without traversing a major vascular structure, neurologic structure, bowel, or infected soft tissue; (3) large body habitus rendering available instruments too short to reach the lesion via the available safe access pathways; (4) uncorrected coagulopathy, especially for spinal lesions, if postprocedural hematoma formation would put the patient at risk for subsequent cord compression; (5) extremely small lesions, on the order of a few millimeters, for which the chances of a diagnostic sample are slim; and (6) pregnancy.

THE BIOPSY
Methods of Image Guidance

Bone and soft tissue lesions can be biopsied using a variety of imaging modalities. CT guidance allows visualization of the intraosseous and soft tissue components of even small lesions as well as their surrounding structures. If there are substantial cystic or necrotic areas within a lesion, it can be difficult to distinguish these areas from more solid or viable components using CT. Especially for these situations, preprocedural cross-sectional

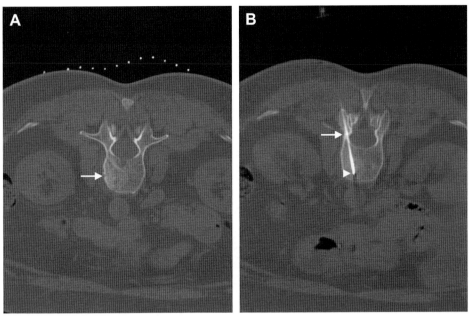

Fig. 9. A 52-year-old woman presented with a parapharyngeal space mass and multiple osseous lesions. Fine-needle aspiration of the parapharyngeal space mass revealed a high-grade malignancy (not shown). Biopsy of one of the osseous lesions was requested for staging. (A) Prone axial image from a CT-guided biopsy shows a primarily sclerotic lesion in the L2 vertebral body (*arrow*). (B) A 14-gauge bone penetration set was used to drill to the posterior aspect of the lesion (*arrow*) using a transpedicular approach. The drill was then exchanged for a 16-gauge trephine-type biopsy needle, which was inserted coaxially through the introducer into the lesion (*arrowhead*). The final diagnosis was metastatic non–small cell carcinoma, consistent with an upper airway primary.

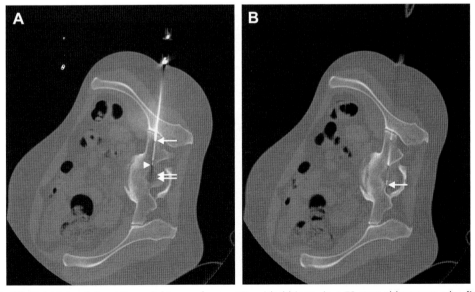

Fig. 10. (A) Right lateral decubitus axial image from a CT-guided biopsy in a 52-year-old woman who first presented with left leg pain and numbness shows a lytic lesion in the midline posterior aspect of the S1 vertebral body (*double arrow*). The inner drill (*arrowhead*) and the outer introducer (*arrow*) of a 14-gauge bone penetration set were advanced in tandem through the left sacroiliac joint. (B) Once the drill tip penetrated the lytic lesion, it was exchanged for an 18-gauge, spring-loaded, side-cutting biopsy needle (*arrow*), which was advanced through the introducer into the lesion to obtain multiple core samples (a 16-gauge, spring-loaded, side-cutting biopsy needle was not available at that time). The final diagnosis was plasmacytoma.

imaging using another modality, such as MR, is helpful for correlation with the biopsy CT to ensure a diagnostic result. CT fluoroscopic guidance is available at many institutions, and its use for image-guided biopsy can reduce overall procedure time. When combined with the quick-check technique described by Paulson and colleagues,[25] radiation doses to the patient and operator can be minimized. Conventional fluoroscopic guidance is particularly suitable for moderate-to-large intraosseous lesions in the extremities. Advantages of fluoroscopy include decreased radiation dose to the patient if the beam is collimated to the region of interest and less dependence of the image quality on the patient's ability to remain still. Disadvantages of fluoroscopy include difficulty visualizing small intraosseous lesions and the soft tissue components of any sized intraosseous lesions, decreased ability to discern soft tissue structures both along the trajectory of the biopsy needle and adjacent to the targeted lesion, and accessing lesions within complex-shaped bones. Ultrasound guidance is well suited for soft tissue lesions or the accessible soft tissue components of intraosseous lesions. Advantages of ultrasound guidance include lack of exposure to ionizing radiation, real-time visualization of the relationship between the needle tip and the lesion, direct visualization of

blood flow and purely cystic or necrotic areas, and hence the ability to avoid these areas. Ultrasound cannot be used to biopsy a purely intraosseous lesion. Ultrasound guidance is particularly useful for very superficial lesions in which it would be difficult to position the biopsy instruments in a stand-alone stationary fashion if the patient were to undergo CT. MR guidance is less commonly used for musculoskeletal biopsies because of issues related to MR compatibility of biopsy instruments as well as limited availability of scanner time.

Needle Types and Biopsy Techniques

Familiarity with the particulars of the biopsy devices typically used is instrumental in obtaining high-quality core specimens. Each needle type is intended to be used in particular ways and for particular types of lesions, and the various components of a biopsy system are meant to be used in a particular order.

For lesions with an accessible soft tissue component (either the lesion arises entirely within soft tissue, or it has arisen in bone but has grown through the cortex and presents with an accessible extraosseous soft tissue component; **Fig. 11**) a spring-loaded side-cutting biopsy

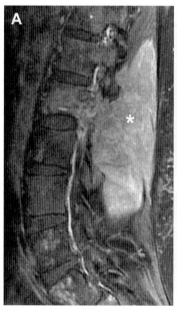
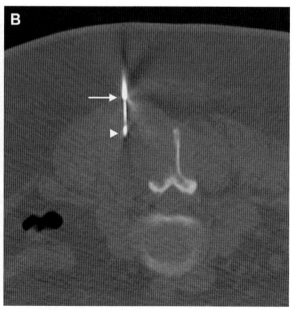

Fig. 11. (*A*) Sagittal T1-weighted, fat-suppressed, postgadolinium MR image of the lumbar spine in a 27-year-old woman who presented with back pain shows an enhancing lesion essentially occupying the entire L2 vertebral body. There is a large soft tissue component of the lesion within the posterior paraspinal muscles (*asterisk*). (*B*) Prone axial image from a CT-guided biopsy shows a 13.5-gauge introducer advanced to the edge of the lesion (*arrow*). A 14-gauge, spring-loaded, side-cutting biopsy needle (*arrowhead*) was inserted coaxially through the introducer to obtain multiple core samples. The final diagnosis was diffuse large B-cell lymphoma.

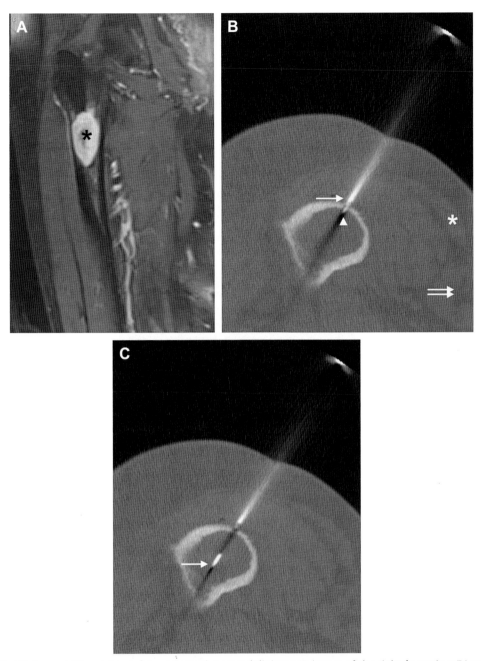

Fig. 12. (*A*) Coronal T1-weighted, fat-suppressed, postgadolinium MR image of the right femur in a 74-year-old man obtained 2 years after resection of a grade 2/3 pleomorphic fibrosarcoma from the ipsilateral medial thigh shows an enhancing lesion in the subtrochanteric region of the femur (*asterisk*). (*B*) Axial image from a CT-guided biopsy with the patient in the left lateral decubitus position. A bone penetration introducer (*arrow*) was inserted to the femoral cortex using an anterolateral approach. The needle traveled posterior to the tensor fascia lata (*asterisk*) and avoided the rectus femoris, which contained an intramuscular lipoma in this case (*double arrow*). The bone penetration drill was inserted coaxially through the introducer to penetrate the cortex (*arrowhead*). (*C*) The drill was then exchanged for a 16-gauge, spring-loaded, side-cutting biopsy needle (*arrow*), which was inserted coaxially through the introducer and the drill hole into the lesion to obtain multiple core samples. The final diagnosis was metastatic grade 3/3 pleomorphic fibrosarcoma with histologic features similar to the initial lesion.

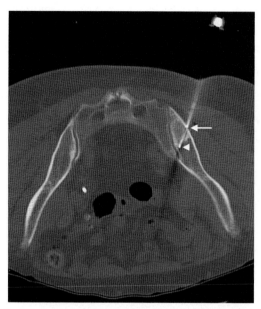

Fig. 13. Prone axial image from a CT-guided biopsy in a 60-year-old woman with a history of endometrial cancer shows a sclerotic lesion in the right iliac bone. A 14-gauge bone penetration set was inserted to the surface of the iliac bone using a posterior oblique approach (*arrow*). A more posterior approach along the long axis of the lesion was not used because the bone penetration set would have a tendency to slide off the curved posterior surface of the iliac bone. Available instruments were not long enough to approach the iliac bone perpendicular to its surface. A 16-gauge trephine-type biopsy needle (*arrowhead*) was then inserted coaxially through the introducer to obtain a core sample. The final diagnosis was metastatic endometrial adenocarcinoma.

needle can be used. Examples include Temno (Cardinal Health, Dublin, OH), Tru-Cut (Cardinal Health, Dublin, OH), and Quick-Core (Cook Medical, Bloomington, IN). These needles are usually packaged with an introducer, which is first inserted up or just inside the edge of the lesion. The introducer serves as a sheath and protects the tissues external to the lesion by minimizing soft tissue trauma and contamination by tumor cells. The biopsy needle proper is coaxially inserted through the introducer to take multiple core samples. Large core samples (14-gauge or larger) can be taken depending on the size and location of the lesion. Many spring-loaded side-cutting needles consist of a tray or trough that captures the biopsy specimen once the device is fired. The distal-most 7 to 8 mm of the tips of these needles do not have any ability to cut or capture tissue. This dead space needs to be taken into account when planning the biopsy, particularly of a small lesion. If the

lesion is small enough, it is possible that, once the needle is deployed, the entire lesion or nearly the entire lesion is occupied by the dead space, and the tray lies external to, or nearly completely external to, the lesion.

For intraosseous lesions without an easily accessible extraosseous soft tissue component, a bone penetration set can be used to traverse cortical bone and gain access into the lesion. Examples include Bonopty (Apriomed, Uppsala, Sweden), T-Lok (Angiotech, Vancouver, British Columbia, Canada), and Jamshidi (CareFusion, San Diego, CA). The Bonopty system consists of an outer cannula containing an inner stylet that is inserted to the bone cortex. Once the cannula reaches the bone surface, local anesthetic can be injected through it to anesthetize the periosteum in anticipation of the drilling of bone.[26] The stylet is then exchanged for a drill with an eccentric tip, which is inserted coaxially through the cannula to drill a hole through the cortex. Because the drill is eccentric, the diameter of the hole that is created is larger than the outer diameter of the cannula. This permits insertion of the cannula into the newly created opening in the cortex, where it can function as an introducer sheath. If the intraosseous lesion is lytic and of primarily soft tissue attenuation, then a spring-loaded side-cutting biopsy needle can be coaxially inserted through the penetration cannula to obtain multiple core samples (**Fig. 12**). If the intraosseous lesion is primarily sclerotic or otherwise too firm to allow insertion of a side-cutting biopsy needle, which has a blunt tip, then a trephine-type biopsy needle can be inserted coaxially through the penetration cannula to obtain the core samples (**Fig. 13**). Examples of trephine-type biopsy needles include Ostycut (Bard, Murray Hill, NJ) and Ackerman (Cook Medical, Bloomington, IN). The T-Lok and Jamshidi needles contain their own components for extraction of the core biopsy samples.

For lesions suspicious for spondylodiscitis, the intervertebral disc can be targeted from a parasagittal approach in the lumbar spine or a transcostotransverse approach in the thoracic spine using a spring-loaded side-cutting biopsy needle (**Fig. 14**). If this cannot be manipulated into the disc, a trephine-type biopsy needle of the appropriate gauge can be inserted coaxially through the introducer sheath to obtain samples of the vertebral endplate and usually adjacent disc material.

To reiterate, an individual bone or soft tissue lesion often has heterogeneous imaging features, and prebiopsy imaging is often helpful for selection of an area of the lesion that is most likely to yield diagnostic tissue. Thus, areas of enhancement or

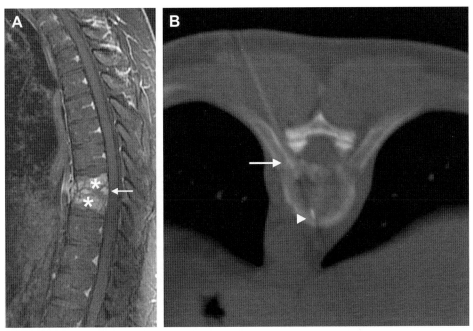

Fig. 14. (A) Sagittal T1-weighted, fat-suppressed, postgadolinium MR image of the thoracic spine in a 25-year-old intravenous drug user who presented with back pain shows enhancement of the T8 to T9 intervertebral disc (*arrow*) and T8 and T9 vertebral bodies (*asterisks*), and erosions of the T8 vertebral body inferior endplate and T9 vertebral body superior endplate. Constellation of findings suggests spondylodiscitis. (B) Prone axial CT image through the T8 to T9 intervertebral disc level. A 14-gauge bone penetration set was advanced through the left costotransverse junction into the periphery of the disc (*arrow*). Then, a 16-gauge spring-loaded side-cutting biopsy needle (*arrowhead*) was inserted coaxially through the introducer into the disc to obtain multiple core samples. The final histology showed acute and chronic osteomyelitis. No organism could be cultured from the samples, possibly related to administration of intravenous antibiotics the day before the biopsy.

increased blood flow, areas of increased radiotracer activity, and areas that appear solid rather than cystic or necrotic are favored for biopsy (**Fig. 15**). It is desirable for the biopsy needle to traverse as few compartments as possible, preferably only 1. The needle track should be located within the anticipated surgical resection bed (see **Fig. 3**). If a bone biopsy is requested to evaluate for osteomyelitis, a biopsy route is selected that does not require the needle to pass through soft tissue that appears inflamed before entering the osseous lesion so as to minimize the possibility of iatrogenically inoculating sterile bone with infected material. For lesions that are more oblong or ovoid than they are spherical, it is preferable to enter the lesion along its long axis, if possible, to ensure capture of the maximal amount of tissue with each pass or throw of the needle.

Because the surfaces of bones typically have curved cross sections, it is important when biopsying intraosseous lesions for the cannula or penetration device to arrive at the surface of the bone at an angle as close to perpendicular to the surface as possible. When the instrument lands on the bone surface at an obliquity, it is liable to slip off the bone surface once any substantial forward pressure is applied.[27] This can be particularly dangerous if there are important structures (eg, blood vessels, solid organs, lung parenchyma, spinal cord, and nerves) deep to the targeted bone.

Handling of Specimens

Handling of specimens varies by institution, tissue type, and even the suspected diagnosis; therefore, the radiologist and pathologist should communicate so that the specimen is processed appropriately. Specimens are typically placed in saline or formalin before delivery to surgical pathology. When it is feasible to obtain multiple core samples, the first specimens can be delivered to the frozen section laboratory for immediate evaluation of the diagnostic adequacy of the tissue while the patient remains on the biopsy table with the needle in place. If the specimens are deemed not to contain diagnostic tissue, which could be for myriad

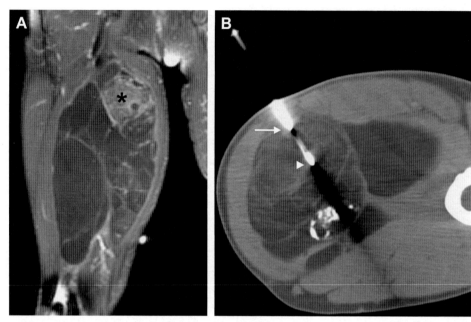

Fig. 15. (*A*) Coronal T1-weighted, fat-suppressed, postgadolinium MR image of the right thigh in a 73-year-old man who presented with a palpable mass shows a predominantly fat signal intensity mass with scattered, thin, enhancing septations, consistent with a fatty tumor. An area of more pronounced enhancement in the most superior aspect of the mass (*asterisk*) was targeted for biopsy. (*B*) Axial image from a CT-guided biopsy through the most superior aspect of the mass. A 13.5-gauge introducer was inserted to the edge of the lesion (*arrow*). A 14-gauge, spring-loaded, side-cutting biopsy needle (*arrowhead*) was inserted coaxially through the introducer to obtain multiple core samples from the anterior, higher-attenuation area of the mass, corresponding with the area of increased enhancement in (*A*). The final diagnosis was atypical lipoma.

reasons, including but not limited to an acellular sample, a predominantly hemorrhagic sample, and extensive crush artifact, then additional core samples can be obtained without creating a new needle entry site. If a lesion is such that, once the sample or samples are obtained, it is difficult or impractical to acquire additional specimens, then the biopsy is terminated once imaging confirms that the needle is within the lesion, and the retrieved samples are submitted to surgical pathology without frozen section interpretation. Frozen section evaluation may be difficult for lesions that are small, sclerotic, intraosseous, and in a difficult access location, such as a vertebral pedicle.

The presence of a cytopathologist can accelerate the biopsy and minimize the number of passes into the lesion before arriving at a diagnosis. In this situation, once the biopsy sample is obtained and before it is placed in saline or formalin, a touch prep slide is made by injecting or touching the specimen to a glass slide and smearing it with a second slide placed on top. This slide is then delivered to the cytopathologist for immediate analysis. A positive diagnosis could allow termination of the biopsy at this time. If the diagnosis is indeterminate or negative, then additional core samples are retrieved and submitted to surgical pathology, with or without frozen section evaluation, using the protocol described earlier.

If there is clinical concern for infection, additional samples are obtained and submitted in separate containers to microbiology for culture and analysis.

Complications

Complications of percutaneous core needle biopsies of bone and soft tissue lesions are similar to other procedures in which a needle punctures the skin, and can be divided into medication-related and technical complications. Patients can have allergies to any of the medications administered and can undergo adverse events as a result of conscious sedation. Technical complications include bleeding requiring transfusion, infection, and damage to adjacent structures (eg, nerve roots near paraspinal lesions, cord compression following postprocedural epidural hematoma formation). Pneumothorax can occur following biopsies in the region of the thoracic spine or rib cage. Rarely, needles can break, and fragments can be left within the patient, even after seemingly minor force (**Fig. 16**). Our group reports one case in which postprocedural hematoma formation in a lower extremity required enlargement of the originally planned pretreatment radiation field because of presumed contamination of the additional tissue by blood from the biopsy site.

Complication rates are less than 10%, and most studies report a complication rate less than 5%.[8–12,15,28,29] Our group is currently performing a prospective study to establish the incidence of complications following percutaneous CT-guided biopsies of bone and soft tissue lesions. To date, of nearly 400 adult patients referred to our group for biopsy, there have been no cases of post-biopsy infection. Less than 15% of patients report bruising after biopsy, and the average diameter of the reported bruises is 2 cm. One percent of patients have reported a bruise of 5 cm or greater following biopsy. There have been no major complications as a result of conscious sedation (Huang AJ, unpublished data).

THERAPEUTIC APPLICATIONS

Knowledge of the biopsy techniques detailed earlier is also valuable for various therapeutic applications, including alcohol injection, ultrasound therapy, laser coagulation, radiofrequency (RF) ablation, microwave therapy, cryogenic ablation, and vertebroplasty/kyphoplasty. These percutaneous treatment options are alternatives to surgery and are available for benign and malignant, primary and secondary, bone and soft tissue lesions, including osteoporotic compression fractures, osseous metastatic disease with or without compression fracture, bone and soft tissue hemangiomas, eosinophilic granulomas,[30] and simple and aneurysmal bone cysts.[31–33]

Pain relief following RF ablation of bone metastases is superior to conventional treatment methods in small series[34] and multicenter trials.[35,36] Vertebroplasty and kyphoplasty are well-established techniques for treating painful osteoporotic compression fractures[37] and painful bone metastases.[38]

Symptomatic hemangiomas in the soft tissues and vertebral bodies have been treated with direct intralesional injection of alcohol with good results.[39,40] We have treated many patients with painful bone and soft tissue hemangiomas with alcohol injections in our division as well.

Although observation is considered adequate for some eosinophilic granulomas, symptomatic granulomas have been treated with steroids successfully (see **Fig. 7**). Complete resolution and healing of the lesions was seen in 17 out of 19 patients with eosinophilic granuloma treated by intralesional corticosteroid injection.[41] Aneurysmal bone cysts are also treated with various materials, including alcohol and sclerosing agents (**Fig. 17**).

There are numerous treatment options for osteoid osteomas, and they include conservative management, medical management, open surgical excision, and several minimally invasive techniques.[42] RF ablation is a well-established therapy for osteoid osteomas and is considered the treatment of choice because of its high success rate and low complication rate. The procedure is usually performed under general anesthesia. Once the lesion is biopsied, typically using a coaxial technique with a bone penetration set followed by a trephine-type biopsy needle, the biopsy needle is exchanged for an RF probe with a 5-mm tip, which is also inserted coaxially through the introducer into the lesion (**Fig. 18**). The RF generator

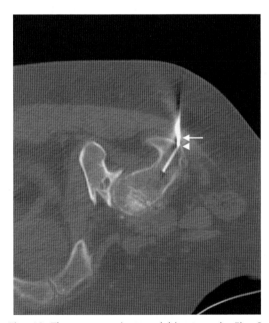

Fig. 16. The same patient and biopsy as in Fig. 3. During the procedure, the patient moved on the CT table, which resulted in a visible change in the orientation of the part of the needle external to the skin surface. Prone axial CT image immediately following the patient motion shows backing out of the introducer (*arrow*) and the biopsy needle as well as acute angulation of the biopsy needle where it enters the femoral cortex (*arrowhead*), which was presumably related to sudden flexion of the patient's gluteal muscles while moving. All instruments were subsequently removed from the patient, and postprocedural imaging (not shown) showed no retained foreign body.

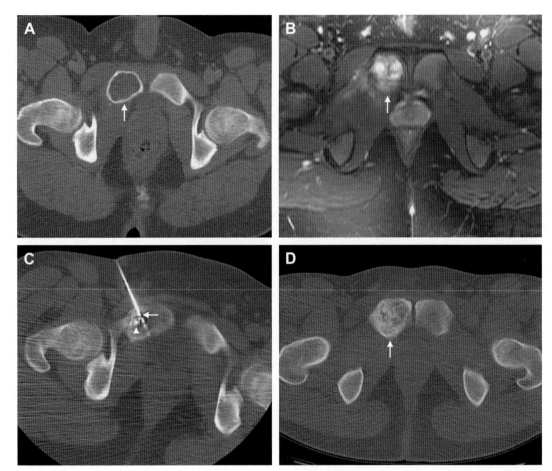

Fig. 17. (*A*) Axial CT image of the lower pelvis in a 15-year-old boy who presented with right groin pain shows a lytic lesion in the right superior pubic ramus that enlarges the contour of the bone (*arrow*). (*B*) Axial, T2-weighted, fat-suppressed MR image through the lesion shows multiple T2-hyperintense cystic spaces within the lesion (*arrow*), suggesting an aneurysmal bone cyst. (*C*) A 14-gauge bone penetration set was used to gain access to the lesion (*arrow*), and a spring-loaded side-cutting biopsy needle was inserted coaxially through the introducer to obtain multiple core samples (not shown). The biopsy needle was exchanged for a spinal needle, through which a mixture of 100 mg of triamcinolone and nonionic contrast was injected into the lesion (*arrowhead*). (*D*) Axial CT image from a follow-up examination 4 years later shows that the lesion is no longer cystic and has filled in with new bone formation (*arrow*). The final diagnosis was a collection of fibrous walled cysts, consistent with aneurysmal bone cyst.

increases the temperature of the tip to 90°C, where it is maintained for 4 to 6 minutes.[27,43,44] This process induces a spherical volume of necrosis slightly more than 1 cm in diameter.[45] Therefore, the tip is ideally positioned such that every part of the lesion is less than or equal to 5 mm away from the tip. If this is not possible, then multiple successive ablations are performed to ensure complete coverage of the tumor. Similarly, the electrode should be placed at least 1 cm away from vital neurovascular structures to prevent their damage.[43,46] This criterion excludes most spinal lesions. Long-term clinical success rates (ie, patient is pain free

and is not taking any pain medications) range from 89% to 94% after 1 treatment and range from 60% to 100% after 2 or more treatments.[27,43,47,48] Complication rates in larger series are less than 5%.[27,43,47,48] Most complications involve burns to the skin.[47,49,50] Cantwell and colleagues[51] reported an ablation of deep muscular tissue adjacent to the osteoid osteoma. Venbrux and colleagues[50] reported 1 case of transient paresthesia, which resolved after 2 weeks. Rosenthal and colleagues[27] reported 1 case of vasomotor instability, 1 case of cellulitis, and 2 cases of anesthesia-related complications.

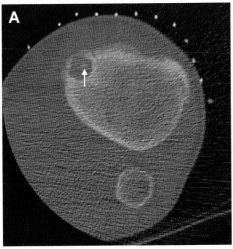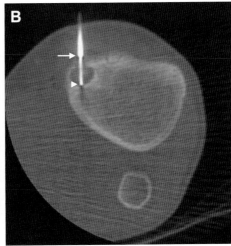

Fig. 18. (*A*) Left lateral decubitus axial image from a CT-guided biopsy of the left proximal tibia in a 15-year-old boy who presented with medial knee pain shows a lytic lesion with a thick sclerotic margin and a focus of central mineralization (*arrow*). Findings are virtually diagnostic of an osteoid osteoma. (*B*) A 14-gauge bone penetration set was used to gain access into the lesion (*arrow*). A 16-gauge trephine-type biopsy needle was inserted coaxially through the introducer into the lesion to obtain a core sample (*arrowhead*). Subsequently, a radiofrequency electrode was inserted coaxially through the introducer into the lesion for ablation (not shown). The final diagnosis was osteoid osteoma.

SUMMARY

Biopsy can be an important step in the workup of a bone or soft tissue lesion. Percutaneous core needle biopsy and fine-needle aspiration are safe and cost-effective methods of performing these procedures and should be performed in collaboration with the orthopedic oncologist who performs the definitive surgery. In the extremities, attention to and knowledge of compartmental anatomy is paramount. With concomitant use of frozen section evaluation at the time of biopsy, the chances of a nondiagnostic specimen necessitating rebiopsy are minimized. A solid understanding of the principles underlying the percutaneous approach to various lesions is extremely valuable and can be applied to the growing field of minimally invasive percutaneous therapy for bone and soft tissue lesions.

REFERENCES

1. Parikh J, Hyare H, Saifuddin A. The imaging features of post-traumatic myositis ossificans, with emphasis on MRI. Clin Radiol 2002;57(12):1058–66.
2. Ragunanthan N, Sugavanam C. Pseudomalignant myositis ossificans mimicking osteosarcoma: a case report. J Orthop Surg (Hong Kong) 2006;14(2):219–21.
3. Cottle L, Riordan T. Infectious spondylodiscitis. J Infect 2008;56(6):401–12.
4. Mankin HJ, Lange TA, Spanier SS. The hazards of biopsy in patients with malignant primary bone and soft-tissue tumors. J Bone Joint Surg Am 1982;64(8):1121–7.
5. Bickels J, Jelinek JS, Shmookler BM, et al. Biopsy of musculoskeletal tumors. Current concepts. Clin Orthop Relat Res 1999;(368):212–9.
6. Ashford RU, McCarthy SW, Scolyer RA, et al. Surgical biopsy with intra-operative frozen section. An accurate and cost-effective method for diagnosis of musculoskeletal sarcomas. J Bone Joint Surg Br 2006;88(9):1207–11.
7. Skrzynski MC, Biermann JS, Montag A, et al. Diagnostic accuracy and charge-savings of outpatient core needle biopsy compared with open biopsy of musculoskeletal tumors. J Bone Joint Surg Am 1996;78(5):644–9.
8. Heslin MJ, Lewis JJ, Woodruff JM, et al. Core needle biopsy for diagnosis of extremity soft tissue sarcoma. Ann Surg Oncol 1997;4(5):425–31.
9. Altuntas AO, Slavin J, Smith PJ, et al. Accuracy of computed tomography guided core needle biopsy of musculoskeletal tumours. ANZ J Surg 2005;75(4):187–91.
10. Jelinek JS, Murphey MD, Welker JA, et al. Diagnosis of primary bone tumors with image-guided percutaneous biopsy: experience with 110 tumors. Radiology 2002;223(3):731–7.
11. Hau A, Kim I, Kattapuram S, et al. Accuracy of CT-guided biopsies in 359 patients with musculoskeletal lesions. Skeletal Radiol 2002;31(6):349–53.
12. Stoker DJ, Cobb JP, Pringle JA. Needle biopsy of musculoskeletal lesions. A review of 208 procedures. J Bone Joint Surg Br 1991;73(3):498–500.

13. Wu JS, Goldsmith JD, Horwich PJ, et al. Bone and soft-tissue lesions: what factors affect diagnostic yield of image-guided core-needle biopsy? Radiology 2008;248(3):962–70.

14. Kattapuram SV, Khurana JS, Rosenthal DI. Percutaneous needle biopsy of the spine. Spine (Phila Pa 1976) 1992;17(5):561–4.

15. Welker JA, Henshaw RM, Jelinek J, et al. The percutaneous needle biopsy is safe and recommended in the diagnosis of musculoskeletal masses. Cancer 2000;89(12):2677–86.

16. Bommer KK, Ramzy I, Mody D. Fine-needle aspiration biopsy in the diagnosis and management of bone lesions: a study of 450 cases. Cancer 1997; 81(3):148–56.

17. Kattapuram SV, Rosenthal DI. Percutaneous biopsy of the cervical spine using CT guidance. AJR Am J Roentgenol 1987;149(3):539–41.

18. McDonald DJ. Limb-salvage surgery for treatment of sarcomas of the extremities. AJR Am J Roentgenol 1994;163(3):509–13 [discussion: 514–6].

19. Liu PT, Valadez SD, Chivers FS, et al. Anatomically based guidelines for core needle biopsy of bone tumors: implications for limb-sparing surgery. Radiographics 2007;27(1):189–205 [discussion: 206].

20. Toomayan GA, Robertson F, Major NM. Lower extremity compartmental anatomy: clinical relevance to radiologists. Skeletal Radiol 2005;34(6):307–13.

21. Toomayan GA, Robertson F, Major NM, et al. Upper extremity compartmental anatomy: clinical relevance to radiologists. Skeletal Radiol 2006;35(4): 195–201.

22. Enneking WF, Spanier SS, Goodman MA. Current concepts review. The surgical staging of musculoskeletal sarcoma. J Bone Joint Surg Am 1980; 62(6):1027–30.

23. Kattapuram SV, Rosenthal DI. Percutaneous biopsy of skeletal lesions. AJR Am J Roentgenol 1991; 157(5):935–42.

24. Sucu HK, Bezircioglu H, Cicek C, et al. Computerized tomography-guided percutaneous transforaminodiscal biopsy sampling of vertebral body lesions. J Neurosurg 2003;99(Suppl 1):51–5.

25. Paulson EK, Sheafor DH, Enterline DS, et al. CT fluoroscopy–guided interventional procedures: techniques and radiation dose to radiologists. Radiology 2001;220(1):161–7.

26. Espinosa LA, Jamadar DA, Jacobson JA, et al. CT-guided biopsy of bone: a radiologist's perspective. AJR Am J Roentgenol 2008;190(5):W283–9.

27. Rosenthal DI, Hornicek FJ, Torriani M, et al. Osteoid osteoma: percutaneous treatment with radiofrequency energy. Radiology 2003;229(1):171–5.

28. Murphy WA, Destouet JM, Gilula LA. Percutaneous skeletal biopsy 1981: a procedure for radiologists–results, review, and recommendations. Radiology 1981;139(3):545–9.

29. Olscamp A, Rollins J, Tao SS, et al. Complications of CT-guided biopsy of the spine and sacrum. Orthopedics 1997;20(12):1149–52.

30. Mavrogenis AF, Rimondi E, Ussia G, et al. Successful treatment of a bifocal eosinophilic granuloma of the spine with CT-guided corticosteroid injection. Orthopedics 2011;34(3):230.

31. Adamsbaum C, Kalifa G, Seringe R, et al. Direct Ethibloc injection in benign bone cysts: preliminary report on four patients. Skeletal Radiol 1993;22(5): 317–20.

32. Guibaud L, Herbreteau D, Dubois J, et al. Aneurysmal bone cysts: percutaneous embolization with an alcoholic solution of zein–series of 18 cases. Radiology 1998;208(2):369–73.

33. Garg NK, Carty H, Walsh HP, et al. Percutaneous Ethibloc injection in aneurysmal bone cysts. Skeletal Radiol 2000;29(4):211–6.

34. Callstrom MR, Charboneau JW, Goetz MP, et al. Painful metastases involving bone: feasibility of percutaneous CT- and US-guided radio-frequency ablation. Radiology 2002;224(1):87–97.

35. Goetz MP, Callstrom MR, Charboneau JW, et al. Percutaneous image-guided radiofrequency ablation of painful metastases involving bone: a multicenter study. J Clin Oncol 2004;22(2):300–6.

36. Dupuy DE, Liu D, Hartfeil D, et al. Percutaneous radiofrequency ablation of painful osseous metastases: a multicenter American College of Radiology Imaging Network trial. Cancer 2010;116(4): 989–97.

37. Kobayashi K, Shimoyama K, Nakamura K, et al. Percutaneous vertebroplasty immediately relieves pain of osteoporotic vertebral compression fractures and prevents prolonged immobilization of patients. Eur Radiol 2005;15(2):360–7.

38. Jakobs TF, Trumm C, Reiser M, et al. Percutaneous vertebroplasty in tumoral osteolysis. Eur Radiol 2007;17(8):2166–75.

39. Heiss JD, Doppman JL, Oldfield EH. Brief report: relief of spinal cord compression from vertebral hemangioma by intralesional injection of absolute ethanol. N Engl J Med 1994;331(8):508–11.

40. Doppman JL, Oldfield EH, Heiss JD. Symptomatic vertebral hemangiomas: treatment by means of direct intralesional injection of ethanol. Radiology 2000;214(2):341–8.

41. Rimondi E, Mavrogenis AF, Rossi G, et al. CT-guided corticosteroid injection for solitary eosinophilic granuloma of the spine. Skeletal Radiol 2011;40(6):757–64.

42. Simon CJ, Dupuy DE. Percutaneous minimally invasive therapies in the treatment of bone tumors: thermal ablation. Semin Musculoskelet Radiol 2006;10(2):137–44.

43. Woertler K, Vestring T, Boettner F, et al. Osteoid osteoma: CT-guided percutaneous radiofrequency

ablation and follow-up in 47 patients. J Vasc Interv Radiol 2001;12(6):717–22.

44. Barei DP, Moreau G, Scarborough MT, et al. Percutaneous radiofrequency ablation of osteoid osteoma. Clin Orthop Relat Res 2000;(373):115–24.

45. Tillotson CL, Rosenberg AE, Rosenthal DI. Controlled thermal injury of bone. Report of a percutaneous technique using radiofrequency electrode and generator. Invest Radiol 1989;24(11):888–92.

46. Rosenthal DI, Springfield DS, Gebhardt MC, et al. Osteoid osteoma: percutaneous radio-frequency ablation. Radiology 1995;197(2):451–4.

47. Sung KS, Seo JG, Shim JS, et al. Computed-tomography-guided percutaneous radiofrequency thermoablation for the treatment of osteoid osteoma-2 to 5 years follow-up. Int Orthop 2009;33(1):215–8.

48. Cribb GL, Goude WH, Cool P, et al. Percutaneous radiofrequency thermocoagulation of osteoid osteomas: factors affecting therapeutic outcome. Skeletal Radiol 2005;34(11):702–6.

49. Finstein JL, Hosalkar HS, Ogilvie CM, et al. Case reports: an unusual complication of radiofrequency ablation treatment of osteoid osteoma. Clin Orthop Relat Res 2006;448:248–51.

50. Venbrux AC, Montague BJ, Murphy KP, et al. Image-guided percutaneous radiofrequency ablation for osteoid osteomas. J Vasc Interv Radiol 2003;14(3):375–80.

51. Cantwell CP, O'Byrne J, Eustace S. Radiofrequency ablation of osteoid osteoma with cooled probes and impedance-control energy delivery. AJR Am J Roentgenol 2006;186(Suppl 5):S244–8.

Posttherapy Imaging of Musculoskeletal Neoplasms

Hillary Warren Garner, MD*, Mark J. Kransdorf, MD,
Jeffrey J. Peterson, MD

KEYWORDS

• Musculoskeletal • Sarcoma • Posttherapy • Imaging

Survival rates for patients with bone and soft tissue sarcomas have steadily improved in the last few decades because of improved surgical techniques and the use of adjuvant therapy. However, recurrence continues to plague long-term prognosis, in the form of both local recurrence and metastatic disease. Large studies of extremity soft tissue sarcomas have shown local recurrence rates of 17% to 29% and distant metastatic rates of 22% to 36%.[1,2] In cases of osteosarcoma, lung metastasis occurs in 28% by 5 years[3]; bone metastasis and local recurrence are less common, affecting 8% to 10% and 4% to 7% of patients, respectively.[4,5] These statistics emphasize the importance of both systemic and local surveillance. Because recurrences usually develop within the first 2 years following therapy,[6] with only 5% developing after 5 years,[5,7–9] follow-up imaging is most aggressive during this early posttreatment period. Although there is debate and variation in optimal surveillance strategies, imaging is commonly performed at shorter intervals in patients with high-grade, large, and deep tumors, all factors that portend higher risk.[1,2] Regardless of the time interval used, magnetic resonance (MR) imaging is the primary imaging modality used for local surveillance, with chest computed tomography (CT) most often used for metastatic lung surveillance. More recently, positron emission tomography (PET) CT has gained attention as an accurate surveillance tool for both local and distant recurrence.

Although posttreatment changes can mimic or obscure local recurrence on MR imaging, a systematic approach to and knowledge of the features of recurrence versus therapeutic change allows differentiation in almost all cases. This article presents a systematic approach to posttherapy MR imaging, emphasizing fundamental concepts and discussing potentially confounding posttreatment changes. We also highlight the recent advent of PET-CT in local and metastatic surveillance.

FUNDAMENTAL CONCEPTS

A systematic approach to the imaging of patients following therapy is essential and is applicable to patients with either bone or soft tissue sarcoma. It begins with a thorough understanding of the clinical history, including previous therapy, continues with a review of previous radiographic and imaging studies, and concludes with protocol and interpretation of the posttherapy imaging.

Preimaging evaluation of the patient's clinical history, including the pathology report(s), details of surgery and/or adjuvant therapy, and an assessment of the surgical site, is fundamental to obtaining a useful posttreatment MR imaging examination and essential in distinguishing expected posttherapy changes and posttherapy complications from local tumor recurrence. Review of previous imaging studies, most importantly the imaging obtained at the time of initial diagnosis, is also essential. In our experience, the imaging appearance of local recurrence most often simulates the appearance of the initial lesion (Fig. 1). Awareness of the expected appearance of local recurrence also makes it easier to identify.

The authors have nothing to disclose.
Department of Radiology, Mayo Clinic Florida, 4500 San Pablo Road, Jacksonville, FL 32224, USA
* Corresponding author.
E-mail address: garner.hillary@mayo.edu

Radiol Clin N Am 49 (2011) 1307–1323
doi:10.1016/j.rcl.2011.07.011

radiologic.theclinics.com

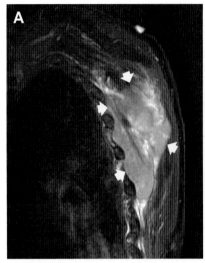
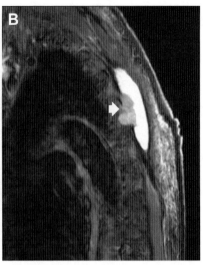

Fig. 1. An 87-year-old man with a left periscapular leiomyosarcoma who underwent surgical resection and post-operative radiation therapy. Preoperative sagittal short-tau inversion recovery (STIR) image (*A*) shows a heterogeneous hyperintense mass (*arrows*) in the periscapular region abutting multiple upper ribs. Sagittal STIR image performed 3 months after surgical resection (*B*) shows a recurrent tumor nodule (*arrow*) with T2 signal characteristics identical to the initial tumor. Note radiation change in the surrounding soft tissues.

Inspection of the surgical site and marking the surgical scars ensures adequate coverage of the tumor bed (**Fig. 2**). Preimaging evaluation allows imaging protocols to be modified appropriately

Fig. 2. A 65-year-old woman with a history of liposarcoma in the posterior right thigh who underwent surgical resection and postoperative radiation (6660 cGy), then suffered a recurrence 12 years later that was treated with reresection and 2500 cGy brachytherapy. Photograph shows a well-healed longitudinal scar with skin markers placed at the proximal and distal extents of the scar (*arrows*). Note well-demarcated rectangular area of radiation dermatitis with skin discoloration.

for each individual patient. For example, special CT or MR imaging techniques may be required for metal suppression in patients with indwelling hardware.

Preparation and coordination between imaging and ordering personnel can ensure that the appropriate information is available and greatly reduce potential interpretation delays and call-backs, which most often occur because of a lack of clinical and prior imaging data and incomplete coverage of the surgical site.

Preimaging Evaluation

Clinical history
A detailed knowledge of the previous surgery is imperative and should include an understanding of the tumor type, histologic grade, location, extent, and adequacy of surgical margins. Each of these factors significantly affects the risk for recurrence of both bone and soft tissue sarcomas. Poor cell differentiation, axial skeletal location, and positive or close surgical margins all portend a higher risk. Large, deep lesions also carry a higher risk of recurrence in patients treated for soft tissue sarcoma.[2]

Reconstructive surgery for limb salvage and/or soft tissue coverage is often necessary following treatment of musculoskeletal neoplasms. Progressive advancements in imaging and surgical techniques have afforded more patients the option of limb salvage rather than amputation in the treatment of malignant bone and soft tissue tumors, with equivalent long-term patient survival. Current limb salvage reconstruction techniques include modular/megaprostheses, allograft-prosthesis composite (APC), bone autograft/allograft and cementation. The 2 most commonly performed procedures for malignant and aggressive benign bone tumors of the extremities are APC and megaprostheses, which show equivalent long-term component longevity.[10–13] Familiarity with the appearance of these prostheses and an understanding of their respective potential complications is important to provide a detailed assessment during follow-up imaging. Patients opting for limb salvage undergo radiographs at regular intervals to evaluate for mechanical complications, such as loosening or prosthesis fracture, whereas the oncological complications of local recurrence and metastatic disease often require more advanced imaging techniques.

The patient's history should also be examined for neoadjuvant chemotherapy or radiation therapy. Chemotherapy alters tumor size, morphology, and enhancement pattern. Assessment of tumor response to neoadjuvant therapy can help further stratify recurrence risk, because poor response is associated with more aggressive tumors and increased risk of local recurrence and metastatic disease. Familiarity with a patient's radiation treatment history, including total dose and time course, is also useful, because radiation causes predictable time-dependent changes to the skin and soft tissues within the treatment bed.[14] Radiation changes also occur in the bone marrow, more commonly when radiation is used in combination with chemotherapy.[15] Similar time-dependent changes occur within rotation and free myocutaneous flaps used for reconstructive soft tissue coverage.[16]

Review of previous imaging

Review of the radiographic and CT/MR imaging obtained at the time of initial diagnosis is invaluable, because it familiarizes the radiologist with the imaging characteristics of the original tumor, which are likely to be the imaging characteristics of recurrent disease. Obtaining the initial diagnostic imaging is frequently difficult, often performed at outside imaging centers/hospitals, or provided on incompatible media. Staff members can inform or remind patients of the need to provide their outside imaging studies, pathology reports, and other pertinent data at the time of their imaging appointment, or even in advance, to help streamline care.

POSTTREATMENT IMAGING: TIMING AND FREQUENCY

A consensus review regarding the optimal timing and frequency of follow-up imaging of malignant or aggressive musculoskeletal tumors was reported by Roberts and colleagues[17] as part of the American College of Radiology (ACR) Appropriateness Criteria. This review covers both bone and soft tissue sarcomas, and emphasizes the need for frequent local and systemic surveillance in high-risk patients. The investigators reference the follow-up recommendations of a retrospective analysis[18] of data derived from a review of 1500 patients with soft tissue sarcoma from Memorial Sloan-Kettering and the MD Anderson Cancer Center. These patients were stratified based on tumor size, with those at high risk having extremity tumors larger than 5 cm. This analysis advocates local and systemic surveillance intervals of every 3 months for 2 years, every 4 months for the next 2 years, every 6 months for the fifth year, and then annually for years 5 to 10 in high-risk patients. Similar intervals are recommended for trunk and retroperitoneal tumors, regardless of size. Surveillance of low-risk patients with extremity tumors less than 5 cm could be individualized for the patient and location of tumor.[18]

Optimal surveillance strategies in bone sarcoma have not been scientifically established, but because of the risk of lung metastases, chest CT is advocated every 3 to 6 months for at least 5 years. Local surveillance strategies for patients with bone sarcoma include radiographs, also performed every 3 to 6 months for at least 5 years, and then annually thereafter up to 10 years. For higher risk lesions or where physical examination may be limited, MR imaging may also be performed at close intervals for local surveillance.

Current literature supports the use of PET/CT as a problem-solving tool in patients with equivocal MR imaging, chest CT, or technetium bone scan findings and as a primary evaluation tool in patients with extensive metallic hardware.[17] However, limitations of MR imaging from metallic artifact have decreased in recent years because of improvements in metal suppression software.

Local Surveillance

Radiography

Radiographs are an essential tool for the assessment of mechanical postoperative complications as well as local recurrence in patients with bone tumors. They are performed at regular intervals, and are reliable for evaluation of instability, dislocation, loosening, fracture/nonunion (**Fig. 3**), and infection. In addition, radiographs accurately

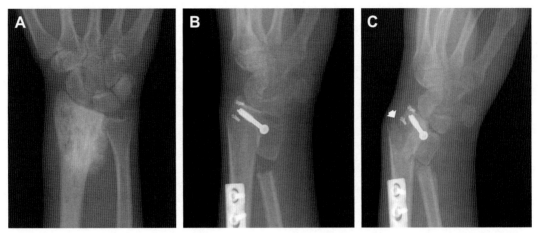

Fig. 3. A 24-year-old woman with a low-grade intramedullary osteosarcoma of the distal radius. Preoperative anteroposterior (AP) radiograph of the right wrist (*A*) shows a sclerotic, partially exophytic, osseous mass in the distal radius. Oblique radiograph obtained 3 months after en bloc resection with allograft and plate and screw fixation (*B*) shows anatomic alignment and intact hardware. Oblique radiograph obtained 7 months after distal radial resection (*C*) shows a comminuted displaced fracture (*arrow*) of the distal radial allograft.

characterize soft tissue and osseous mineralization and provide an assessment of bone contour and structure, which is useful in identifying recurrence in patients with both bone and soft tissue sarcoma. When oncology complications are suspected clinically, radiographs are an important comparison study to ensure that MR imaging findings are not misconstrued.

MR and CT protocol modification

Both MR and CT imaging protocols may require modification in patients following sarcoma treatment. MR imaging is highly accurate and is currently the most widely used modality for detection of local recurrence in patients with treated bone and soft tissue tumor. Routine protocols as well as several helpful modifications for posttreatment tumor imaging, including subtraction imaging and gradient echo imaging, have been described previously.[14] More recently, improvements in metal suppression software have greatly improved CT and MR imaging evaluation of the treatment bed in limb salvage patients with prostheses. Despite the potential risks of routine contrast use in posttreatment follow-up, contrast-enhanced sequences are usually included as part of the tumor protocol at many tertiary care centers in the United States. Recent attention to the risks of contrast may necessitate better triage of patients to select those who would most benefit from its use.

Metal susceptibility artifacts have been a major limitation in the usefulness of MR imaging for follow-up of patients with bone sarcoma. Recent advances in metal artifact suppression have greatly improved visualization of the periprosthetic tissues. Bandwidth, echo time, echo train length, gradient strength, and voxel size are a few of the parameters that can be adjusted to optimize metal suppression.[19–22] Although availability is limited on commercial scanners, special sequences such as view angle tilt (VAT) and metal artifact reduction sequence (MARS)[23,24] also exist for metal suppression. A newer work-in-progress (WIP) application developed by Siemens for the Magnetom Avanto machine is currently being tested at our institution with promising results. This application effectively reduces metallic artifact on T1-weighted imaging by increasing the bandwidth and reduces metallic artifact on short-tau inversion recovery (STIR) imaging by matching the excitation bandwidth of the inversion pulse to the bandwidth of the refocusing pulses (**Fig. 4**). Signal-to-noise ratio can suffer when parameters or techniques are used to optimize metal suppression, but a balance between factors can usually be achieved to provide the best diagnostic quality image.

CT can also be limited by metallic hardware because of photon starvation and beam hardening artifact. As with MR imaging, several parameters can be adjusted to reduce metallic hardware–related artifact, including higher peak voltage and tube charge, narrow collimation, thick section and soft tissue/smooth kernel reconstruction, and extended CT scale.[20] Recently, dual-energy CT has shown efficacy in reducing beam hardening artifact by extrapolating an image with beam

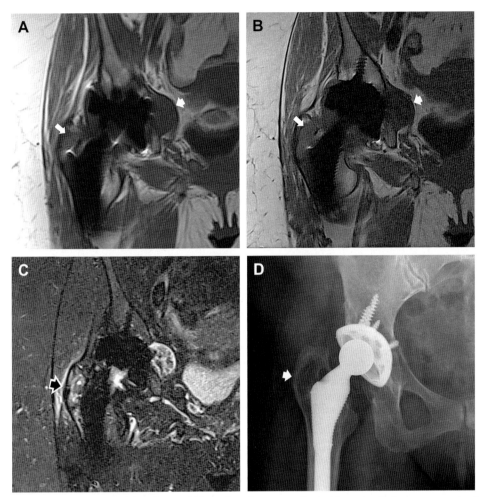

Fig. 4. A 58-year-old woman with right total hip arthroplasty complicated by polyethylene wear and osteolysis. Routine coronal T1-weighted image of the pelvis (*A*) shows metallic susceptibility artifact in the right hip region caused by arthroplasty components with areas of intermediate T1 intensity in zone III of the acetabulum and zone I of the proximal femur (*arrows*), compatible with areas of osteolysis. Coronal T1-weighted image of the right hemipelvis obtained at a higher bandwidth (*B*) allows for better delineation of the marrow around the prosthesis and improved visualization of the areas of osteolysis (*arrows*). Coronal STIR image of the right hemipelvis optimized for metal suppression (*C*) shows the T2 hyperintense areas of osteolysis as well as a small transverse linear area of high signal in the lateral cortex of the greater trochanter (*arrow*) with overlying soft tissue edema, compatible with a subtle nondisplaced fracture confirmed on radiographs (*arrow*) (*D*).

hardening properties at very high photon energies from the information acquired from the dual-energy acquisition.[25]

COMMON POSTTREATMENT CHANGES

There are several imaging features that are commonly seen following treatment of bone and soft tissue tumor. Knowledge of these imaging features minimizes the likelihood that they will be misconstrued for recurrent tumor. Posttreatment changes include the effects of chemotherapy, preoperative or postoperative radiation on bone

and soft tissue, postsurgical fluid collections, hemorrhage, and reconstructive myocutaneous flaps.

Chemotherapy

The effects of chemotherapy are often believed to be inconsequential; however, significant increase in tumor size secondary to chemotherapy-induced hemorrhage has been reported.[26] In other cases, chemotherapy may significantly reduce tumor size, with only necrotic, fibrotic, and reactive tissue identified at subsequent surgery.[27] We find contrast-enhanced imaging to be useful in determining the degree of intralesional necrosis; a feature that may be useful in establishing the effectiveness of chemotherapy and tumor biologic potential (**Fig. 5**). In cases with spontaneous or chemotherapy-induced hemorrhage, we have found the subtraction technique to be a useful method of distinguishing hemorrhage from enhancing viable tumor (**Fig. 6**).

Radiation therapy

It has long been recognized that resection of high-grade soft tissue sarcomas without adjuvant therapy results in unacceptably high rates of local recurrence. In the 1970s, this motivated oncologists to evaluate the use of adjuvant radiation therapy and chemotherapy in patients with soft tissue sarcoma undergoing limb-sparing surgery.[28] The usefulness of radiation in patients with bone sarcoma varies by tumor type, with radiation playing an important role in treatment of Ewing sarcoma of bone,[29,30] but a more limited role in osteosarcoma.[31] In current practice, radiation may be administered before, during, or following surgical tumor resection.[32]

Radiation changes are readily identified in both bone and soft tissue. Osseous changes following radiation have been well-documented; however, the current discussion focuses on those changes primarily identified on MR imaging. MR imaging can detect radiation-induced marrow changes as early as 8 days following onset of therapy.[33] In between 3 and 6 weeks, the marrow shows increasingly heterogeneous signal intensity, with increasing fat signal. In most patients, complete fatty replacement usually occurs within 6 to 8 weeks.[33,34] Uncommonly, a band of peripheral intermediate signal surrounding central fat may be seen.[34] About half of those patients receiving radiation will show changes in the marrow immediately adjacent to the radiated field. These changes are milder and are more common in patients with highly cellular pretreatment marrow.[33,35] In radiated extremities, poorly-defined areas of nonspecific nonadipose tissue can develop within the marrow in approximately 40% of patients. usually several months following the completion of radiation, becoming more prominent in the succeeding months before stabilizing (**Fig. 7**).[15]

As a result of the cellular damage caused by radiation, irradiated bone is at increased risk for fracture.[36] The pelvis is the most likely area to be involved and the incidence of pelvis-associated injury is small at 0.1% to 0.3%.[37] This percentage is considerably less than the 1.8% estimated incidence of sacral insufficiency fractures in women aged 55 years and older.[38]

Soft tissue changes are more variable and differ with the type of radiotherapy. Richardson and colleagues [39] characterized the soft tissue changes following radiation and noted that irradiated soft tissue showed abnormal edemalike signal intensity. The signal intensity showed great variability,

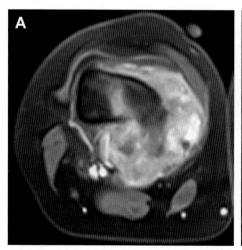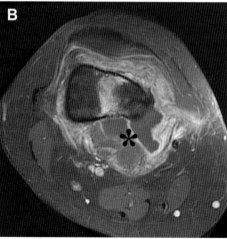

Fig. 5. A 16-year-old girl with high-grade osteosarcoma of the right distal femur treated with 4 cycles of preoperative chemotherapy consisting of doxorubicin, ifosfamide, and cisplatin, followed by distal femoral resection and prosthesis placement with a rotating hinge knee arthroplasty. Pretreatment axial fat-saturated postgadolinium T1-weighted image of the distal right thigh obtained at an outside institution (*A*) shows a heterogeneously enhancing mass in the medial aspect of the distal femoral metadiaphysis with a large soft tissue component. Axial fat-saturated postgadolinium T1-weighted image obtained after 4 cycles of 3-drug chemotherapy (*B*) shows extensive necrosis of the tumor, especially in the soft tissue component (*asterisk*). There was 5% to 10% of viable high-grade osteosarcoma at surgery.

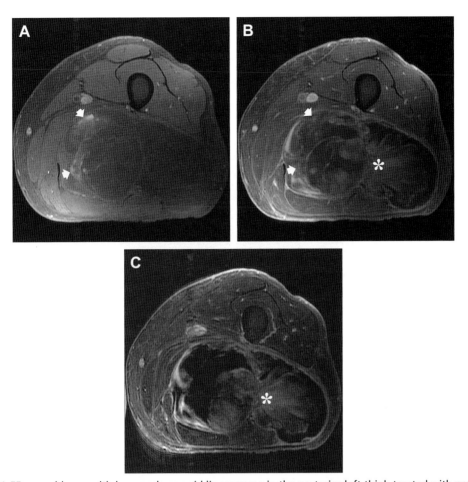

Fig. 6. A 55-year-old man with low-grade myxoid liposarcoma in the posterior left thigh treated with preoperative radiation therapy (5040 cGy). Axial fat-saturated T1-weighted image obtained 1 month after completion of neoadjuvant radiation (*A*) shows wispy T1 hyperintensity (*arrows*) compatible with internal hemorrhage at the medial aspect of the mass. Axial fat-saturated postgadolinium T1-weighted image (*B*) shows lobular areas of T1 hyperintensity not evident on the precontrast image, compatible with enhancing viable tumor (*asterisk*), with signal intensity similar to that of preexisting hemorrhage (*arrows*). Axial subtraction image (*C*) discriminates between enhancing viable tumor (*asterisk*) and the areas of nonenhancing internal hemorrhage.

but was generally greater on STIR images than on T2-weighted spin-echo images. Signal alterations increase with time, being greatest in photon-treated patients at 12 to 18 months and returning to normal in about half of these in 2 to 3 years. In neutron-treated patients, signal intensity increases to a maximum at 6 months; however, return to normal is slower and less frequent, requiring 3 to 4 years and occurring in less than 20% of patients. The edema signal in the subcutaneous tissue appears as a trabecular or lattice like pattern of low to intermediate signal intensity on T1-weighted spin-echo images and high signal intensity on fluid-sensitive sequences.[26] Radiation-induced changes in muscle are more diffuse with minimal enhancement following

contrast administration and preservation of muscle shape and texture.[26,40,41]

MR imaging signal abnormalities are greater and persist longer in the intermuscular septa than in the fat or muscle. The size of the fat and intermuscular septa increase mildly, whereas muscle shows a decrease in size following treatment.[39]

Following radiation therapy, patients may also develop inflammatory pseudotumors.[42] There is scant documentation of this rare phenomenon in the literature, but Vanel and colleagues[41] noted 2 such cases in a review of follow-up imaging of 182 patients with aggressive soft tissue tumors. Both lesions presented as masses with high signal intensity, one 1 year following and the other 12 years following radiation and surgery. Both of

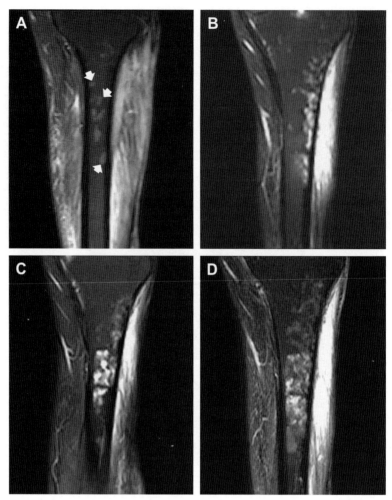

Fig. 7. A 58-year-old man with history of intermediate-grade undifferentiated pleomorphic sarcoma of the lateral aspect of the proximal left lower leg who received 5040 cGy of preoperative radiation. Coronal STIR image obtained 5 months after the completion of radiation therapy (*A*) shows patchy areas of increased signal (*arrows*) in the marrow within the upper aspect of the radiation field. Coronal STIR images obtained 13 months (*B*), 27 months (*C*), and 32 months (*D*) after completion of radiation therapy show progressive increase in radiation osteitis with time.

these lesions were investigated with dynamic contrast enhancement and showed delayed enhancement (4–7 minutes), compared with tumor recurrence (1–3 minutes).

Postoperative fluid and hemorrhage
Postoperative fluid collections and hemorrhage following sarcoma surgery show a similar appearance to that seen following nononcology procedures. In the oncology patient, the masslike appearance of these complications may mimic local tumor recurrence and vice versa, and the distinction may be especially difficult in selected cases, such as in tumors with myxoid features. In these instances, contrast imaging is helpful in making this distinction (**Fig. 8**).

Uncomplicated postoperative fluid collections are more readily distinguished from tumor recurrence. Recurrent tumor is usually more heterogeneous and the margins are usually more irregular than those in simple postoperative hygroma. Contrast-enhanced imaging may prove helpful in cases in which seromas show increased (intermediate) signal intensity on T1-weighted images. Most seromas seem to resolve in 3 to 18 months,[26,43] although this time is variable, and they may persist for an extended period of time.

Reconstructive surgery
The extensive tissue resection required to achieve adequate surgical margins in oncological surgery often requires soft tissue reconstructive surgery.

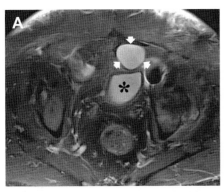 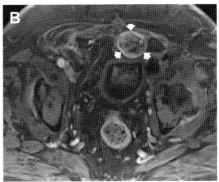

Fig. 8. A 79-year-old man with history of myxoid liposarcoma of the left inguinal region treated with preoperative radiation (4500 cGy) and wide local excision. Axial fat-saturated T2-weighted image of the lower pelvis obtained 6 years after surgery (*A*) shows a rounded high-intensity structure (*arrows*) immediately anterior to the bladder (*asterisk*). This nodule has a seromatous appearance on T2-weighted images. Corresponding axial fat-saturated postcontrast T1-weighted image (*B*) shows heterogeneous enhancement of the nodule (*arrows*), similar in appearance to the original tumor (not shown) and compatible with a delayed local recurrence.

Myocutaneous flaps are used in more than two-thirds of extremity sarcoma surgeries.[44]

Myocutaneous flaps contain both muscle and overlying skin. Rotational flaps are rotated into position, covering the soft tissue defect and preserving the native neurovascular supply via a pedicle. Free flaps are completely detached, placed into the soft tissue defect, and the vascular pedicle is reanastomosed using a microvascular technique. Although most flaps are used for coverage only, rotational flaps using muscles such as the latissimus dorsi may provide both coverage and function when they are used for the upper arm.

As the MR imaging appearance of radiated tissue will change with time, so will the appearance of myocutaneous flaps. A recent report by Fox and colleagues[16] reviewed the MR imaging findings in 30 myocutaneous flaps. They noted that all flaps show time-dependent changes in size, signal intensity, and enhancement. All flaps atrophy with time, showing decreased muscle mass and progressive fatty replacement. However, the amount of atrophy is variable, ranging from mild to marked, but is less in flaps providing coverage and function. In addition, all flaps initially show increased signal intensity on T2-weighted images, which return to baseline (similar to the signal intensity of the surrounding muscle) in one-third of cases in between 5 and 21 months. Enhancement is seen in about three-quarters of cases, returning to baseline in about one-third, in 18 months. Postoperative radiation therapy increased the likelihood that a flap will exhibit increased signal on T2-weighted images and enhancement.

Local Recurrence

Soft tissue tumors

MR imaging and ultrasonography have both been shown to be useful in detecting local recurrence.[45] Recurrent tumor is characterized by the presence of a discrete nodule or mass, typically with prolonged T1 and T2 relaxation times, usually showing prominent contrast enhancement (**Fig. 9**). However, tumor recurrence is usually well seen without enhanced imaging. When identification of a discrete high–signal intensity nodule on fluid-sensitive images is used as a criterion for local recurrence, MR imaging is accurate.[41]

Postsurgical changes are more variable and usually show areas of low or intermediate signal intensity or fluid collections, without a discrete nodule.[41,45] When a mass with high signal intensity on T2-weighted images is found, tumor must be differentiated from postoperative hygroma. In most cases, this differentiation is straightforward with fluid characterized by a homogeneous, well-defined mass with intermediate to low T1 and high T2 signal relative to muscle on spin-echo MR images.

As noted previously, comparison with pretreatment images is essential. For example, myxoid tumors may mimic cysts on MR imaging; hence, differentiation between a postoperative fluid collection and recurrent tumor would be more difficult if the patient's original tumor was a myxoid liposarcoma. When there is question as to whether an area of high signal intensity on T2-weighted images represents fluid, ultrasound examination is an ideal method for further evaluation. It is easy, inexpensive, and highly accurate. Alternatively, gadolinium-enhanced MR imaging may be used.

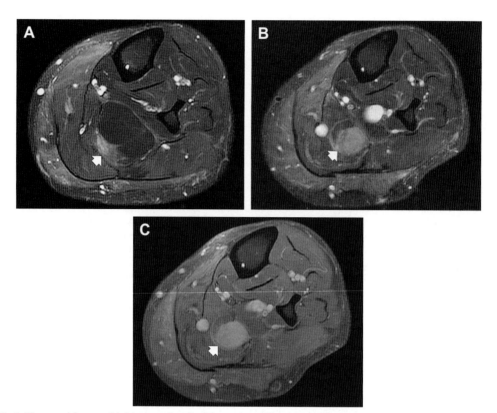

Fig. 9. A 62-year-old man with history of well-differentiated liposarcoma centered in the deep posterior compartment of the left lower leg, treated with marginal excision. Pretreatment axial fat-saturated T2-weighted image of the left lower leg (*A*) shows a fatty mass with a focal peripheral area of high signal posteromedially (*arrow*). Posttreatment axial fat-saturated T2-weighted (*B*) and axial fat-saturated postcontrast T1-weighted image (*C*) obtained 19 months after (*A*) show a discrete nodular focus of T2 hyperintensity with diffuse homogeneous enhancement (*arrows*), compatible with recurrent dedifferentiated liposarcoma.

Ultrasound may be used as the primary modality to follow patients for recurrence, with a discrete hypoechoic mass considered to be recurrent tumor.[45] Doppler imaging is helpful to identify internal hypervascularity (**Fig. 10**). However, ultrasound is operator dependent, and of limited value in cases where the osseous anatomy is complex, such as in the shoulder girdle or pelvis. Consequently, we prefer MR imaging for identification of recurrent tumor.

Bone tumors

As stated previously, radiographs are performed at regular intervals in the postoperative patient with bone tumor and are highly reliable for detection of mechanical complications. Manifestations of tumor recurrence, including osteolysis, periostitis, and/or matrix mineralization, are also readily detectable with radiography (**Fig. 11**). However, routine interval CT or MR imaging is reasonable in high-risk patients because recurrence can typically be identified earlier with

advanced techniques than with radiography (**Fig. 12**). In addition, CT or MR imaging can discriminate between fluid collections and tumor and better evaluate the extent of disease.[46] Metallic artifact can be reduced sufficiently to provide good-quality diagnostic information in most cases. As with soft tissue sarcoma, the MR imaging characteristics of local bone sarcoma recurrence typically mimic the characteristics of the original tumor, usually with a nodular focus of intermediate to high T2 signal noted in the soft tissues or marrow. Ultrasound is a useful modality for discriminating solid recurrent tumor from an abscess or seroma and is a highly efficient method for biopsy guidance.

PET/CT: Local and Metastatic Surveillance

In the past decade, PET has shown value in musculoskeletal tumor imaging for specific indications.[47–49] Although PET is of limited benefit for screening purposes or in aiding the diagnosis of various musculoskeletal tumors, it has proved

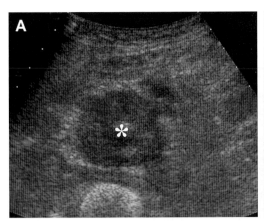

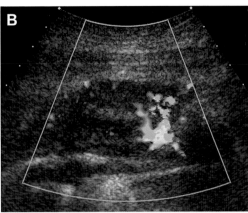

Fig. 10. A 70-year-old man with history of undifferentiated pleomorphic sarcoma of the right medial thigh treated with wide local excision and postoperative radiation (5040 cGy). Targeted transverse sonographic image (A) in the area of palpable concern within the treatment bed of the right medial thigh shows a discrete rounded hypoechoic nodule (*asterisk*). Hypervascularity of the nodule is noted on the Doppler image (B). Ultrasound-guided biopsy of this nodule confirmed recurrent tumor.

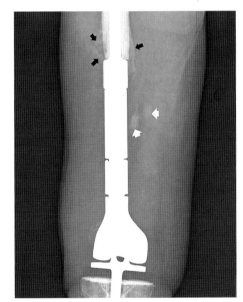

Fig. 11. A 69-year-old man with history of high-grade osteoblastic osteosarcoma of the distal femur complicated by pathologic fracture, treated with preoperative chemotherapy and en bloc resection with placement of a modular distal femoral megaprosthesis and knee arthroplasty. Postoperative course was complicated by 2 local recurrences (the patient declined amputation after the first recurrence). AP radiograph obtained 6 months after initial resection surgery and 2 months after resection of first local recurrence shows periosteal reaction at the distal resection margin with irregular mineralization in the surrounding soft tissue (*black arrows*). Two mineralized soft tissue nodules are noted medial to the megaprosthesis (*white arrows*), compatible with a soft tissue osteosarcoma recurrence.

useful in the evaluation of previously treated musculoskeletal lesions for staging, restaging, and monitoring response to therapy.[50,51] Specifically, PET is a useful tool for restaging of primary bone tumors and soft tissue sarcomas, allowing for simultaneous detection of local recurrence as well as distant metastatic disease.[47] PET imaging can also be efficacious for monitoring response to therapy for both primary osseous lesions and soft tissue tumors, allowing a noninvasive assessment of histologic response to treatment.[52–55]

Fluorine-18 2-fluoro-2-deoxyglucose (FDG) is the most common and readily available radiopharmaceutical used for PET imaging. Acquisition of CT with the FDG PET scan allows accurate depiction of physiologic information from the PET scan superimposed on the anatomic data from the CT examination, which permits precise localization of sites of abnormal glucose uptake. Most musculoskeletal tumors depict accelerated glucose metabolism with uptake of glucose in sufficient quantities to be easily differentiated from the surrounding background activity. FDG PET has proved sensitive for detection and localization of musculoskeletal tumors.[56,57] However, specificity of FDG PET has proved to be less than optimal for musculoskeletal lesions, because both benign and malignant lesions may show significant abnormal metabolic activity, and differentiating the two can be difficult. However, this issue is less of a concern when dealing with restaging and monitoring response to therapy for musculoskeletal tumors. In these clinical scenarios, the histology of the lesion is known and the clinical question concerns the presence or absence of residual or recurrent tumor, or whether previous

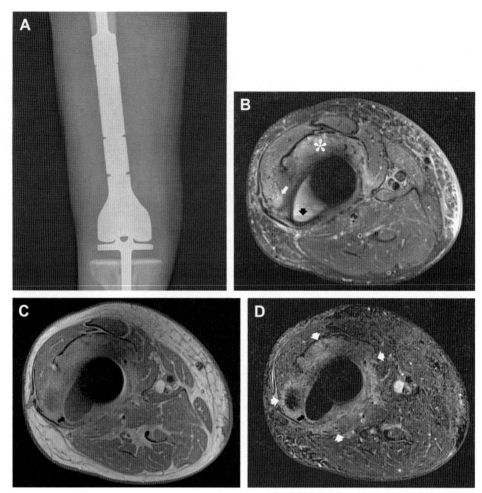

Fig. 12. The same patient as in **Fig. 11**: a 69-year-old man with history of high-grade osteoblastic osteosarcoma of the distal femur complicated by pathologic fracture, treated with preoperative chemotherapy and en bloc resection with placement of a modular distal femoral megaprosthesis and knee arthroplasty. Postoperative course was complicated by 2 local recurrences (the patient declined amputation after the first recurrence). AP radiograph of the distal right femur (*A*) obtained four months after the initial resection surgery (at the time of first recurrence) shows no evidence of recurrence. Axial STIR image with metal artifact optimization (*B*), obtained the same day as the radiograph (*A*), shows a complex fluid collection with fluid-fluid level (*black arrow*) abutting the lateral aspect of the prosthesis. In addition, there is a nodular focus of high signal lateral to the fluid collection (*white arrow*) as well as heterogeneous abnormal high-signal tissue abutting the prosthesis anteriorly (*asterisk*) in the region of the vastus intermedius. Axial postcontrast T1-weighted (*C*) and axial subtraction images (*D*) show thin rim enhancement of the fluid collection (*black arrow*). The nodular focus laterally shows irregular peripheral enhancement and the areas of heterogeneous high T2 signal anteriorly show diffuse enhancement surrounding the prosthesis (*white arrows in D*), confirmed to be a local recurrence (the first of 2). The patient declined amputation in favor of radiation therapy.

therapy has been efficacious. In such cases, FDG PET imaging can prove an invaluable tool.

Restaging

FDG PET imaging can be useful for restaging primary osseous malignancies and soft tissue sarcomas.[50] Obtaining PET following therapy is useful for assessing for residual or recurrent disease at the site of the primary tumor (**Fig. 13**).[49] It can also be helpful in identifying sites of additional involvement or metastases elsewhere within the body.[49] Approximately 20% to 40% of patients with soft tissue sarcomas will develop local or distant recurrence of disease, and accurate and timely detection of sites of both local and distant disease can allow prompt initiation of further treatment, which can have a profound effect on patient prognosis.[48,51]

FDG PET allows whole-body imaging, accurately evaluating both the osseous structures and

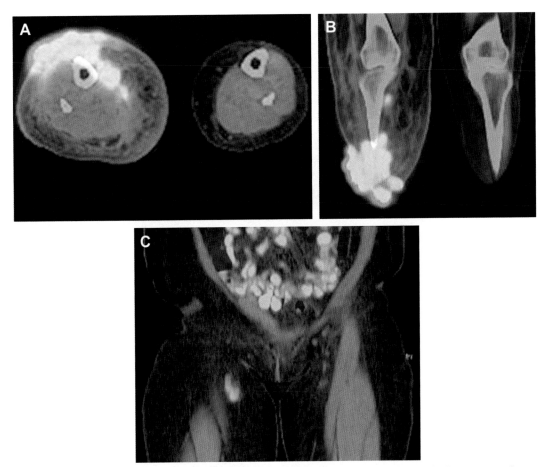

Fig. 13. A 55-year-old woman with a previously treated angiosarcoma involving the right lower extremity presented with obvious recurrence of disease with an ulcerating lesion involving the right anterior calf. FDG PET scan was obtained for restaging purposes. Axial image of the lower legs (*A*) shows the degree of involvement with a large area of abnormal metabolic activity corresponding to the ulcerating lesion. Coronal image of the lower extremities (*B*) depicts a smaller focus of recurrence just proximal to the larger lesion. Discovery of this unsuspected focus altered the original surgical plan and amputation was performed at a higher level. In addition, coronal image through the groin (*C*) shows a focus of abnormal metabolic activity corresponding to a mildly prominent inguinal lymph node. Biopsy confirmed right inguinal nodal metastatic disease.

soft tissues for tumor involvement. PET/CT examinations have the potential to replace multiple other modalities including bone scintigraphy, CT, and MR, which can prove both time efficient and cost-effective.[49] Although sensitivity for small (<8 mm) pulmonary nodules has not surpassed chest CT, PET/CT has proved an excellent modality for detection of pulmonary metastases 8 to 10 mm or larger as well as nodal and other soft tissue tumor involvement, which can obviate the need for separate diagnostic CT examinations (**Fig. 14**). FDG PET also has significant advantages compared with bone scintigraphy for the detection of osseous metastatic disease.[49,58] FDG PET allows earlier detection of osseous lesions compared with bone scintigraphy and provides evaluation

of both soft tissues and the osseous structures in a single examination. Detection of previously unsuspected sites of metastases can have a significant impact on treatment options.[57,59]

Evaluation of sites of prior tumor resection can be challenging because of posttreatment changes in the operative bed. Differentiation of residual or recurrent tumor from posttreatment changes can be difficult with anatomic imaging because of anatomic distortion, disrupted tissue planes, radiation changes, and metal artifact.[48,49,53] FDG PET is useful in such cases by providing a glucose analogue to assess for the presence of tumor in the operative bed. FDG PET imaging can also be useful as an adjunct to anatomic imaging to either identify sites of interest to guide follow-up

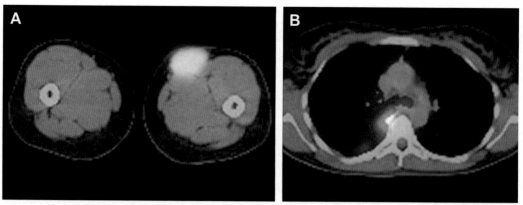

Fig. 14. A 37-year-old woman with history of leiomyosarcoma of the left anterior thigh status postsurgical resection. Restaging FDG PET axial image of the thighs (*A*) depicts a focus of abnormal metabolic activity corresponding to a lesion in the operative bed and compatible with local tumor recurrence. Axial image through the thorax (*B*) shows a peripheral lesion in the posteromedial hemithorax. Biopsy confirmed a pleural metastasis.

anatomic imaging or to further clarify equivocal findings identified on prior MR or CT examinations.[60,61] However, specificity can be an issue with FDG PET from the immediate postoperative period to up to 6 months following surgery because of the hypermetabolism associated with postoperative changes and healing. For this reason, it is suggested to avoid FDG PET imaging for at least 3 months following surgery to allow postoperative uptake to dissipate.[52–55,62]

Monitoring response to therapy
PET has also shown promise in assessing therapy response in musculoskeletal lesions.[52–55] Neoadjuvant chemotherapy and/or radiation therapy is often used before surgical treatment of various

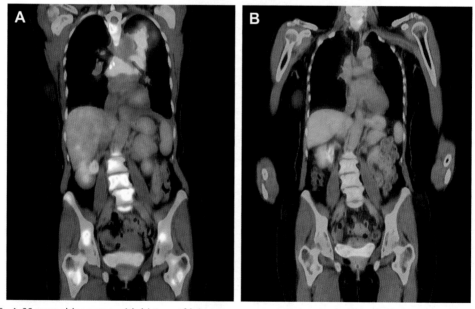

Fig. 15. A 66-year-old woman with history of leiomyosarcoma underwent whole-body FDG PET examination for staging purposes. Coronal whole-body image (*A*) depicts widespread osseous and pulmonary metastatic disease. The patient was aggressively treated with chemotherapy and radiation, and subsequently underwent follow-up FDG PET to monitor response to therapy. Posttreatment coronal whole-body image (*B*) shows an excellent response to therapy. Previously noted foci of abnormal metabolic activity in the lungs and osseous structures show significant interval decrease in uptake, which was considered a good prognostic sign, and therapy was continued.

types of primary bone tumors and soft tissue sarcomas. However, distinguishing viable from nonviable tumor to assess response to therapy can occasionally be challenging with CT and MR imaging.[53] In addition, many lesions do not significantly decrease in size following successful response to therapy, which can also limit evaluation with routine anatomic imaging. In such cases, FDG PET imaging is a valuable alternative, providing a glucose analogue to assess the internal metabolism of the tumor following treatment (Fig. 15). Obtaining FDG PET before initiation of chemotherapy and then following chemotherapy allows comparison between the 2 studies to best assess response to therapy, allowing a noninvasive method for distinguishing viable from nonviable tissue within the treated lesion.[52,53]

Various studies have shown good correlation between PET imaging and histopathologic findings. Benz and colleagues[52] in 2009 studied 50 patients with soft tissue sarcoma treated with neoadjuvant chemotherapy and found that a 35% reduction in FDG uptake with PET imaging was a sensitive indicator of histopathologic tumor response. Findings on posttherapy FDG PET imaging can direct additional therapeutic interventions. Successful response often results in continuation of the previous therapy, whereas a suboptimal response usually results in drastic changes in treatment, which could include a change in chemotherapeutic regimen or more timely surgical intervention. PET can also help guide surgical therapy, helping to ascertain whether limb salvage techniques can be used or helping to circumvent unwarranted surgical resection in the setting of metastatic disease.[53]

SUMMARY

MR imaging is currently the preferred modality for the evaluation of local recurrence, which can be readily differentiated from posttreatment change in most cases. Chest CT is the most widely used and available modality for lung metastatic surveillance, with higher sensitivity for small pulmonary metastases compared with PET/CT. However, PET/CT is gaining attention as an accurate method for both local and metastatic surveillance, and in the future may be incorporated into the standard follow-up protocol of patients with musculoskeletal tumors.

REFERENCES

1. Coindre JM, Terrier P, Bui NB, et al. Prognostic factors in adult patients with locally controlled soft tissue sarcoma. A study of 546 patients from the French Federation of Cancer Centers Sarcoma Group. J Clin Oncol 1996;14(3):869–77.

2. Pisters PW, Leung DH, Woodruff J, et al. Analysis of prognostic factors in 1,041 patients with localized soft tissue sarcomas of the extremities. J Clin Oncol 1996;14(5):1679–89.

3. Aljubran AH, Griffin A, Pintilie M, et al. Osteosarcoma in adolescents and adults: survival analysis with and without lung metastases. Ann Oncol 2009;20(6): 1136–41.

4. Bacci G, Briccoli A, Longhi A, et al. Treatment and outcome of recurrent osteosarcoma: experience at Rizzoli in 235 patients initially treated with neoadjuvant chemotherapy. Acta Oncol 2005;44(7):748–55.

5. Kempf-Bielack B, Bielack SS, Jurgens H, et al. Osteosarcoma relapse after combined modality therapy: an analysis of unselected patients in the Cooperative Osteosarcoma Study Group (COSS). J Clin Oncol 2005;23(3):559–68.

6. Cormier JN, Pollock RE. Soft tissue sarcomas. CA Cancer J Clin 2004;54(2):94–109.

7. Ferrari S, Briccoli A, Mercuri M, et al. Late relapse in osteosarcoma. J Pediatr Hematol Oncol 2006;28(7): 418–22.

8. Hauben EI, Bielack S, Grimer R, et al. Clinico-histologic parameters of osteosarcoma patients with late relapse. Eur J Cancer 2006;42(4):460–6.

9. Strauss SJ, McTiernan A, Whelan JS. Late relapse of osteosarcoma: implications for follow-up and screening. Pediatr Blood Cancer 2004;43(6):692–7.

10. Anract P, Coste J, Vastel L, et al. Proximal femoral reconstruction with megaprosthesis versus allograft prosthesis composite. A comparative study of functional results, complications and longevity in 41 cases. Rev Chir Orthop Reparatrice Appar Mot 2000;86(3): 278–88 [in French].

11. Biau DJ, Larousserie F, Thevenin F, et al. Results of 32 allograft-prosthesis composite reconstructions of the proximal femur. Clin Orthop Relat Res 2010; 468(3):834–45.

12. Farid Y, Lin PP, Lewis VO, et al. Endoprosthetic and allograft-prosthetic composite reconstruction of the proximal femur for bone neoplasms. Clin Orthop Relat Res 2006;442:223–9.

13. Zehr RJ, Enneking WF, Scarborough MT. Allograft-prosthesis composite versus megaprosthesis in proximal femoral reconstruction. Clin Orthop Relat Res 1996;322:207–23.

14. Garner HW, Kransdorf MJ, Bancroft LW, et al. Benign and malignant soft-tissue tumors: posttreatment MR imaging. Radiographics 2009;29(1):119–34.

15. Hwang S, Lefkowitz R, Landa J, et al. Local changes in bone marrow at MRI after treatment of extremity soft tissue sarcoma. Skeletal Radiol 2009; 38(1):11–9.

16. Fox MG, Bancroft LW, Peterson JJ, et al. MRI appearance of myocutaneous flaps commonly used in

orthopedic reconstructive surgery. AJR Am J Roent-genol 2006;187(3):800–6.

17. Fitzgerald JJ, Roberts CC, Daffner RH, et al. Expert panel on musculoskeletal imaging. ACR Appropriate-ness Criteria® follow-up of malignant or aggressive musculoskeletal tumors. Reston (VA): American College of Radiology (ACR); 2011.

18. Patel SR, Zagars GK, Pisters PW. The follow-up of adult soft-tissue sarcomas. Semin Oncol 2003; 30(3):413–6.

19. Eustace S, Goldberg R, Williamson D, et al. MR imaging of soft tissues adjacent to orthopaedic hard-ware: techniques to minimize susceptibility artefact. Clin Radiol 1997;52(8):589–94.

20. Lee MJ, Kim S, Lee SA, et al. Overcoming artifacts from metallic orthopedic implants at high-field-strength MR imaging and multi-detector CT. Radio-graphics 2007;27(3):791–803.

21. Suh JS, Jeong EK, Shin KH, et al. Minimizing arti-facts caused by metallic implants at MR imaging: experimental and clinical studies. AJR Am J Roent-genol 1998;171(5):1207–13.

22. White LM, Kim JK, Mehta M, et al. Complications of total hip arthroplasty: MR imaging-initial experience. Radiology 2000;215(1):254–62.

23. Chang SD, Lee MJ, Munk PL, et al. MRI of spinal hardware: comparison of conventional T1-weighted sequence with a new metal artifact reduction sequence. Skeletal Radiol 2001;30(4):213–8.

24. Olsen RV, Munk PL, Lee MJ, et al. Metal artifact reduc-tion sequence: early clinical applications. Radio-graphics 2000;20(3):699–712.

25. Bamberg F, Dierks A, Nikolaou K, et al. Metal artifact reduction by dual energy computed tomography using monoenergetic extrapolation. Eur Radiol 2011.

26. Varma DG, Jackson EF, Pollock RE, et al. Soft-tissue sarcoma of the extremities. MR appearance of post-treatment changes and local recurrences. Magn Re-son Imaging Clin N Am 1995;3(4):695–712.

27. Pezzi CM, Pollock RE, Evans HL, et al. Preoperative chemotherapy for soft-tissue sarcomas of the extrem-ities. Ann Surg 1990;211(4):476–81.

28. Fuller BG. The role of radiation therapy in the treatment of bone and soft-tissue sarcomas. In: Malawer M, editor. Musculoskeletal cancer surgery. Treatment of sarcomas and allied diseases. Dordrecht: Kluwer; 2001. p. 85–133.

29. Dunst J, Schuck A. Role of radiotherapy in Ewing tumors. Pediatr Blood Cancer 2004;42(5):465–70.

30. Krasin MJ, Rodriguez-Galindo C, Billups CA, et al. Definitive irradiation in multidisciplinary manage-ment of localized Ewing sarcoma family of tumors in pediatric patients: outcome and prognostic factors. Int J Radiat Oncol Biol Phys 2004;60(3): 830–8.

31. Machak GN, Tkachev SI, Solovyev YN, et al. Neoad-juvant chemotherapy and local radiotherapy for high-grade osteosarcoma of the extremities. Mayo Clin Proc 2003;78(2):147–55.

32. Khatri VP, Goodnight JE Jr. Extremity soft tissue sarcoma: controversial management issues. Surg Oncol 2005;14(1):1–9.

33. Blomlie V, Rofstad EK, Skjonsberg A, et al. Female pelvic bone marrow: serial MR imaging before, during, and after radiation therapy. Radiology 1995; 194(2):537–43.

34. Stevens SK, Moore SG, Kaplan ID. Early and late bone-marrow changes after irradiation: MR evalua-tion. AJR Am J Roentgenol 1990;154(4):745–50.

35. Kauczor HU, Dieti B, Brix G, et al. Fatty replacement of bone marrow after radiation therapy for Hodgkin disease: quantification with chemical shift imaging. J Magn Reson Imaging 1993;3(4):575–80.

36. Mumber MP, Greven KM, Haygood TM. Pelvic insuf-ficiency fractures associated with radiation atrophy: clinical recognition and diagnostic evaluation. Skel-etal Radiol 1997;26(2):94–9.

37. Fu AL, Greven KM, Maruyama Y. Radiation osteitis and insufficiency fractures after pelvic irradiation for gynecologic malignancies. Am J Clin Oncol 1994;17(3):248–54.

38. Weber M, Hasler P, Gerber H. Insufficiency fractures of the sacrum. Twenty cases and review of the liter-ature. Spine (Phila Pa 1976) 1993;18(16):2507–12.

39. Richardson ML, Zink-Brody GC, Patten RM, et al. MR characterization of post-irradiation soft tissue edema. Skeletal Radiol 1996;25(6):537–43.

40. Biondetti PR, Ehman RL. Soft-tissue sarcomas: use of textural patterns in skeletal muscle as a diagnos-tic feature in postoperative MR imaging. Radiology 1992;183(3):845–8.

41. Vanel D, Shapeero LG, De Baere T, et al. MR imaging in the follow-up of malignant and aggres-sive soft-tissue tumors: results of 511 examinations. Radiology 1994;190(1):263–8.

42. Moore LF, Kransdorf MJ, Buskirk SJ, et al. Radiation-induced pseudotumor following therapy for soft tissue sarcoma. Skeletal Radiol 2009;38(6):579–84.

43. Poon-Chue A, Menendez L, Gerstner MM, et al. MRI evaluation of post-operative seromas in extremity soft tissue sarcomas. Skeletal Radiol 1999;28(5):279–82.

44. Paz IB, Wagman LD, Terz JJ, et al. Extended indica-tions for functional limb-sparing surgery in extremity sarcoma using complex reconstruction. Arch Surg 1992;127(11):1278–81.

45. Choi H, Varma DG, Fornage BD, et al. Soft-tissue sarcoma: MR imaging vs sonography for detection of local recurrence after surgery. AJR Am J Roent-genol 1991;157(2):353–8.

46. Costelloe CM, Kumar R, Yasko AW, et al. Imaging characteristics of locally recurrent tumors of bone. AJR Am J Roentgenol 2007;188(3):855–63.

47. Charest M, Hickeson M, Lisbona R, et al. FDG PET/CT imaging in primary osseous and soft tissue

sarcomas: a retrospective review of 212 cases. Eur J Nucl Med Mol Imaging 2009;36(12):1944–51.

48. el-Zeftawy H, Heiba SI, Jana S, et al. Role of repeated F-18 fluorodeoxyglucose imaging in management of patients with bone and soft tissue sarcoma. Cancer Biother Radiopharm 2001;16(1): 37–46.

49. Peterson JJ. F-18 FDG-PET for detection of osseous metastatic disease and staging, restaging, and monitoring response to therapy of musculoskeletal tumors. Semin Musculoskelet Radiol 2007;11(3): 246–60.

50. Bastiaannet E, Groen H, Jager PL, et al. The value of FDG-PET in the detection, grading and response to therapy of soft tissue and bone sarcomas; a systematic review and meta-analysis. Cancer Treat Rev 2004;30(1):83–101.

51. Piperkova E, Mikhaeil M, Mousavi A, et al. Impact of PET and CT in PET/CT studies for staging and evaluating treatment response in bone and soft tissue sarcomas. Clin Nucl Med 2009;34(3):146–50.

52. Benz MR, Czernin J, Allen-Auerbach MS, et al. FDG-PET/CT imaging predicts histopathologic treatment responses after the initial cycle of neoadjuvant chemotherapy in high-grade soft-tissue sarcomas. Clin Cancer Res 2009;15(8):2856–63.

53. Bredella MA, Caputo GR, Steinbach LS. Value of FDG positron emission tomography in conjunction with MR imaging for evaluating therapy response in patients with musculoskeletal sarcomas. AJR Am J Roentgenol 2002;179(5):1145–50.

54. Hawkins DS, Rajendran JG, Conrad EU 3rd, et al. Evaluation of chemotherapy response in pediatric bone sarcomas by [F-18]-fluorodeoxy-D-glucose positron emission tomography. Cancer 2002;94(12): 3277–84.

55. Iagaru A, Masamed R, Chawla SP, et al. F-18 FDG PET and PET/CT evaluation of response to chemotherapy in bone and soft tissue sarcomas. Clin Nucl Med 2008;33(1):8–13.

56. Heusner T, Golitz P, Hamami M, et al. "One-stop-shop" staging: should we prefer FDG-PET/CT or MRI for the detection of bone metastases? Eur J Radiol 2009.

57. McCarville MB, Christie R, Daw NC, et al. PET/CT in the evaluation of childhood sarcomas. AJR Am J Roentgenol 2005;184(4):1293–304.

58. Peterson JJ, Kransdorf MJ, O'Connor MI. Diagnosis of occult bone metastases: positron emission tomography. Clin Orthop Relat Res 2003;(415 Suppl): S120–8.

59. Franzius C, Daldrup-Link HE, Wagner-Bohn A, et al. FDG-PET for detection of recurrences from malignant primary bone tumors: comparison with conventional imaging. Ann Oncol 2002;13(1):157–60.

60. Klaeser B, Mueller MD, Schmid RA, et al. PET-CT-guided interventions in the management of FDG-positive lesions in patients suffering from solid malignancies: initial experiences. Eur Radiol 2009; 19(7):1780–5.

61. O'Sullivan PJ, Rohren EM, Madewell JE. Positron emission tomography-CT imaging in guiding musculoskeletal biopsy. Radiol Clin North Am 2008;46(3): 475–86, v.

62. Bestic JM, Peterson JJ, Bancroft LW. Use of FDG PET in staging, restaging, and assessment of therapy response in Ewing sarcoma. Radiographics 2009; 29(5):1487–500.

Advanced Magnetic Resonance Imaging Techniques in the Evaluation of Musculoskeletal Tumors

Flávia Martins Costa, MD[a,b,*], Clarissa Canella, MD[a,b], Emerson Gasparetto, MD, PhD[a,b]

KEYWORDS

- Magnetic resonance imaging • Bone tumors
- Advanced magnetic resonance imaging techniques
- Dynamic contrast-enhanced perfusion imaging
- Proton magnetic resonance spectroscopy imaging
- Diffusion-weighted imaging
- In-phase and opposed-phase imaging

Because of its high resolution, tissue contrast, and multiplanar capabilities, magnetic resonance (MR) imaging is an important imaging modality for the preoperative staging and posttreatment evaluation of musculoskeletal tumors.[1,2] Although radiography, ultrasonography, and computed tomography (CT) are useful for tumor evaluation, MR imaging is the modality of choice to determine the extent of the lesion before intervention.[1]

Conventional MR imaging uses morphologic parameters to evaluate the extent of bone and soft tissue tumors, but it is limited with regard to distinguishing benign from malignant lesions and determining histologic composition.[2,3] Of the various imaging modalities, radiography remains the most reliable predictor of the histologic nature of bone tumors and can help determine whether or not MR imaging is required.[1] Further evaluation of bone tumors with MR imaging is often necessary when the lesion is indeterminate on radiographs, when the lesion requires further staging

(eg, all primary malignant tumors or benign lesions that require local staging), or when biopsy of the lesion is contemplated.[1]

For many patients, conventional MR imaging is unable to provide a specific histologic diagnosis or determine the true extent of tumor necrosis or the presence of viable cells, factors used to assess response to treatment and the prognosis of patients with musculoskeletal tumors (**Fig. 1**A, B, E and F).[2,4] These patients may benefit from advanced MR imaging techniques, such as dynamic contrast-enhanced perfusion imaging (with color-map imaging), proton MR spectroscopy (^{1}H MRS), diffusion-weighted imaging (DWI), and in-phase/opposed-phase MR imaging. These methods are currently used, together with conventional MR imaging, to improve diagnostic accuracy and the evaluation of response to treatment.[2]

This article reviews each of these advanced MR imaging techniques (including their technical aspects and clinical applications) with regard to

[a] Clínica de Diagnóstico por Imagem (CDPI)/DASA, Rio de Janeiro, Brazil
[b] Serviço de Radiologia da, Universidade Federal do Rio de Janeiro, Rio de Janeiro, Brazil
* Corresponding author. Clínica de Diagnóstico por Imagem (CDPI), Avenue. das Américas N°4666 sl 325, Barra da Tijuca, 22631004, Rio de Janeiro, Brazil.
E-mail address: flavia26rio@hotmail.com

Radiol Clin N Am 49 (2011) 1325–1358
doi:10.1016/j.rcl.2011.07.014
0033-8389/11/$ – see front matter © 2011 Elsevier Inc. All rights reserved.

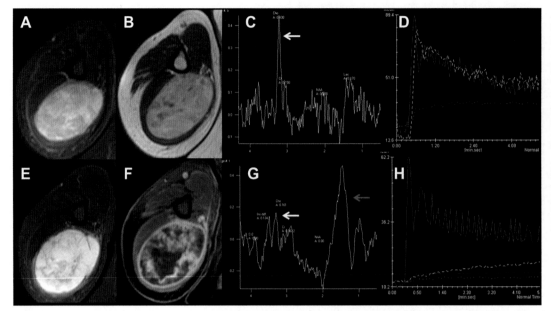

Fig. 1. Malignant fibrous histiocytoma in the right arm of a 50-year-old man. Pretreatment images (*A–D*) and posttreatment images (*E–H*) are shown. Pretreatment (*A*) axial short tau inversion recovery (STIR) MR image shows a large hyperintense tumor in the extensor compartment. (*B*) Axial T1-weighted MR image after intravenous contrast administration shows homogeneous contrast enhancement of the tumor. (*C*) Spectroscopic analysis shows high choline peak (*arrow*), suggesting malignancy. (*D*) The TICs show in red an arterial vessel (type IV curve), in yellow the tumor curve (type IV) with slope value of 286% per minute, suggesting highly perfused tumor, and in green the muscle curve (type III). After treatment, (*E*) axial STIR MR image shows almost the same appearance of the tumor as before treatment, and (*F*) the axial fat-suppressed postcontrast image shows heterogeneous contrast enhancement, making it difficult to analyze the response. However, spectroscopic analysis (*G*) shows reduction in the choline peak (*arrow*) and increase of the lipid peak (*red arrow*), suggesting necrosis. The perfusion study (*H*) shows that the tumor curve (*yellow*) dropped after the treatment (now type II) with a slope value of 8% per minute, suggesting more than 90% necrosis. The histopathologic analysis showed absence of tumoral cells.

detection and characterization of tumors, differentiation of benign from malignant lesions (and tumor tissue from nontumor tissue), and assessment of response to treatment.

DYNAMIC CONTRAST-ENHANCED PERFUSION IMAGING

Dynamic contrast-enhanced perfusion MR imaging is a method of physiologic imaging in which early tumor enhancement is monitored after an intravenous bolus injection of contrast agent.[5] This technique provides physiologic information that cannot be determined from conventional anatomic MR imaging, including information regarding tissue vascularization and perfusion, capillary permeability, and the volume of the interstitial space.[1,5] Dynamic contrast-enhanced perfusion MR imaging has been frequently used in the study of musculoskeletal tumors.[6–12] This technique has several important advantages including:

- tissue characterization;
- staging of local extent;
- identification of areas of viable tumor to guide biopsy;
- monitoring of preoperative chemotherapy;
- detection of residual or recurrent tumor, and distinguishing tumor from fibrosis.

At our institution, routine dynamic contrast enhancement is performed during an intravenous bolus injection of 0.1 mmol/kg of gadolinium (Magnevist; Schering AG, Berlin, Germany), using an infusion pump at a flow rate of 2 mL/s, followed by 20 mL of saline solution. Imaging is performed using a T1-weighted gradient echo sequence, on a total of 5 sections, with slice thickness and spacing between slices varying according to the tumor size (**Table 1**). Total acquisition time is approximately 5 minutes, at the end of which T1-weighted fast spin echo images are acquired with fat suppression in the axial and coronal planes (repetition time (TR)/echo time (TE): 759/10 milliseconds; matrix: 512 × 512).

Table 1
T1-weighted gradient echo sequence protocol used for perfusion imaging

TA (time of acquisition)	5:00
Field of view (cm)	280
TR (ms)	606
Matrix size	256 × 102
TE (ms)	1.34
Flip angle (°0)	20
Section thickness (mm)	7
Intersection gap (mm)	7
TR (ms)	5:00

To evaluate perfusion data, we designate 3 regions of interest (ROIs), of equal size, at 3 different points: (1) within the lesion, in an area where there is intense early contrast uptake; (2) within an artery; and (3) in the contralateral healthy muscle. Inclusion of an artery is useful for evaluating differences between the time of onset of enhancement in the lesion and the time of arrival of the bolus.[5] All ROIs are positioned by an experienced radiologist specializing in musculoskeletal imaging. Based on these ROIs, the perfusion curves can be quantitatively and qualitatively analyzed with Mean Curve software available at the workstation (Leonardo; Siemens Medical Systems, Erlangen, Germany). Besides qualitatively evaluating time intensity curves (TICs), the slope of the curve (% of increase in signal intensity per minute) can be calculated using the formula:

$$\text{Slope} = (SI_{max} - SI_{prior}) \times 100/(SI_{prior} \times T_{max})$$

where SI_{prior} represents the value of the signal intensity before the intravenous gadolinium injection; SI_{max} is the value of signal intensity at T_{max}; and T_{max} is defined as the point at which relative SI (SI/SI_{prior}) at T_{max} + 20 seconds is less than 3% higher than at T_{max}.[6]

An experienced radiologist specializing in musculoskeletal imaging classifies the TIC patterns into 1 of 5 types (**Fig. 2**)[7,9,13]:

- Type I: no enhancement; this type can be found in lipomas and recent hematomas
- Type II: gradual increase of enhancement; more commonly seen in benign tumors as schwannomas
- Type III: rapid initial enhancement followed by plateau phase; this curve can be seen in vascularized benign tumors (eg, desmoid tumors) in abscesses and also in some

malignant tumors and is not particularly helpful to characterize tumors
- Type IV: rapid initial enhancement followed by washout phase; this curve represents highly vascularized lesions with a small interstitial space; it can be seen, for example, in malignant tumors (malignant fibrous histiocytoma, synovial sarcoma, and leiomyosarcoma) and in some benign tumors such as giant cell tumor and in the nidus of osteoid osteoma
- Type V: rapid initial enhancement followed by slow progression of enhancement; this curve can be found in tumors after radiation or chemotherapy treatment or in tumors with a large interstitial space such as myxoid tumors.

Color mapping data are postprocessed using Mean Curve (Leonardo; Siemens, Erlangen, Germany). For the figures in this article, red regions correspond to hypervascular areas with a washout phase (type IV TIC curves) or less commonly tumors with a type III curve.

Tissue Characterization

The first contrast passage in a dynamic study has been used to characterize tissue vascularization and tumor perfusion.[8,11,14–17] Tissues with high vascularization and high capillary permeability tend to have an earlier and more intense contrast uptake than less vascularized tissues.[16] Dynamic contrast-enhanced perfusion MR imaging may be used to qualitatively evaluate tumor and tumorlike lesions over time using TICs and to quantitatively evaluate these lesions by determining the slope value, which is calculated from the percentage increase in signal intensity in the earliest contrast-enhanced part of the tumor (% per minute) (**Fig. 3**).

Quantitative information on lesion enhancement can be assessed graphically on TICs by measuring signal intensities in 1 or more circular or freely determined ROIs.[1] Pixel-by-pixel postprocessing techniques can show physiologic information, such as the maximum rate of contrast agent accumulation (slope value = % increase of signal intensity per minute).[1] The ROI method can yield TICs from regions encircling the entire tumor or the most active region(s) of the tumor.[1]

In general, malignant tumors tend to have greater enhancement as well as a greater rate of enhancement than benign lesions (see **Fig. 3A–C**).[1] However, overlaps in perfusion curve values, both quantitative and qualitative, have been observed between highly vascularized benign lesions (**Fig. 4C, D**) and poorly vascularized malignant tumors (**Fig. 5C, D**). The slope obtained from

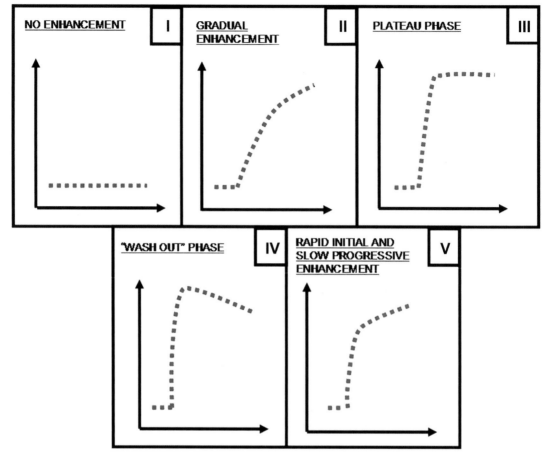

Fig. 2. Types of TICs: type I, no enhancement; type II, gradual increase of enhancement; type III, rapid initial enhancement followed by plateau phase; type IV, rapid initial enhancement followed by washout phase (this curve is the most important curve and represents highly vascularized lesions with a small interstitial space; for example, it can be seen in malignant tumors, in giant cell tumors, and in the nidus of osteoid osteomas); type V, rapid initial enhancement followed by slow progression of enhancement.

dynamic images correlates with the malignant potential of a tumor[6–8,11,18] although high slopes have been observed for highly vascularized or perfused benign lesions (see **Fig. 4C, D**) and low slopes for poorly vascularized malignant tumors (**Box 1**) (see **Fig. 5C, D**).[8,14,19] Thus, the qualitative pattern and quantitative value (slope) of the curves, when used in combination with conventional MR imaging, ^{1}H MRS, and DWI, may be useful for narrowing the differential diagnosis of musculoskeletal tumors.

Staging of Local Extent

The clinical and radiological evaluation of both local extent and distant spread[5] is essential for managing therapy, for planning the ideal approach to the biopsy site, and for determining surgical margins (**Fig. 6D–F**). The most important considerations in staging the local extent of a tumor include:

- Tumor margins and size
- Tumor extension beyond the anatomic compartment
- Tumor invasion of adjacent structures such as bone, joint, muscle, and neurovascular bundle
- Tumor location relative to the deep fascia[1,5]

The initial slopes of tumor and nontumor tissues have been shown to differ significantly.[1,6,8,20] Dynamic study may improve the delineation of tumor margins, because enhancement of tumor tissue is earlier and faster than that of peritumoral edema (see **Fig. 6D–F**).[1,6,8,20]

Identifying Areas of Viable Tumor to Guide Biopsy

Identification of viable areas of tumor tissue is important for biopsy planning, and well-vascularized

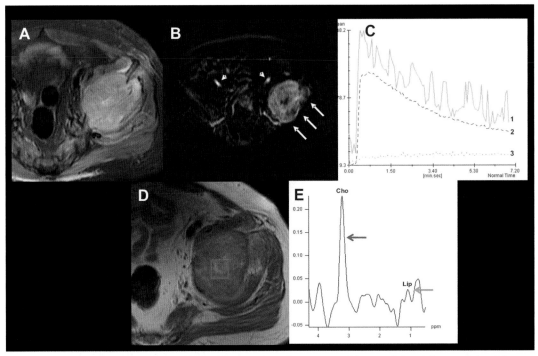

Fig. 3. Leyomiosarcoma, grade III, in the left iliac bone of a 64-year-old man. (*A*) Axial T1-weighted fat-suppressed contrast-enhanced MR image shows the large iliac tumor. (*B*) Axial contrast-enhanced perfusion image with subtraction shows arterial enhancement (*arrowhead*) and tumor enhancement (*long arrows*). (*C*) TICs show type IV curve of the artery (1, *solid blue line*) and type IV curve of the tumor (2, *dashed purple line*) with washout phase. The tumor has a slope of 297% per minute, suggesting highly vascularized and perfused tumor. With spectroscopy (*D*), the voxel (square) is positioned in the solid part of the tumor without surrounding tissue contamination. Analysis (*E*) reveals an increased choline peak (*red arrow*), suggestive of high potential of malignancy, and a small lipid peak (*green arrow*).

areas suggest viable tumor (**Fig. 7**). This finding may not only be of great value for determining tumor type and grade but also it may allow the radiologist to avoid obtaining biopsy specimens that contain mixtures of poorly vascularized tumor tissue, edema, or necrotic material.[1,5]

Monitoring Preoperative Chemotherapy

Accurate determination of tumor response during the initial phase of treatment is essential for assessing the effectiveness of therapy, for planning further treatment, and for predicting patient prognosis.[12] A measurable outcome of preoperative chemotherapy, especially in patients with chemotherapy-sensitive bone tumors (eg, osteosarcoma and Ewing sarcoma) (**Fig. 8**A, D, E, and H) and soft tissue tumors (see **Fig. 1**D, H) (eg, synovial sarcoma), is the percentage of tumor necrosis, which differentiates responders from nonresponders.[1] An increase, no change, or even a slight decrease in amplitude of the TIC and in

the slope of the curve (% of increase of signal intensity per minute) during follow-up indicates a poor response to treatment.[1] Changes in the TIC with a decrease of at least 60% in slope indicate greater than 90% necrosis and, consequently, a good response to treatment (an important factor of prognosis).[21]

Dynamic contrast-enhanced MR imaging has an important role in monitoring the effect of preoperative chemotherapy.[1,8,14] It has an accuracy in distinguishing responders from nonresponders of 85.7% to 100%. This accuracy is likely because of the ability of this method to yield information about tissue vascularization and perfusion.[1,8,14]

To monitor the effects of chemotherapy, dynamic contrast-enhanced MR imaging should be performed before biopsy, during chemotherapy, and immediately before surgery.[1] On the first-pass or slope images, all pixels are displayed at an intensity equal to the highest enhancement rate. Direct visual (qualitative) inspection of these images allows simple recognition of highly

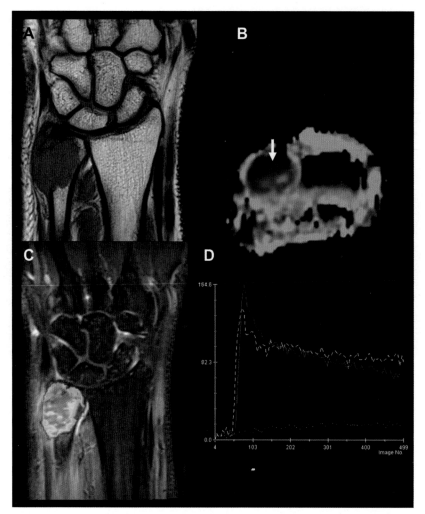

Fig. 4. Giant cell tumor in the ulnar epiphysis of a 29-year-old man. (*A*) Coronal T1-weighted MR image shows the tumor. (*B*) Axial ADC map shows restricted diffusion (*white arrow*) with PIADC = 0.98×10^{-3} mm^2/s, suggesting tissue with more cellularity or a small interstitial space. (*C*) Coronal dynamic contrast-enhanced perfusion imaging with color mapping shows red areas inside the tumor, suggesting hypervascularity. (*D*) TIC shows arterial and tumoral type IV curves in red and yellow, respectively, and a type II curve in green, representing normal muscle.

vascular or highly perfused viable tumor tissue, because these bright areas contrast with less intense (slower enhancing) areas of peritumoral edema, normal tissue, and tumor necrosis.[1] These findings can therefore predict good response of bone tumors to treatment (>90% necrosis), if, at the end of chemotherapy, the first-pass images show no bright areas with high enhancement rates. In contrast, the presence of bright areas suggests that more than 10% of viable tumor tissue is present, which indicates a poor response. In these patients, the first-pass images are useful for guiding a new biopsy or for alerting the pathologist to focus on those particular areas in the resected specimen, which likely have surviving tumor cells.[1]

Detecting Residual or Recurrent Tumors and Distinguishing them from Areas of Fibrosis

Dynamic MR imaging is useful for detecting viable tumor tissue and for differentiating this tissue from reactive changes after therapy. The purpose of MR examination is to detect local tumor recurrence or residual tumor tissue, and to differentiate suspected recurrence from hematopoietic bone marrow reconversion, inflammation, seroma, or reactive tissue.[1]

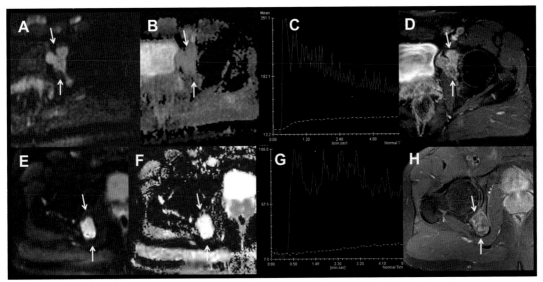

Fig. 5. Differentiation of chondrosarcoma (grade II) and enchondroma. Two different patients: one with a grade II chondrosarcoma (A–D) and another with an enchondroma (E–H). (A) Axial diffusion MR image shows a hyperintense grade II chondrosarcoma in the left acetabulum (*arrows*). (B) ADC map reveals facilitated diffusion with PIADC = 1.9×10^{-3} mm²/s (*arrows*) probably because of high chondroid matrix content. (C) TIC is type III for the tumor (*dashed yellow line*), indicating rapid enhancement; red TIC (type IV) represents artery. (D) Axial fat-suppressed contrast-enhanced MR image shows heterogeneous contrast uptake (*arrows*). (E) Axial diffusion MR image shows a hyperintense enchondroma (*arrows*) in the right ischial tuberosity (*arrows*). (F) ADC map reveals facilitated diffusion with PIADC = 2.1×10^{-3} mm²/s, probably because of high chondroid matrix content. There is facilitated diffusion on the ADC map of benign (F) and malignant (B) cartilaginous tumors (*arrows*), so the diffusion is not useful for differentiation. (G) TIC is type II for the tumor (*dashed yellow line*), suggesting poor vascularity, common in inactive enchondroma; red TIC (type IV) represents artery. (H) Axial fat-suppressed contrast-enhanced MR image shows heterogeneous contrast uptake (*arrows*) in both the enchondroma and the chondrosarcoma (D). They have similar characteristics on conventional MR imaging and DWI but different TICs, so dynamic contrast-enhanced MR imaging may help to differentiate low-grade chondrosarcoma from inactive enchondroma.

With dynamic contrast-enhanced MR imaging, tumor tissue, either residual or recurrent, enhances early and more rapidly during the first-pass of contrast (**Fig. 9**A, B), whereas reactive tissue or a pseudomass resulting from posttherapeutic changes enhances later and more slowly, at a rate equal to that of normal muscle (**Fig. 10**).[1,5]

¹H MRS

¹H MRS imaging can be used as a noninvasive approach to the evaluation of musculoskeletal tumors, providing a means of molecular characterization of bone and soft tissue malignancies.[3,22,23] Clinically, ¹H MRS is more frequently used in brain examinations.[24] This method can characterize lesions based on their metabolic constituents, such as choline, a phospholipid constituent of cell membranes.[23] Diagnostically, ¹H MRS is used to detect increased levels of choline compounds, which are markers of increased cell membrane turnover, a feature of malignancy (see **Fig. 3**D,

E).[3,23,25] The choline/creatine ratio obtained by in vivo ¹H MRS has been shown to distinguish malignant tumors of the extracranial head and neck from uninvolved muscle.[26] In vivo ¹H MRS has been used to analyze bone and soft tissue tumors, breast carcinoma, prostate cancer, and cervical carcinoma.[22,25,27] In vivo ¹H MRS has been shown to differentiate benign from malignant musculoskeletal tumors,[3,22,23] providing further evidence that ¹H MRS is useful for assessing the malignant potential of a lesion (see **Fig. 6**A–C).

¹H MRS can map relative metabolite signal intensity in tissues by obtaining signals from water, choline (cho), creatine, and lipids, using both multivoxel and single-voxel techniques. Multivoxel ¹H MRS has been shown to be feasible for characterizing musculoskeletal tumors.[23] In our experience, the single-voxel technique can be used to analyze cho peaks (see **Fig. 3**D, E).

At our institution, ¹H MRS is performed on a 1.5-T Avantoimager (Siemens Medical Systems, Erlangen, Germany), with surface coils, and, for the

Box 1
Highly vascularized benign lesions and poorly vascularized malignant tumors

Benign Lesions with High Slope

Aneurysmal bone cyst

Eosinophilic granuloma

Giant cell tumor

Osteoid osteoma

Acute osteomyelitis

Abscess

Myositis ossificans

Enchondroma (occasionally)

Fibrous dysplasia (occasionally)

Neurinoma (occasionally)

Aggressive fibromatosis (occasionally)

Angioma/hemangioma

Malignant Lesions with Low Slope

Highly necrotic tumor

Late recurrences after chemotherapy or radiation therapy

Low-grade chondrosarcomas

Osteosarcomas with low vascularity (occasionally)

single-voxel technique, with a point-resolved spectroscopy sequence and echo time (TE) = 135 milliseconds. Volumes of interest (ranging from 3.4 cm^3 to 8 cm^3) are positioned by an experienced radiologist on areas showing early and intense contrast uptake (see **Fig. 7**B arrow), while avoiding the inclusion of bone structures, areas of necrosis or calcification, blood products, fat and muscles. In patients presenting with tumors with subtle or slow contrast uptake or an absence of uptake after perfusion for 5 minutes, the voxel is positioned on areas showing contrast uptake on delayed images.

Spectroscopy data are postprocessed using standard MR imaging software (Spectroscopy Siemens, Erlangen, Germany). The cho peak within a lesion is located at the 3.2 ppm peak on the spectral curve[22] and the lipid peak at the 1.2 ppm peak. The cho peak is used to differentiate benign and malignant tumors. At our institution, the presence of a cho peak (identified visually at 3.2 ppm in a spectrum obtained with TE = 135 milliseconds) is supportive of malignancy (see **Fig. 3**D, E), although some metabolically active benign tumors and abscesses may also show

a cho peak.[3,22,24] The presence of a lipid peak at 1.2 ppm is usually detected in the wall of abscesses, in the solid part of highly malignant lesions, and in tumors during treatment response (see **Fig. 1**C, G), probably related to cell membrane turnover. This peak has to be carefully analyzed, because of the excessive lipid contamination caused by surrounding tissue; we avoid analyzing spectra containing too much noise without identifiable peaks.

DWI

DWI allows quantitative and qualitative analyses of tissue cellularity and cell membrane integrity and has been widely used for tumor detection and characterization, and for monitoring response to treatment. Thus, DWI complements the morphologic information obtained with conventional MR imaging.[2,28]

DWI measures the random motion of water molecules in the body (Brownian motion).[28] In vivo, DWI signal is derived from motion of water molecules in the extracellular, intracellular, and transcellular space, as well as in the intravascular space (microcirculation-perfusion fraction).[28–30] In the intravascular space, because of the blood flow, the water molecules have greater diffusion distance than those in the extracellular and intracellular spaces. The contribution of intravascular water diffusion to the DWI signal is variable among different tissues. In tumors with high vascularity, the contribution of intravascular water diffusion to MR signal can be significant.[28] The degree of restriction of water diffusion in biologic tissue is inversely correlated with tissue cellularity and cell membrane integrity.[28,31–34] The motion of water molecules is more restricted in tissues with high cellularity, intact cell membranes, and reduced extracellular space. In contrast, the motion of water molecules is more facilitated or less restricted in tissues with low cellularity, defective cell membranes, and considerable extracellular space.[28]

Tumors differ in their cellularity characteristics, a difference useful in determining the histologic composition of these tumors. Malignant tumors have higher cellularity (**Fig. 11**) than benign tumors (**Fig. 12**) and tend to have a more restricted diffusion.[2,35] However, not all benign tumors have a large extracellular space (see **Fig. 4**) and not all malignant tumors are more cellular than benign tumors (see **Fig. 5**A, B; **Fig. 13**A–C).[36]

Qualitative Assessment of DWI

DWI is performed by using a conventional T2-weighted pulse sequence with diffusion weighting gradients to filter out the signal from high-mobility

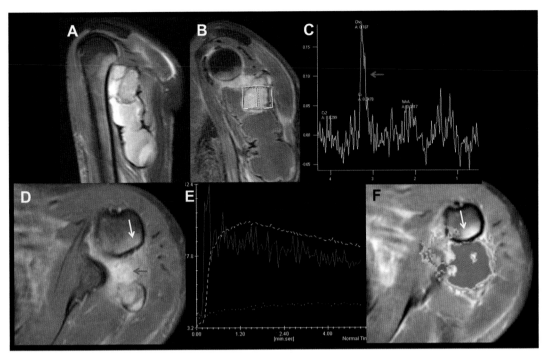

Fig. 6. Soft tissue angiomatoid malignant fibrous histiocytoma in a 27-year-old woman. (A) Coronal oblique STIR MR image shows a large hyperintense soft tissue mass abutting the proximal humerus. (B) Sagittal oblique T1-weighted fat-suppressed contrast-enhanced MR image shows solid and cystic components of the mass with spectroscopy voxel (*square*) placed over the enhancing component. (C) Spectroscopic analysis shows an increased choline peak (*red arrow*), suggesting malignancy. (D) Axial T1-weighted fat-suppressed contrast-enhanced MR image shows contrast uptake in the bone marrow (*white arrow*) adjacent to the solid malignant tumor component (*red arrow*), concerning for osseous invasion. (E) TICs of the artery (*red*) and the tumor (*yellow*) are type IV (slope of the tumor = 183% per minute) with washout phase, suggesting a highly vascularized and perfused lesion. The TIC of the enhancing bone marrow (*green line*) is type II with slope = 8% per minute, suggesting reactive edema (histopathologic analysis showed normal bone marrow with reactive edema). (F) Axial dynamic contrast-enhanced with color mapping MR image shows red hypervascular areas in the solid part of the tumor, but not in the enhancing part of the bone marrow (*white arrow*).

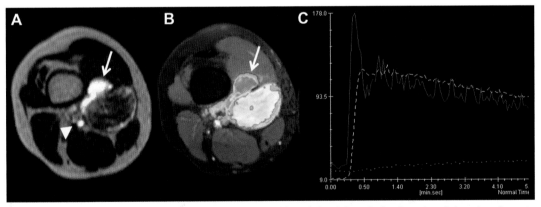

Fig. 7. Synovial sarcoma of the right thigh in a 17-year-old boy. (A) Axial perfusion imaging shows that the anterior part of the tumor enhances early (*white arrow*) at the same time as the artery (*arrowhead*). (B) Axial color-map perfusion imaging shows the most vascularized and perfused part of the tumor (*white arrow*), indicating viable tumor tissue; this tissue has a yellow type IV curve with washout on (C). This region represents the best place to biopsy and to position the spectroscopy voxel. The red type IV curve on (C) indicates the artery. The green curve represents normal muscle.

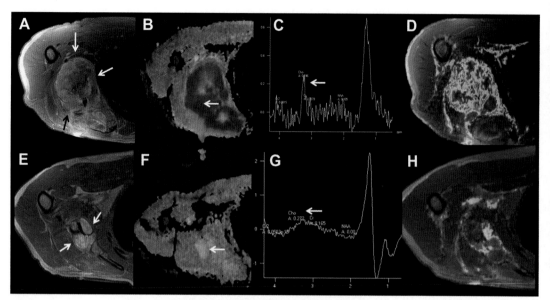

Fig. 8. Evaluation of response to Ewing sarcoma treatment by using DWI, spectroscopy, and dynamic contrast-enhanced imaging with color mapping in a 28-year-old man. Pretreatment images (*A–D*) and posttreatment images (*E–G*) are shown. Pretreatment (*A*) axial T1-weighted contrast-enhanced MR image, (*B*) axial ADC map, (*C*) spectroscopic analysis, and (*D*) dynamic contrast-enhanced with color mapping image show a large tumor in the scapular region with heterogeneous contrast enhancement (*A, arrows*), restricted diffusion on the ADC map (*B, arrow*) with PIDC = 0.61×10^{-3} mm^2/s, suggesting hypercellular tumor, a choline peak in (*C*), and multiple red regions in (*D*), suggesting highly perfused areas. Posttreatment (9 months later) (*E*) axial T1-weighted contrast-enhanced MR image, (*F*) axial ADC map, (*G*) spectroscopic analysis, and (*H*) dynamic contrast-enhanced with color mapping MR image show that the tumor reduced in size, now with heterogeneous contrast enhancement (*E, arrows*), facilitated diffusion on ADC map (*F, arrow*), a reduced choline peak (*G, arrow*), and disappearance of the highly perfused areas on color mapping, suggesting significant necrosis. The histopathologic analysis showed more than 90% necrosis. PIDC, perfusion insensitive ADC.

water molecules and enhance the sensitivity of the method for depicting molecular diffusion and mobility.[37] Different DWI sequences have been described including spin echo DWI, echo-planar imaging (EPI), and steady-state free precession sequences.[30] The most commonly used acquisition strategy for DWI imaging is single or multishot EPI because of its efficiency in terms of scan time. This technique is fast and less sensitive to motion artifacts. However, it is prone to susceptibility artifacts. It is usually performed using at least 2 b values (eg, b = 0 s/mm^2 and b = 1000 s/mm^2), to allow a more accurate interpretation.[28] The b value represents the diffusion strength and provides diffusion weighting for DWI images as TE provides T2 weighting for T2 images.[2,30] When the b value is changed, it is usually the gradient amplitude that is altered.[28] At our institution, DWI is routinely performed using 6 different b values (**Table 2**). By analyzing the relative attenuation of signal intensity on images obtained at different b values, tissues may be characterized based on differences in water diffusion.[28] Cystic tumors show greater signal attenuation on high

b value images because water diffusion is less restricted,[28] whereas more solid or cellular tumors maintain high signal intensities.[28] Visual assessment of relative tissue signal reduction on DWI is being used to detect and characterize tumors and to evaluate response to anticancer therapy.

Quantitative Assessment of DWI

DWI at different b values can enable quantitative analysis, using a workstation to obtain apparent diffusion coefficients (ADCs).[28] The ADC is calculated as an exponential function of the signal intensities of the tumor on images with different b values. An ADC is calculated for each pixel of the image and is displayed as a parametric map. It is possible to differentiate tissues on these maps by drawing ROIs. Highly cellular areas with restricted diffusion have lower ADCs (**Fig. 14**) than less cellular areas with higher ADCs (see **Fig. 13**). Areas of restricted diffusion (ie, because of high cellularity) have higher signal intensity on the DWI images but lower signal intensity on ADC maps (see **Fig. 14**).[28] Areas of facilitated

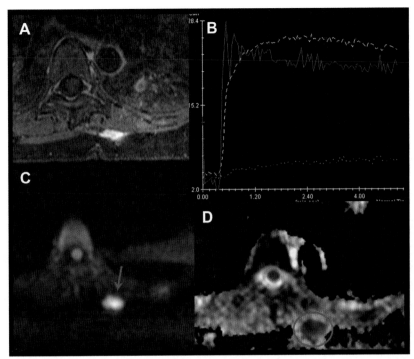

Fig. 9. Follow-up examination of a synovial sarcoma, 1 year after surgery, in a 53-year-old woman. (*A*) Axial T1-weighted fat-suppressed postcontrast MR image shows a small mass (*red arrow*) in the subcutaneous fat of the back with contrast enhancement; (*B*) TIC shows the tumor to have a type III curve (*dashed yellow line*), indicating rapid enhancement, more common in tumor recurrence. The type IV curve (*red*) and type II curve (*green*) represent the artery and normal muscle, respectively. (*C*) Axial DWI shows the hyperintense mass (*red arrow*). (*D*) Axial ADC map image shows the small mass (*red circle*) with restricted diffusion (PIADC = 0.86×10^{-3} mm^2/s), suggesting tumor recurrence.

diffusion show relatively increased signal intensity on ADC maps compared with areas of restricted diffusion. However, in addition to diffusion of water molecules in the extracellular space contributing to ADC values, the ADC values of soft tissue tumors are increased by the degree of tumor perfusion.[36] The perfusion fraction (microcirculation) tends to be higher in malignant than benign

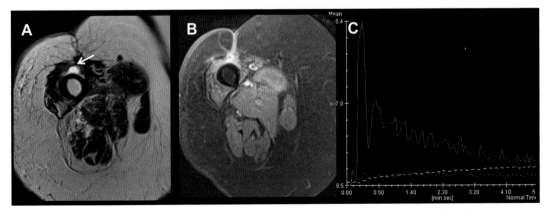

Fig. 10. Follow-up examination of pleomorphic undifferentiated sarcoma in the right thigh in a 74-year-old woman, 2 years after surgery and radiation therapy. (*A*) Axial T2-weighted MR image shows a small lesion (*arrow*) along the anterior femoral shaft in the surgical bed, with ill-defined contrast enhancement on the axial T1-weighted postcontrast fat-suppressed (*B, arrow*) image, suggesting tumor recurrence. (*C*) The qualitative analysis of the dynamic study shows that the type II TIC of the lesion (*yellow*) is similar to the TIC of normal muscle (*green*), suggesting a pseudomass confirmed on surgical biopsy. TIC of the artery is shown in red.

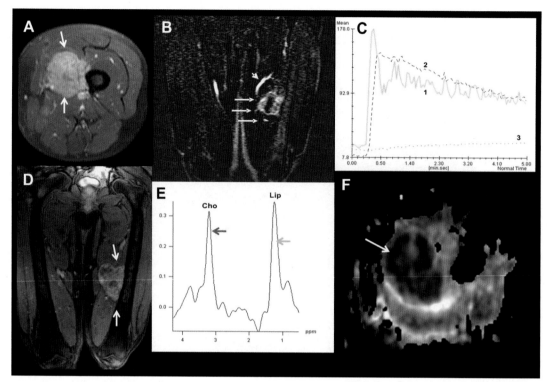

Fig. 11. Malignant fibrous histiocytoma of the left thigh in a 67-year-old man. (*A*) Axial STIR MR image shows a large hyperintense solid mass adjacent to the vessels. (*B*) Coronal contrast-enhanced perfusion study with subtraction MR image shows arterial enhancement (*small arrow*) and enhancement inside the tumor (*long arrows*). (*C*) TICs show arterial (1) and tumoral (2) type IV curves with washout phase. (*D*) Coronal T1-weighted fat-suppressed contrast-enhanced MR image shows tumor with heterogeneous contrast enhancement in the delayed phase (*arrows*). (*E*) Spectroscopy shows cho peak (*red arrow*) and lipid peak (*green arrow*), suggesting highly malignant tumor. (*F*) Axial ADC map shows restricted diffusion (*arrow*) with PIADC = 0.89×10^{-3} mm^2/s, suggesting malignant tissue.

soft tissue tumors, and therefore contributes more to increasing ADC values in malignant soft tissue tumors than it does in benign soft tissue lesions. Hence, perfusion could increase the ADC value more in malignant tumors than in benign tumors, ultimately resulting in overlap in ADC values between benign and malignant tumors.[2] Perfusion-corrected DWI may be able to differentiate benign from malignant soft tissue masses.[36] To differentiate benign from malignant musculoskeletal tumors, we always obtain the perfusion-insensitive ADC value (PIADC) (**Fig. 15**). Conventional ADC is calculated with b values of 0 s/mm^2 and 600 s/mm^2, whereas PIADC is calculated only with high b values (300 s/mm^2, 450 s/mm^2, or 600 s/mm^2). The reduction in signal intensity on DWI images with small b values is probably caused by vascular capillary perfusion; thus, when using PIADC the perfusion effects tend to be minimized. Water molecules with a large degree of motion or a large diffusion distance (as in the intravascular space) show signal attenuation with small b values

(b = 50–100 s/mm^2). On the other hand, slow-moving water molecules or water molecules with small diffusion distances show more gradual attenuation with increasing b values (b = 1000 s/mm^2).[28] We assessed 44 patients with musculoskeletal tumors of the trunk and extremities, with no previous surgical procedures or adjuvant treatment, who underwent MR examination and biopsy. We excluded patients with lesions that had a classic appearance on MR imaging (ie, lipomas, hemangiomas, ganglia, and synovial cysts) and patients with highly necrotic lesions surrounded by edema, because the edema probably contaminates tumor tissue and consequently increases the diffusion coefficient. After qualitative (ADC map) and quantitative (PIADC value) analyses, we found that PIADC was significantly higher in benign than in malignant tumors ($1.67 \pm 0.18 \times 10^{-3}$ mm^2/s vs $1.07 \pm 0.46 \times 10^{-3}$ mm^2/s, P = .0011).[36] We found that a PIADC value of 1.1×10^{-3} mm^2/s separated malignant from benign solid tumors with sensitivity of 90% and specificity of 96%. This value, together

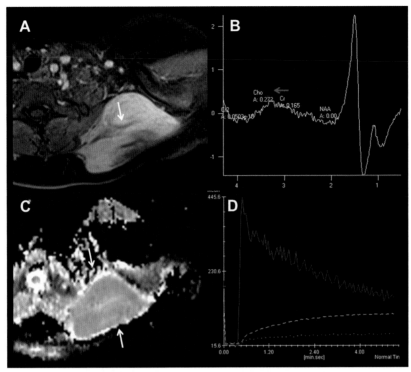

Fig. 12. Desmoid tumor in the left shoulder of a 26-year-old woman with contrast enhancement on axial T1-weighted fat-suppressed contrast-enhanced MR image (A). Observe within the tumor a low signal intensity band without contrast enhancement (*white arrow*), suggesting collagen bands. (B) Spectroscopic analysis shows no cho peak. (C) Axial ADC map shows facilitated diffusion (PIADC = 1.65 × 10^{-3} mm^2/s), suggesting a benign tumor. (D) TICs show the type II curve of the tumor in yellow commonly seen in benign tumors, the type IV curve of the artery in red, and the type I curve of normal muscle in green.

with morphologic characteristics obtained on conventional MR imaging, has been useful for differentiating benign from malignant tumors in our clinical practice.

PIADC may provide more accurate information about tumor tissue cellularity by minimizing vascular contribution, which is higher in malignant tumors.[2,28] DWI can also be used to monitor and to predict tumor response to treatment, because effective anticancer therapy results in changes in the tumor microenvironment, including tumor lysis, loss of membrane integrity, and increased extracellular space. This situation can result in an increase in the diffusion of water molecules and an increase in ADC (see **Fig. 8B, F**).[2,28]

IN-PHASE AND OPPOSED-PHASE IMAGING

Chemical shift MR imaging, which can assess the relationship between the amounts of fat and water coexisting in the same voxel of tissue, has been shown to be effective in differentiating malignant from benign processes and has been extensively used in the adrenal glands and liver.[38,39] The chemical shift MR technique may also be used to assess potentially neoplastic lesions in bone marrow.[40] Differences in changes in signal intensity between in-phase and opposed-phase imaging have been observed in neoplastic versus nonneoplastic lesions of the spine,[40,41] suggesting that this technique may be useful for differentiating acute benign compression fractures from malignant infiltration and pathologic fractures. The technique may also be used to provide an early assessment of response to anticancer treatment.[39]

Normal bone marrow is rich in fat and water, but the difference in the amounts of lipid and water is the main factor affecting signal intensity of marrow on MR imaging (**Fig. 16**).[40] The presence of both fat and water in normal marrow results in the suppression of signal intensity on opposed-phase images (**Fig. 17**). Infiltrative processes in the bone marrow (eg, neoplasms) tend to replace the fatty marrow components completely, resulting in a lack of suppression of signal intensity on opposed-phase images (**Fig. 18A–C**).[38,39] Water and fat protons have different precession

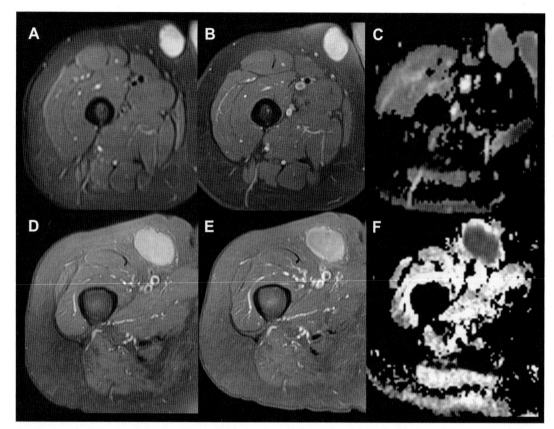

Fig. 13. Similar masses in the subcutaneous fat of the right inguinal region in 2 different patients. *A–C* represent patient 1; *D–F* represent patient 2. Both tumors are hyperintense on axial STIR MR images (*A* and *D*). Both masses show enhancement on the axial T1-weighted fat-suppressed postcontrast images (*B* and *E*), suggesting a solid component. Axial ADC map of the mass in patient 1 (*C*) shows facilitated diffusion with PIADC = 2.66×10^{-3} mm^2/s, suggesting hypocellular tumor. Axial ADC map of the mass in patient 2 in (*F*) shows restricted diffusion with PIADC = 0.58×10^{-3} mm^2/s, suggesting hypercellular tumor. The histopathologic analyses showed myxofibrosarcoma in patient 1 and non-Hodgkin lymphoma in patient 2. In (*C*) the myxoid component increases the ADC value, despite the fact that the tumor is malignant.

Table 2 DWI sequence protocol	
TA (time of acquisition)	3:36
Field of view (cm)	250
TR (ms)	2200
Matrix size	128 × 128
TE (ms)	75
EPI factor	128
b factors (s/mm)	0/50/150/300/450/600
Parallel imaging factor	2 GRAPPA (generalized autocalibrating partially parallel acquisitions)
Number of signal average	3
Section thickness (mm)	5

frequencies because of differences in their molecular environments (see **Fig. 17**). In our protocol (**Table 3**), water and fat protons are in phase with each other at a TE of 4.6 milliseconds, with signal intensity as a result of voxels containing both tissue types. At a TE of 2.4 milliseconds, the water and fat protons are 180° opposed, and the signal intensity from one cancels that of the other. Thus, voxels that contain both tissue types have reduced signal intensity (see **Fig. 17**).[39]

At our institution, the routine in-phase and opposite-phase sequences are performed as shown in **Table 3**. All images are analyzed at a workstation, and areas that seem to have abnormal signal intensity on conventional MR images are identified.[39] ROIs of equal size are drawn over the abnormal areas on both the in-phase and opposed-phase images. The signal intensity ratio (SIR) of the marrow on the opposed-phase image to that of the in-phase image is calculated.[39] Using

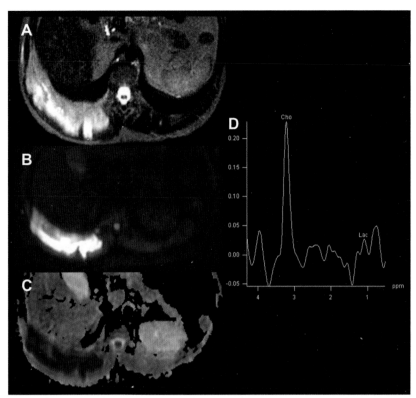

Fig.14. Non-Hodgkin lymphoma in the 10th right rib in a 50-year-old man with pain for 6 months. (*A*) Axial T2-weighted MR image shows a large hyperintense tumor in the right thoracic wall; (*B*) Axial DWI shows a hyperintense mass, suggesting high nuclear/cytoplasm ratio. (*C*) Axial ADC map shows restricted diffusion, PIADC = 0.65 × 10⁻³ mm²/s, suggesting hypercellular tumor. (*D*) Spectroscopic analysis shows an increased cho peak, further supporting malignancy.

an SIR of 0.80 as a cutoff, an SIR greater than 0.80 is typical of a neoplastic process and an SIR less than 0.80 is typical of a nonneoplastic process.[39,41]

CLINICAL APPLICATIONS OF ADVANCED MR IMAGING TECHNIQUES

In the following sections, we discuss the application of all advanced MR imaging techniques in patients with different musculoskeletal tumor types.

Osteoid Osteoma

Osteoid osteoma is a benign bone tumor that occurs most frequently in young patients, aged 7 to 25 years, with a slight male predominance.[42,43] Most patients experience pain that worsens at night and is rapidly relieved by the administration of nonsteroidal antiinflammatory drugs.[42] In most patients, radiographs and CT are diagnostic, showing a nidus with a variable quantity of calcification, as well as adjacent cortical thickening and sclerosis. However, some of these tumors may display misleading imaging findings, making it difficult to differentiate these tumors from other diseases.[42,43] A vascular groove sign is a moderately sensitive and highly specific sign for distinguishing osteoid osteoma from other radiolucent bone lesions on CT.[44]

Although MR imaging has been reported to be of limited value, compared with CT, in depicting the nidus[42,45–47] we have had excellent experience in using advanced MR imaging techniques, especially dynamic contrast-enhanced MR imaging with color mapping and in-phase/opposed-phase sequences, to identify the nidus and to differentiate these tumors from other conditions such as infection (Brodie abscess), inflammatory and noninflammatory arthritis, and other tumors (**Fig. 19**).

Dynamic contrast-enhanced MR imaging was found to more clearly show the nidus in osteoma osteoid than nonenhanced MR imaging, with the

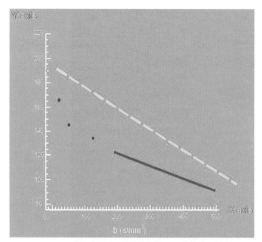

Fig. 15. DWI graph shows signal attenuation with increasing b values. Conventional ADC (*dashed yellow line*) calculated with b values of 0 and 600 mm²/s; PIADC (*solid red line*) calculated with high b values (300, 450, and 600 mm²/s). The initial reduction (*dots*) in signal intensity is probably caused by vascular capillary perfusion. For large b values, perfusion effects tend to be canceled out. The PIADC may provide more accurate information about tumor tissue cellularity by minimizing vascular contribution, which is higher in malignant tumors. (y-axis: logarithm of relative signal intensities; x-axis: different b values).

former as effective as thin-section CT.[44] Most osteoid osteomas show arterial phase enhancement and rapid partial washout (TIC IV) as a result of hypervascularity of the nidus (**Fig. 20F, G, and H**).[44] We routinely use dynamic contrast enhancement after an intravenous bolus injection of 0.1 mmol/kg of gadolinium (Magnevist; Schering AG, Berlin, Germany), with an infusion pump at a flow rate of 2 mL/s, followed by 20 mL of saline solution. MR imaging is performed with a T1-weighted three-dimensional sequence, with 3.5-mm slices used to analyze the nidus (**Table 4**). Color-mapped data are postprocessed by Mean Curve. The presence of red regions corresponds to hypervascular areas with a washout phase found in the nidus of most osteoid osteomas (see **Fig. 20F, G, and H**).

Chemical shift MR imaging is another tool that may be useful in the diagnosis of osteoid osteoma, especially when clinical and radiological features are unclear. We retrospectively analyzed 7 consecutive patients (**Table 5**) who underwent chemical shift MR imaging for the evaluation of osteoid osteoma (manuscript in preparation). For all patients, the signal intensity on in-phase and out-of-phase images was measured using ROIs drawn over the nidus, over areas of abnormal bone marrow signal intensity surrounding the nidus, and over the contralateral normal-appearing bone marrow. The relative SIRs for each region were calculated as values on opposed-phase divided by values on in-phase images, with SIRs greater than 1 considered to indicate neoplastic lesions. Statistical analysis showed that the mean relative SIRs were 1.15 (range 1.04–1.26) for the nidus and 0.36 (range 0.15–0.59) for the surrounding tissue ($P = .0001$).

Some osteoid osteomas have extensive peritumoral edema that can simulate tumor infiltration, especially on MR imaging. In these patients, fat and water are present in the bone marrow, resulting in a suppression of signal intensity of these regions on opposed-phase relative to in-phase images (see **Fig. 20**). Hence, chemical shift MR imaging may be useful for the diagnosis and evaluation of osteoid osteomas.

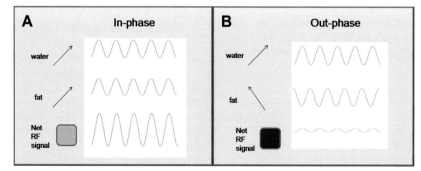

Fig. 16. The physical principles of in-phase and opposed-phase imaging. (*A*) At TE = 4.6 milliseconds, both fat and water protons are in phase, and signal intensity is received from voxels containing both tissue types. (*B*) At TE of 2.4 milliseconds, the fat and water protons are 180° opposed, and the signal intensity from one cancels that of the other. Thus, voxels that contain both tissue types have reduced signal intensity.

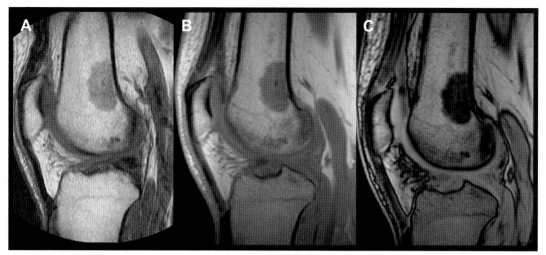

Fig. 17. Focal hematopoietic marrow. (*A*) Sagittal T1-weighted MR image shows an oval focus of intermediate signal intensity in the distal femur. (*B*) Sagittal in-phase MR image shows that the focus remains intermediate in signal intensity. (*C*) Sagittal out-of-phase MR image shows that the focus decreases in signal intensity, with SIR less than 0.80, indicating a benign lesion (an island of hematopoietic marrow).

Giant Cell Tumor

The histologic makeup of giant cell tumors contributes to their low ADCs.[2,48] These tumors typically show high first-pass enhancement, followed by an early washout phase (type IV curve) (see **Fig. 4**). Dynamic contrast-enhanced MR imaging is useful for detecting recurrences or residual tumor tissue after surgery (**Fig. 21**) from granulation tissue and bone grafts. Bone grafts and granulation tissue show fast enhancement within the first months after surgery, but do not show an early washout phase.[1]

Cho peaks have been detected in both malignant hypercellular giant cell tumors and nonmalignant giant cell tumors with proliferative activity (**Fig. 22**).[22,49] The reappearance of cho after radiation therapy is useful for detecting tumor recurrence, and a reduction in cho level is recognized as an indicator of response to treatment.[49] We have found that these parameters are useful in diagnosis and in management of local recurrence after surgery by helping to differentiate residual or recurrent tumor tissue from postsurgical fibrosis.

Fibroblastic/Myofibroblastic and Fibrohistiocytic Tumors

In adults, fibrous tumors are among the most common soft tissue lesions encountered in clinical practice.[50] These mesenchymal tumors are characterized histologically by the proliferation of fibroblasts and myofibroblasts, with marked production of intercellular collagen, and biologic behavior intermediate between that of benign lesions (see

Fig. 12) and malignant tumors (see **Fig. 11**).[51] MR imaging findings that point toward the diagnosis of a benign fibrous tumor such as aggressive fibromatosis include bands of low signal intensity across all sequences and moderate to intense enhancement after contrast administration (see **Fig. 12**).[2,51] However, malignant fibrous tumors can also have these characteristics on MR imaging.

In accordance with the World Health Organization (WHO) classification of soft tissue tumors, myositis ossificans is classified as a fibroblastic/myofibroblastic tumor. This lesion is a benign, solitary, self-limiting, ossifying soft tissue mass usually occurring within skeletal muscle. A history of trauma is frequently elicited, but is often absent.[52] Its MR appearance changes with the age of the lesion. During its early active phase, the immature lesion may show high perfusion as a result of neovascularity and may mimic a malignant neoplasm (**Fig. 23**).[52] We have found that myositis ossificans presents with facilitated diffusion on DWI, and a high ADC (see **Fig. 23**; **Fig. 24**), compatible with a benign tumor. In accordance with clinical history, follow-up examination after 2 to 4 weeks is suggested to confirm the diagnosis, avoiding unnecessary biopsy (see **Fig. 24**).

We used MR imaging to assess 21 patients with histologically proven fibroblastic/myofibroblastic and fibrohistiocytic soft tissue tumors (trunk and extremities), who had received no previous adjuvant treatment (**Table 6**). In accordance with WHO guidelines, 5 tumors were classified as benign, 9 as intermediate, and 8 as malignant. Statistical analysis was performed by assessing

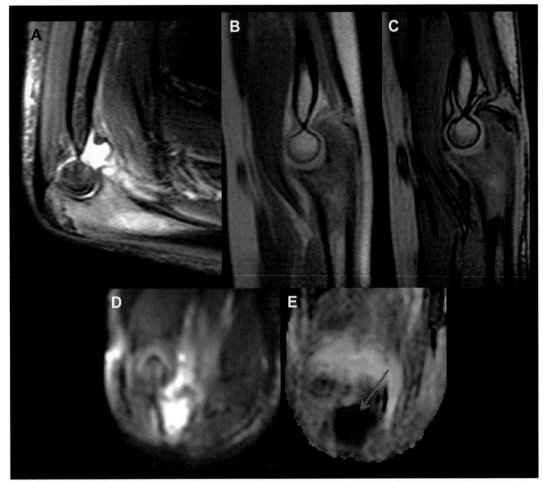

Fig. 18. (*A*) Sagittal STIR MR image of a 16-year-old boy with pain after recent trauma reveals a hyperintense area in the proximal ulna with articular effusion, suggesting traumatic edema. In the ulna the hypointensity seen on the T1-weighted in-phase image (*B*) shows mild increase in signal intensity on the opposed-phase image (*C*) with SIR greater than 0.80, suggesting tumoral infiltration. Axial DWI (*D*) shows hyperintensity; ADC map (*E*) shows restricted diffusion (*red arrow*) with PIADC = 0.68 × 10^{-3} mm^2/s, suggesting hypercellularity. Histologic analysis revealed Ewing sarcoma.

Table 3	
In-phase and out-of-phase sequence protocol	
TA (time of acquisition)	1:14/3:36
Field of view (cm)	300
TR (ms)	185
Matrix size	128 × 128
TE (ms)	In: 4.6
TE (ms)	Out: 2.4
Phase oversampling	80
Slices	9
Slice thickness (mm)	3.5

the value of each advanced MR imaging technique for differentiating benign/intermediate and malignant tumors (with $P<.01$ considered significant). We found that these advanced MR imaging techniques are useful, together with conventional MR imaging, for the differential diagnosis of an indeterminate mass with morphologic characteristics of a fibrous tissue tumor.[2]

Abscesses, Hematomas, and Necrotic Tumors

Detection of an abscess with certainty influences management, leading to surgical drainage.[53] Abscesses may be highly vascularized, perfused lesions with slopes similar to those of malignant

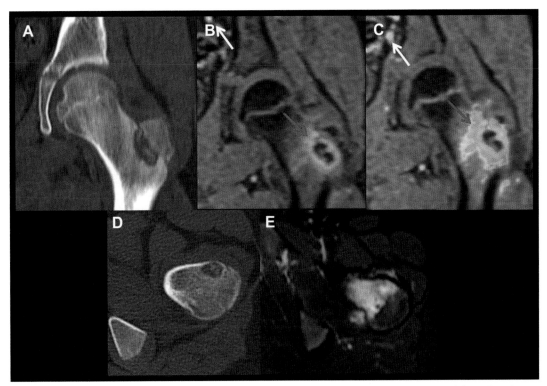

Fig. 19. Brodie abscess in an 8-year-old girl with pain at night for 2 months. (*A*) Coronal and (*D*) axial CT images show a small hyperlucent lesion with sclerotic margins and internal mineralization, mimicking osteoid osteoma adjacent to the apophyseal growth plate. (*B*) Coronal dynamic contrast-enhanced perfusion MR imaging shows arterial enhancement (*white arrow*) together with enhancement along the periphery of the femoral lesion (*red arrow*). (*C*) Coronal perfusion color-map imaging shows red regions along the periphery of the lesion (*red arrow*), suggesting hypervascularity, and in arterial vessels (*white arrow*). (*E*) Axial STIR MR image shows edema in the bone marrow with extension to the periosteal region and into the adjacent musculature. Although the CT and axial STIR MR images suggest osteoid osteoma as a possible diagnosis, the lack of perfusion in the center of the lesion argues against a nidus, supporting instead an abscess.

tumors.[8] In contrast, highly necrotic malignant tumors may have a low slope, similar to that of benign lesions.[8] Moreover, benign lesions with inflammatory cells, like abscesses, may have cho peaks without harboring a malignancy.[22]

DWI analysis of brain abscesses usually reveals markedly reduced ADC in the necrotic center.[2,54,55] Abscesses contain inflammatory cells, a matrix of proteins, cellular debris, and bacteria in high-viscosity pus, with all of these factors restricting the motion of water., Hence, the abscess cavity is characterized by high signal intensity on DWI and decreased ADCs.[53] Necrotic neoplasms tend to have more facilitated diffusion in their necrotic centers than do abscess cavities. Highly malignant tumors tend to have more restricted diffusion on the ADC map in the solid wall of the tumor, which has higher cellularity.[2]

Care must be taken during diagnostic imaging to differentiate hemorrhagic malignant tumors from hematomas.[2] DWI may differentiate chronic expanding hematomas (CEHs) from malignant tumors, with 1 report showing that the mean ADC value of CEHs was significantly higher than that of malignant soft tissue tumors.[56] On the other hand, acute and subacute hematomas have typical morphologic characteristics on conventional MR imaging and present with restricted diffusion on ADC maps of the central part of the lesion. Contrast enhancement in benign hematomas is rare.[56] The spectroscopic analysis of hematomas is complicated by the susceptibility artifacts caused by red blood cell products; however, necrotic hemorrhagic malignant tumors tend to have a cho peak detected in the solid part of the tumor, indicating cellular proliferation (**Fig. 25**).

After conventional MR imaging and determination of clinical history, advanced MR imaging techniques may be superior in differentiating abscesses and hematomas from malignant tumors. This process may include a determination of the ADC of the necrotic portion of the tumor on the DWI sequence.

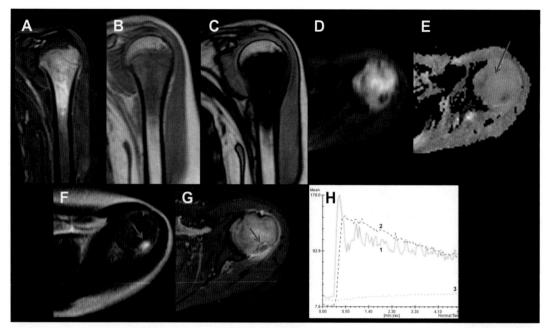

Fig. 20. Coronal oblique STIR MR image (*A*) of a 22-year-old woman with pain for 1 year shows a hyperintense area in the bone marrow of the proximal humerus, with a nonspecific appearance. (*B*) T1-weighted in-phase image shows hypointensity with significant reduction in signal intensity on the opposed-phase image (*C*) with SIR less than 0.8, suggesting edema. Axial DWI (*D*) shows hyperintensity. Axial ADC map (*E*) shows facilitated diffusion (*red arrow*) with PIADC = 2.3×10^{-3} mm²/s. Histologic evaluation revealed a benign bone tumor (osteoid osteoma). (*F*) Axial dynamic contrast-enhanced perfusion MR imaging shows arterial enhancement (*red arrow*) in the posterior part of the humeral head, suggesting osteoid osteoma. (*G*) Axial perfusion color-map MR imaging shows red region in the osteoid osteoma nidus (*red arrow*), and contrast enhancement in bone marrow surrounding the nidus. (*H*) TIC shows type IV curve of the artery (1) similar to the type IV curve of the nidus (2) with washout phase, suggesting hypervascularity.

Small Round Blue Cell Tumors

Small round blue cell tumors (SRBCTs) are a group of undifferentiated embryonal tumors with aggressive behavior, including neuroblastoma, rhabdomyosarcoma, non-Hodgkin lymphoma, and the family of Ewing sarcomas. These tumors have similar histologic features and immunohistochemistry, and other molecular techniques are required for their diagnosis. Moreover, diagnosis, which is often based on the clinical features of the tumors, may be difficult in patients presenting in an unusual clinical context.[2] Accurate diagnosis of these cancers is important for the administration of appropriate therapy and for avoiding unnecessary procedures. Currently there is no widely available tool for real-time noninvasive diagnosis.[2]

Because cho level increases in proportion to cellular proliferation and tumor malignancy, ^{1}H MRS, which assesses the biochemical characteristics and metabolites of tumor tissue, may be a useful method of diagnosis.[24] Cho peaks have been observed in malignant lymphomas (see **Fig. 14**).[22,24]

Malignant lymphomas in the brain, head, and neck, and retroperitoneal regions have low ADCs. Pathologically, these tumors are more cellular, larger, and have more angulated nuclei and less extracellular space than other solid tumors.[48] Because of

Table 4	
Dynamic study osteoid osteoma protocol	
TA (time of acquisition)	6:14
Field of view (cm)	240
TR (ms)	3.46
TE (ms)	1.35
Slabs	1
Slices per slab	24
Phase oversampling (%)	0
Slice oversampling (%)	16.7
Slice thickness (mm)	3.50
Averages	1

Table 5
MR evaluation of 7 patients using in-phase/opposed-phase with histologically proven osteoid osteoma. The table shows relative ratios (SIR) of the nidus, the edematous bone marrow surrounding the nidus and in normal contralateral bone marrow on the opposed-phase image to that of the in-phase image

Patients	SIR of the Nidus	SIR of the Edematous Bone Marrow Surrounding the Nidus	SIR of Normal Bone Marrow
Patient 1	1.08	0.27	0.88
Patient 2	1.26	0.15	1.10
Patient 3	1.21	0.52	0.98
Patient 4	1.04	0.14	0.84
Patient 5	1.17	0.38	0.80
Patient 6	1.10	0.59	0.80
Patient 7	1.18	0.45	0.81

their high cellularity and high nuclear/cytoplasm ratio, lymphomas have high signal intensity on DWI images and a lower ADC than other tumor types in the body (**Fig. 26**).[54,57–59]

We have found that these tumors tend to have lower PIADC values and more restricted diffusion on ADC maps than other malignant musculoskeletal tumors (see **Fig. 18**D, E). In a study of 12 patients with histologically proven SRBCTs, including soft tissue and bone tumors of the trunk and extremities, and 15 other patients with malignant non-SRBCTs, none of whom had undergone previous surgical procedures or adjuvant treatment, MR examination and biopsy showed that the PIADC was significantly higher in malignant non-SRBCTs than in SRBCTs ($0.98 \pm 0.21 \times 10^{-3}$ mm^2/s vs $0.64 \pm 0.18 \times 10^{-3}$ mm^2/s). Furthermore, SRBCTs tended to contain tissue

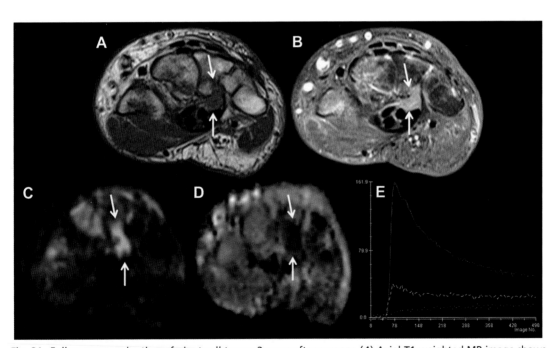

Fig. 21. Follow-up examination of giant cell tumor 2 years after surgery. (A) Axial T1-weighted MR image shows a small hypointense lesion (*arrows*) with intense contrast uptake on (B) axial T1-weighted FS contrast-enhanced MR image. Axial diffusion-weighted MR image (C) shows hyperintensity. Axial ADC map (D) shows restricted diffusion with PIADC = 0.98×10^{-3} mm^2/s, suggesting tumor recurrence. (E) TIC shows type IV curve of the artery in red and the type IV curve of the recurrent tumor in yellow.

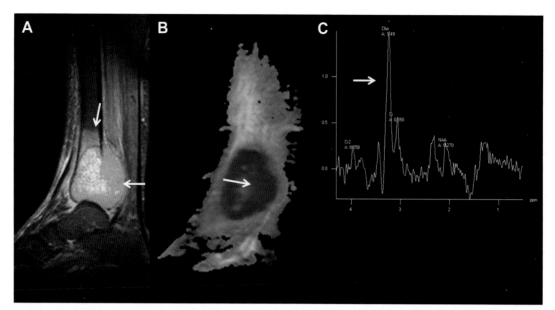

Fig. 22. Giant cell tumor in the distal tibia, hyperintense on sagittal STIR MR image (*A*), with restricted diffusion on sagittal ADC map image (*white arrow, B*) with PIADC = 0.97×10^{-3} mm²/s and increased cho peak at spectroscopy (*white arrow, C*).

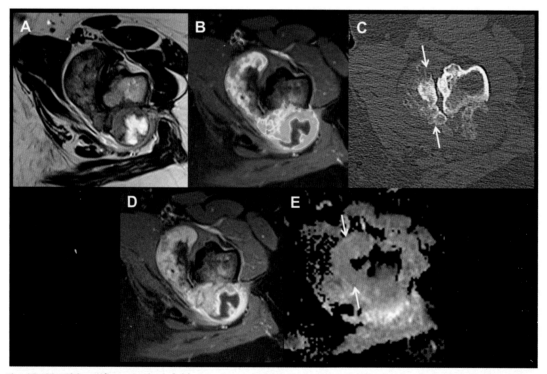

Fig. 23. Myositis ossificans in the left hip in a 51-year-old woman. (*A*) Axial T2-weighted MR image shows a large heterogeneous mass partially surrounding the left femur. (*B*) Axial dynamic contrast-enhanced with color mapping MR image shows red regions posteriorly, suggesting hypervascularity. (*C*) Axial CT shows ossification of most of the lesion (*white arrows*), but nonossified areas (*red arrow*) are noted in the hypervascular region, suggesting immature tissue. Heterogeneous contrast uptake with a hypovascular area posteriorly is noted on the axial T1-weighted contrast-enhanced MR image (*D*). The lesion shows facilitated diffusion on the axial ADC map image (*white arrows, E*) with PIDC = 1.78×10^{-3} mm²/s.

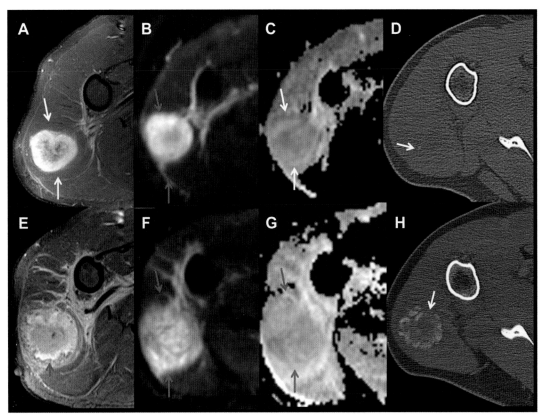

Fig. 24. Myositis ossificans in right deltoid muscle in an 18-year-old man with pain for 2 weeks. (*A*) and (*E*) axial T1 fat-suppressed postcontrast MR images; (*B*) and (*F*) axial diffusion images; (*C*) and (*G*) axial ADC images; (*D*) and (*H*) axial CT images. There is a soft tissue mass with contrast enhancement after gadolinium administration (*A, white arrows*), hyperintensity on DWI (*B, red arrows*), facilitated diffusion on the ADC map (*C, white arrows*) with PIADC = 1.78×10^{-3} mm²/s, suggesting a benign lesion, and a small focus of calcification on CT (*D, white arrow*). After 3 weeks (*E–H*), the lesion grew with enlargement (*red arrow*) of surrounding edema seen on MR imaging (*E*), hyperintensity on DWI (*F, red arrows*), facilitated diffusion on the ADC map (*G, red arrows*) with PIADC = 1.69×10^{-3} mm²/s, suggesting a benign lesion, and zonal ossification seen on CT (*H, white arrow*).

Table 6
The statistical analysis of the value of each advanced MR imaging technique for fibroblastic/myofibroblastic and fibrohistiocytic tumors

	Benign (n = 5)	Intermediate (n = 9)	Malignant (n = 8)
PIADC value[a]	Mean + SD = 1.56 (+0.25) × 10^{-3} mm²/s		Mean + SD = 0.89 (+0.15) × 10^{-3} mm²/s
ADC map[a]	Facilitated diffusion	Facilitated diffusion	Restricted diffusion
Slope value[a] %/min	Mean + SD = 32.5 (+16)%/min		Mean + SD = 88 (+21)%/min
¹H MRS[a]	Absent	Present	Present
Cho peak		1	7

Abbreviation: SD, standard deviation.
 [a] The statistical analysis was performed by assessing the value of each advanced MR imaging technique for differentiating benign/intermediate and malignant tumors with $P<.001$ considered significant.

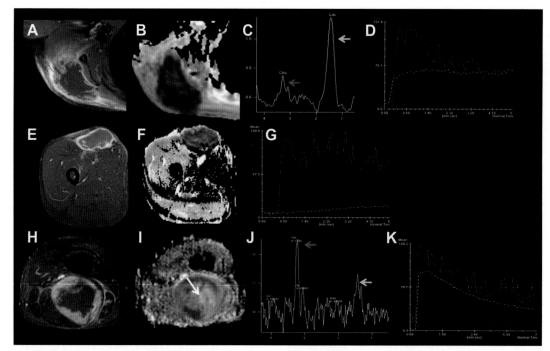

Fig. 25. Differentiation between abscess (*A–D*) and hematoma (*E–G*) from necrotic malignant tumor (*H–K*) using advanced MR imaging techniques. Axial T1-weighted fat-suppressed contrast-enhanced MR images of an abscess in the right shoulder (*A*), of a hematoma in the thigh (*E*), and of a necrotic malignant tumor posteriorly in the thigh (*H*) all show peripheral contrast enhancement. ADC maps show restricted diffusion in the central portion in the abscess (*B*) and in the hematoma (*F*). The ADC map of the necrotic tumor shows facilitated diffusion in the necrotic portion (*I, white arrow*) and restricted diffusion in the solid wall (*I, red arrow*), suggesting hypercellularity. Spectroscopic analyses show cho and lipid peaks in the solid wall of the abscess (*C, red* and *green arrows,* respectively) and in the wall of the malignant tumor (*J, red* and *green arrows,* respectively), suggesting high cell membrane turnover. TIC plots show that the abscess has a type III curve (*D, yellow curve*) and a slope of 43% per minute. The hematoma has a type II TIC (*G, yellow curve*) and a slope of 2% per minute (indicating hypovascularity). The malignant tumor has type IV curve (*K, yellow curve*), with a slope of 87% per minute and a washout phase, suggesting hypervascularity. The red and green curves represent the artery and normal muscle.

with a relatively uniform population of SRBCs, which have less extracellular space and typically smaller PIADC values than non-SRBC malignant tumors (see **Fig. 26**).

Whole-body DWI with ADC mapping can potentially be used for lesion detection and staging in patients with diffuse large B-cell lymphoma (DLBC). ADC values are decreased in DLBC lesions.[60]

SRBC tumors should be the main consideration in the differential diagnosis of tumors with restricted diffusion on ADC maps and low PIADCs.

Myxoid Tumors

Myxoid tissue is present in myxomas, myxoid liposarcomas, myxoid components of myxoid chondrosarcomas, and myxoid malignant fibrous histiocytomas.[1] Myxoid tumors have higher diffusion coefficients than nonmyxoid tumors; this is true for both benign and malignant soft tissue myxoid tumors (see **Fig. 13**).[2,35,36,48,61] These high values reflect their high mucin and low collagen contents, with these lesions being composed of large amounts of water, as confirmed by histologic analyses.[2,35] ADC values of benign and malignant myxoid tumors show substantial overlap because both contain myxoid matrix.[35]

Myxoid liposarcoma is a type of malignant fatty tumor, accounting for approximately one-third of all liposarcomas. These tumors have low signal intensities on T1-weighted sequences and high signal intensities on T2-weighted sequences, occasionally resembling cysts. Moreover, these tumors may be indistinguishable from most benign and malignant soft tissue masses.[1,2,62] Perfusion methods are useful for distinguishing cysts from myxoid tumors, because fluid does not enhance, whereas myxoid tissue in a sarcoma shows intense and fast enhancement.[1]

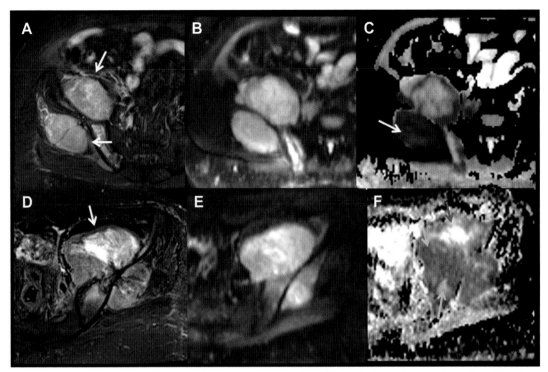

Fig. 26. Two similar tumors in right iliac bone (patient 1, *A–C*) and left iliac bone (patient 2, *D–F*). Patient 1: (*A*) axial STIR MR image shows a large hyperintense mass (*white arrows*) with extension into the adjacent muscle with hyperintensity on DWI (*B*) and restricted diffusion on the ADC map (*C, white arrow*) in the posterior portion with PIADC = 0.57×10^{-3} mm^2/s, suggesting hypercellular tumor. Histologic analysis revealed non-Hodgkin lymphoma. Lymphomas tend to have lower ADCs than other tumor types. Patient 2: (*D*) axial STIR MR image shows a large hyperintense mass similar in appearance to that of patient 1, with a necrotic area in the anterior part (*white arrow*), and extension into the adjacent muscle. (*E*) The tumor shows hyperintensity on DWI and restricted diffusion on the ADC map (*F, green arrows*) with PIADC = 0.98×10^{-3} mm^2/s, suggesting malignant tumor, but not so hypercellular as that of patient 1. On (*F*) observe the necrotic portion with facilitated diffusion (*red arrow*). Histologic analysis revealed melanoma metastasis.

Intramuscular myxoma is a benign tumor characterized by the presence of abundant, almost completely avascular myxoid stroma and, in perfusion studies, slow enhancement. These tumors also show gradual fill-in during the first few minutes after bolus injection because of the large interstitial space and slow perfusion.[1] If a myxoid tumor shows rapid fill-in, then a myxoid-containing malignancy, such as a myxoid liposarcoma or synovial sarcoma, should be suspected.[1]

An understanding of the morphologic MR imaging appearance as well as the perfusion and DWI characteristics of myxoid tumors may permit more accurate diagnosis of these often indeterminate soft tissue masses.[2]

Cartilaginous Lesions

The differentiation of enchondroma from low-grade chondrosarcoma is crucial for planning treatment because enchondromas do not require further workup, whereas chondrosarcomas must be completely resected.[1] Plain radiography, CT, and even conventional MR imaging cannot always differentiate these 2 types of tumor,[1] and scintigraphic patterns alone cannot always distinguish between benign or malignant variants.[63] However, fast contrast-enhanced MR imaging, may be used to differentiate benign cartilage neoplasms from chondrosarcoma, because, in adults, both early and exponential enhancement are predictors of malignancy (see **Fig. 5**).[64] Dynamic contrast-enhanced MR imaging may differentiate low-grade chondrosarcoma and active enchondroma from inactive enchondroma. Inactive enchondromas have slow enhancement and perfusion, whereas active enchondromas and chondrosarcomas have similar, earlier and faster enhancement.[1] However, an active enchondroma cannot be distinguished from a low-grade chondrosarcoma when the perfusion study shows early and fast enhancement.[1] Thus, these patients must be treated as having a low-grade chondrosarcoma.

Malignant cartilaginous tumors can have higher ADCs than benign tumors.[2,61] We have observed high PIADC values and facilitated diffusion on ADC maps of benign and malignant cartilaginous tumors, perhaps because of their high chondroid matrix content. However, the usefulness of diffusion in the diagnosis of cartilaginous tumors requires further evaluation (see **Fig. 5**).

Osteosarcoma and Ewing Sarcoma

Osteosarcoma and Ewing sarcoma represent more than 90% of all primary malignant bone tumors in children. The current treatment of localized forms consists of neoadjuvant chemotherapy to treat micrometastatic disease and to reduce primary tumor volume, thus facilitating subsequent surgery.[65] Accurate determination of tumor response during the initial phase of treatment is vital for assessing the effectiveness of neoadjuvant therapy, for planning further treatment, and for predicting patient prognosis (see **Fig. 8**).[12]

The efficacy of preoperative chemotherapy can be assessed precisely by histologic evaluation of tumor specimens after resection. In general, an effective response is defined as the death of more than 90% of tumor cells. Patients who respond to chemotherapy have a significantly higher disease-free survival rate than nonresponders.[21] Consequently, a noninvasive method capable of assessing intracellular necrosis and viable cells is essential for the evaluation of response to treatment (see **Fig. 8**).

Conventional imaging techniques, including radiography, CT, and static postcontrast MR imaging, cannot accurately quantitate tumor response.[1] Conventional MR imaging is limited in assessing tumor viability, because on T2-weighted imaging, both viable and necrotic tumor tissue show high signal intensities, and the morphologic changes induced by chemotherapy may be associated with hemorrhage, necrosis, edema, and inflammatory fibrosis without specific MR imaging patterns.[2,6,12,66–68] In addition, osteosarcoma size is often not diminished significantly during successful chemotherapy, because therapy has limited impact on the mineralized matrix of these tumors (**Fig. 27**).

TICs derived from perfusion studies have been used to more precisely assess the response of osteosarcomas and Ewing sarcomas to treatment.[12,21] A 60% reduction in slope in regions with maximal slope before chemotherapy was found to be the most reliable criterion of tumor response (see **Fig. 8**).[21] Dynamic contrast-enhanced MR imaging should not be performed until 4 to 6 weeks after preoperative chemotherapy to avoid the misclassification of a good responder as a poor responder. Tumor tissue with low vascularity, including chemotherapy-resistant chondroblastic areas in osteosarcomas, may mimic tumor necrosis, whereas newly formed granulation tissue replacing areas of tumor necrosis may simulate viable tumor areas (**Fig. 28**).[1] The assessment of a patient as a responder or nonresponder, based on dynamic contrast-enhanced MR examination, should be performed about 3 months after the first round of chemotherapy, because at this time perfusion in the granulation tissue replacing the tumor has been reduced, whereas residual tumor tissue is still highly vascularized and perfused (see **Figs. 27** and **28**).[1]

ADC values of viable tumor tissue and necrotic areas on DWI differ significantly; DWI may be used to evaluate treatment response by analyzing changes in tumor cellularity over time.[68] DWI may provide earlier information about therapeutic results, because cellular changes usually precede reduction in tumor size, as observed on conventional MR imaging.[68] DWI MR imaging may be used to distinguish highly cellular regions of a tumor from regions in which cellularity is altered in response to treatment.[69] In patients with osteosarcoma, a direct relationship has been observed between treatment-induced increase of ADC and the extent of tumor necrosis.[70] A significant difference in minimum ADC of solid tumor components was observed between patients with osteosarcoma with good and poor responses to chemotherapy (see **Fig. 28**).[71]

DWI may be useful for evaluating the response of osteosarcomas to chemotherapy and is considered a promising method for monitoring the therapeutic response of primary bone sarcomas.[2,66,68,71]

Miscellaneous Malignant Bone Disease

Diffusion-weighted MR imaging performed regionally or as whole-body imaging has been shown to have a high diagnostic accuracy for the identification of bone metastases when combined with conventional MR imaging.[72] DWI was found to detect more metastatic lesions and smaller metastases that positron emission tomography (PET) or bone scintigraphy.[73] The detection of bone metastasis is crucial for cancer staging and for determining the appropriate treatment strategy (**Fig. 29**).[73]

Acute vertebral collapse is a common clinical problem in elderly patients and usually results from osteoporosis or metastasis.[30] An investigation

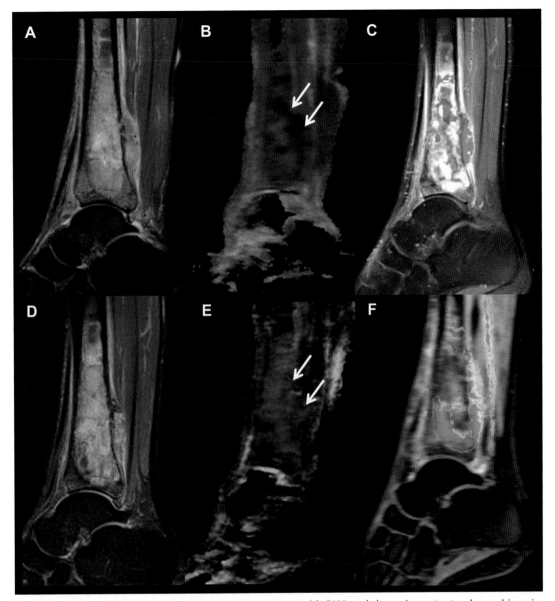

Fig. 27. Evaluation of response to osteosarcoma treatment with DWI and dynamic contrast-enhanced imaging with color mapping in a 27-year-old man with pain in the left ankle after trauma. Before treatment: (*A*) sagittal STIR MR image shows a large hyperintense lesion with soft tissue extension, suggesting malignancy. (*B*) Sagittal ADC map image shows areas with restricted diffusion (*white arrows*) with PIDC = 0.91×10^{-3} mm^2/s, suggesting malignant tissue. (*C*) Sagittal dynamic contrast-enhanced imaging with color mapping shows many red regions in the periphery of the tumor, suggesting hypervascularity. After treatment: sagittal STIR (*D*) MR image shows no change in tumor characteristics. On the sagittal ADC map image (*E*) the areas with restricted diffusion are reduced in size (*white arrows*), but perfusion color mapping (*F*) shows persistence of red regions, suggesting viable cells with hypervascularity and consequently poor response to treatment, confirmed on histologic analysis.

of the percentage of peak contrast enhancement, enhancement slope, and TIC patterns in the first passage of contrast into vertebral bodies showed that the type IV curve, with rapid contrast washin followed by a washout phase, had a high positive predictive value for metastatic collapsed vertebral bodies, whereas the type V curve, with a rapid washin and a second slower rising slope had a high positive predictive value for benign spinal compression fractures.[74] In-phase/opposed-phase imaging may also be useful for differentiating acute benign compression fractures from malignant

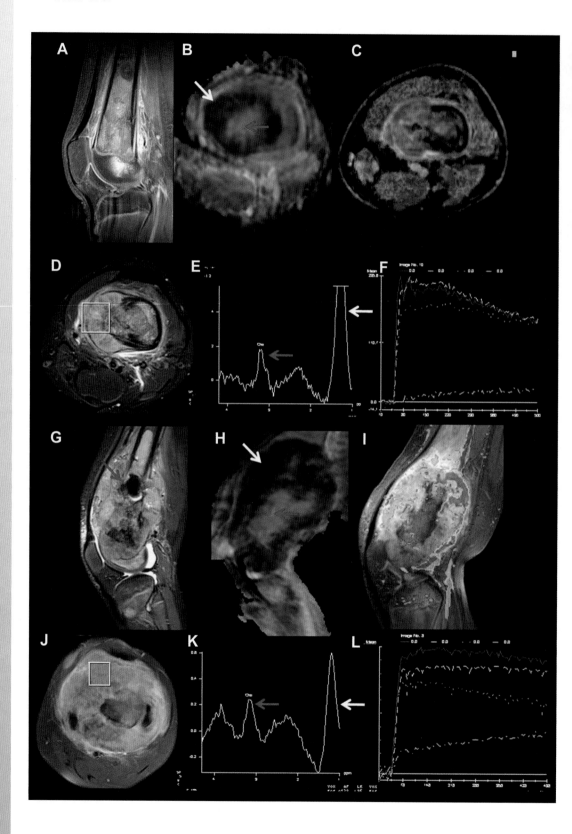

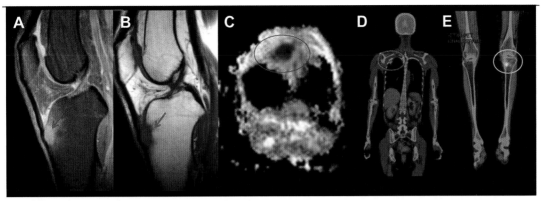

Fig. 29. Metastatic adenocarcinoma of the lung in the left tibia in a 55-year-old woman with knee pain for 4 months. (*A*) Sagittal STIR MR image and (*B*) sagittal T1-weighted MR image show a small lesion in the tibia, with restricted diffusion on axial ADC map image (*C, red circle*); PIADC = 0.97×10^{-3} mm^2/s, suggesting malignant tumor. (*D, E*) PET/CT shows focal activity in the right lung (*D, red circle*), and (*E*) in the proximal left tibia (*green circle*).

infiltration and pathologic fractures.[39] Decreases in signal intensity greater than 35% on out-of-phase compared with in-phase images may be a cutoff value for differentiating between osteoporotic and neoplastic vertebral collapse.[39] This cutoff may also be an early indicator of response to radiation therapy for the spine.[39]

^{1}H MRS may also be useful for analyzing the presence of a cho peak, which reflects the potential malignancy of a lesion.[23] Both qualitative and quantitative diffusion-weighted MR imaging have been shown to be additional tools for differentiating malignant from benign vertebral fractures.[30,72]

Monitoring Treatment Response

The use of follow-up conventional MR imaging after treatment of musculoskeletal soft tissue masses is traditionally based on anatomic approaches, such as measurements of tumor size and the degree of contrast enhancement. However, this type of anatomic imaging has significant limitations, including poor measurement reproducibility and (nonneoplastic) mass lesions that persist after therapy.[75]

Because cellular death and vascular changes in response to treatment precede changes in lesion size, functional imaging such as DWI may result in the earlier identification of patients with a poor

◄─────────────────────────────────

Fig. 28. Evaluation of response to osteosarcoma treatment with DWI, dynamic contrast-enhanced imaging with color mapping and spectroscopy in a 12-year-old boy. Before treatment: a large tumor in the distal femur with heterogeneous contrast enhancement is shown on the sagittal fat-suppressed T1-weighted contrast-enhanced MR image (*A*), with restricted diffusion peripherally on the ADC map (*B*) (*white arrow*), a PIADC = 0.89×10^{-3} mm^2/s, suggesting hypercellular tissue, and facilitated diffusion in the central part (*red arrow*), which could represent necrosis or a cartilaginous component. Axial dynamic contrast-enhanced MR image with color mapping (*C*) shows highly perfused areas in red along the peripheral part of the lesion. (*D*) shows an axial fat-suppressed T1-weighted contrast-enhanced MR image with a spectroscopy voxel placed on enhancing tissue. Spectroscopic analysis in (*E*) shows a cho peak (*red arrow*) and lipid peak (*white arrow*), suggesting highly malignant tumor. (*F*) Yellow and green type IV TICs represent the tumor, the red type IV TIC represents the artery, and the blue type II curve represents normal muscle. After the treatment (6 months): (*G*) sagittal fat-suppressed T1-weighted contrast-enhanced MR image shows that the lesion grew and now has a pathologic metaphyseal fracture (*red arrow*) at the site of previous biopsy, with continued peripheral restricted diffusion on the ADC map (*H, white arrow*) and facilitated diffusion (*red arrow*) in the center. (*I*) On the sagittal dynamic contrast-enhanced MR image with color mapping, note the highly perfused areas in the peripheral part of the tumor and hypovascularity in the central part of the lesion, suggesting necrosis or a cartilaginous component, the same appearance as before treatment; (*J*) shows an axial fat-suppressed T1-weighted contrast-enhanced MR image with a spectroscopy voxel placed on enhancing tissue. Spectroscopic analysis (*K*) shows a cho peak (*red arrow*) and lipid peak (*white arrow*), suggesting poor response to treatment. (*L*) Yellow and green type IV TICs represent the tumor, the red type IV TIC represents the artery, and the blue type II TIC represents normal muscle. The histologic analysis showed Huvos grade 2 neoplasm, with a cartilaginous component in the central part of the tumor.

response to treatment and those with tumor recurrence (**Fig. 30**).[76,77] Functional imaging therefore provides the opportunity to adjust individual treatment regimens more rapidly, sparing patients unnecessary morbidity, expense, and delay in initiation of effective treatment modalities.[74]

Effective anticancer therapy should result in:

- tumor lysis
- loss of membrane integrity
- increased extracellular space
- increased diffusion of water molecules, all of which increase ADC values (see **Fig. 8**)[28,78]

Preclinical[37,79] and clinical studies have shown the usefulness of DWI as a sensitive biomarker capable of detecting early cellular changes in treated tumors, changes preceding morphologic responses. In musculoskeletal tumors, successful therapy has been associated with increased ADC values (see **Fig. 8**).[66,69,70]

The DWI technique is also being used to assess the activity of residual disease after treatment and to detect early recurrence at a time when a salvage therapy may still be effective.[75] Differentiating between posttherapeutic soft tissue changes and residual or recurrent tumor is a common diagnostic problem, because these pathologies have the same appearance on morphologic imaging (high signal intensity on T2-weighted and short tau inversion recovery (STIR) images and low signal intensity on T1-weighted spin echo images) (see **Fig. 9**).[80]

With DWI evaluation of the signal characteristics of recurrent solid soft tissue tumors and nonneoplastic posttherapeutic soft tissue changes, the latter shows significantly greater diffusion than viable recurrent tumors.[80] It is expected to occur because solid tumors show high cellularity and intact cell membranes, whereas successful treatment results in decreased tumor cellularity and loss of cell membrane integrity.[81]

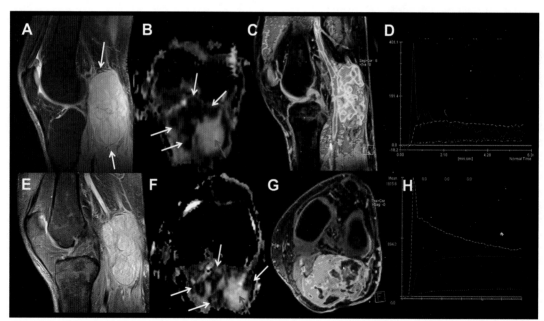

Fig. 30. Evaluation of response to leiomyosarcoma treatment by using DWI and dynamic contrast-enhanced imaging with color mapping in a 50-year-old man. (*A*) and (*E*) Sagittal STIR MR images before and after treatment, respectively; (*B*) and (*F*) axial ADC maps before and after treatment, respectively; (*C*) and (*G*) dynamic contrast-enhanced with color mapping images before and after treatment, respectively; (*D*) and (*H*) TICs before and after treatment, respectively. Before treatment: there is a large hyperintense tumor in the popliteal fossa (*A, arrows*) with restricted diffusion in the solid portions (*B, white arrows*), PIDC = 0.93 × 10^{-3} mm^2/s, and facilitated diffusion in necrotic areas (*B, red arrow*). (*C*) shows red regions, suggesting high vascularity; note the type III yellow curve in (*D*), representing the tumor. The red curve in (*D*) represents the artery and the green curve represents normal muscle. After the treatment: the tumor did not change on the STIR MR image (*E*). Note restricted diffusion (*white arrows*) in solid areas on (*F*), PIDC = 0.98 × 10^{-3} mm^2/s, and facilitated diffusion in necrotic areas (*red arrow*) with many red regions on (*G*), suggesting viable tissue. The red type III curve in (*H*), representing the tumor, did not change. In (*H*) the yellow curve (type IV) represents the artery and the green curve (type II) represents normal muscle.

Dynamic contrast-enhanced MR imaging is the method of choice to monitor preoperative response to chemotherapy. Poor and good responders to chemotherapy can easily be detected on first-pass or subtraction images, or by evaluation of changes in slopes using the ROI method.[1] The purpose of MR examination is to detect local tumor recurrence or residual tumor tissue, and to differentiate recurrence from reactive tissue. Tumor enhances fast during the first pass, whereas reactive tissue enhances later and more slowly (see **Fig. 21**).[1] All recurrences of all bone tumors (except chondral components) enhance faster and earlier than reference tissue (normal muscle).

In soft tissue sarcomas, focal areas of early and rapidly progressive enhancement correspond to residual viable or recurrent tumor (see **Fig. 30**). In contrast, dynamic studies showing no areas of early enhancement indicate a good response (see **Fig. 8**).[1]

Radiation therapy can induce neovascularization, resulting in increased perfusion in the irradiated area. Differentiation of a reactive mass with young granulation tissue from residual tumor tissue or tumor recurrence may be difficult in the first 3 to 6 months after irradiation of a sarcoma.[1] Follow-up examinations are necessary because perfusion of a reactive mass decreases, whereas residual tumor tissue grows and remains highly vascularized (see **Fig. 9**).[1]

SUMMARY

These advanced MR imaging techniques, together with conventional MR imaging, the clinical history of the patient, and other imaging methods, are important tools for analyzing and diagnosing musculoskeletal tumors, avoiding unnecessary biopsies, facilitating early and efficient treatment, and consequently enhancing patient outcomes.

ACKNOWLEDGMENTS

The authors thank Evandro Miguelote Vianna MD, Walter Meohas MD, José Francisco Rezende MD and Ierecê Lins Aymoré for technical support.

REFERENCES

1. Verstraete KL, Lang P. Bone and soft tissue tumors: the role of contrast agents for MR imaging. Eur J Radiol 2000;34(3):229–46.

2. Costa FM, Ferreira EC, Vianna EM. Diffusion-weighted magnetic resonance imaging for the evaluation of musculoskeletal tumors. Magn Reson Imaging Clin N Am 2011;19(1):1–22, 159–80.

3. Fayad LM, Barker PB, Jacobs MA, et al. Characterization of musculoskeletal lesions on 3-T proton MR spectroscopy. Am J Roentgenol 2007;188(6): 1513–20.

4. Kransdorf MJ, Murphey MD. Radiologic evaluation of soft-tissue masses: a current perspective. Am J Roentgenol 2000;175(3):575–87.

5. De Schepper AM, De Beuckerleer PM, Vanhoenacker F. Imaging of soft tissue tumors. 2nd edition. Edegem (Belgium): Springer; 2001. p. 83, 86, 101 and 107.

6. Erlemann R, Reiser MF, Peters PE, et al. Musculoskeletal neoplasms: static and dynamic Gd-DTPA–enhanced MR imaging. Radiology 1989;171(3): 767–73.

7. Van Rijswijk CS, Geirnaerdt MJ, Hogendoorn PC, et al. Soft-tissue tumors: value of static and dynamic gadopentetate dimeglumine-enhanced MR imaging in prediction of malignancy. Radiology 2004;233(2): 493–502.

8. Verstraete KL, De Deene Y, Roels H, et al. Benign and malignant musculoskeletal lesions: dynamic contrast-enhanced MR imaging–parametric "first-pass" images depict tissue vascularization and perfusion. Radiology 1994;192(3):835–43.

9. Tokuda O, Hayashi N, Taguchi K, et al. Dynamic contrast-enhanced perfusion MR imaging of diseased vertebrae: analysis of three parameters and the distribution of the time-intensity curve patterns. Skeletal Radiol 2005;34(10):632–8.

10. Kajihara M, Sugawara Y, Sakayama K, et al. Evaluation of tumor blood flow in musculoskeletal lesions: dynamic contrast-enhanced MR imaging and its possibility when monitoring the response to preoperative chemotherapy – work in progress. Radiat Med 2007;25(3):94–105.

11. Öztekin O, Argin M, Oktay A, et al. Musculoskeletal tumors: does fast dynamic contrast-enhanced subtraction MR imaging contribute to the characterization? Radiology 1998;208(3):821–8.

12. Fletcher BD, Hanna SL, Fairclough DL, et al. Pediatric musculoskeletal tumors: use of dynamic, contrast-enhanced MR imaging to monitor response to chemotherapy. Radiology 1992;184(1):243–8.

13. Van Herendael BH, Heyman SR, Vanhoenacker FM, et al. The value of magnetic resonance imaging in the differentiation between malignant peripheral nerve-sheath tumors and non-neurogenic malignant soft-tissue tumors. Skeletal Radiol 2006;35(10):745–53.

14. Verstraete KL, Van der Woude HJ, Hogendoorn PC, et al. Dynamic contrast-enhanced MR imaging of musculoskeletal tumors: basic principles and clinical applications. J Magn Reson Imaging 1996; 6(2):311–21.

15. Fletcher BD, Hanna SL. Musculoskeletal neoplasms: dynamic Gd-DTPA-enhanced MR imaging. Radiology 1990;177(1):287–8.

16. Verstraete KL, Vanzieleghem B, De Deene Y, et al. Static, dynamic and first-pass MR imaging of

musculoskeletal lesions using gadodiamide injection. Acta Radiol 1995;36(1):27–36.

17. Daldrup H, Shames DM, Wendland M, et al. Correlation of dynamic contrast-enhanced MR imaging with histologic tumor grade: comparison of macromolecular and small-molecular contrast media. AJR Am J Roentgenol 1998;171(4):941–9.

18. Öztekin Ö, Argin M, Oktay A, et al. Intraosseous lipoma: radiological findings. Radiol Bras 2008; 41(2):81–6.

19. Hawighorst H, Libicher M, Knopp MV, et al. Evaluation of angiogenesis and perfusion of bone marrow lesions: role of semiquantitative and quantitative dynamic MRI. J Magn Reson Imaging 1999;10(3):286–94.

20. Lang P, Honda G, Roberts T, et al. Musculoskeletal neoplasm: perineoplastic edema versus tumor on dynamic postcontrast MR images with spatial mapping of instantaneous enhancement rates. Radiology 1995;197(3):831–9.

21. Erlemann R, Vassallo P, Bongartz G, et al. Musculoskeletal neoplasms: fast low-angle shot MR imaging with and without Gd-DTPA. Radiology 1990;176(2): 489–95.

22. Wang CK, Li CW, Hsieh TJ, et al. Characterization of bone and soft-tissue tumors with in vivo 1H MR spectroscopy: initial results. Radiology 2004; 232(2):599–605.

23. Fayad LM, Bluemke DA, McCarthy EF, et al. Musculoskeletal tumors: use of proton MR spectroscopic imaging for characterization. J Magn Reson Imaging 2006;23(1):23–8.

24. Doganay S, Altinok T, Alkan A, et al. The role of MRS in the differentiation of benign and malignant soft tissue and bone tumors. Eur J Radiol 2011;20(2): 219–25.

25. Bartella L, Morris EA, Dershaw DD, et al. Proton MR spectroscopy with choline peak as malignancy marker improves positive predictive value for breast cancer diagnosis: preliminary study. Radiology 2006;239(3):686–92.

26. Mukherji SK, Schiro S, Castillo M, et al. Proton MR spectroscopy of squamous cell carcinoma of the upper aerodigestive tract: in vitro characteristics. AJNR Am J Neuroradiol 1996;17(8):1485–90.

27. Allen JR, Prost RW, Griffith OW, et al. In vivo proton (H1) magnetic resonance spectroscopy for cervical carcinoma. Am J Clin Oncol 2001;24(5):522–9.

28. Koh DM, Takahara T, Imai Y, et al. Practical aspects of assessing tumors using clinical diffusion-weighted imaging in the body. Magn Reson Med Sci 2007; 6(4):211–24.

29. Latour LL, Svoboda K, Mitra PP, et al. Time-dependent diffusion of water in a biological model system. Proc Natl Acad Sci U S A 1994;91(4):1229–33.

30. Baur A, Reiser MF. Diffusion-weighted imaging of the musculoskeletal system in humans. Skeletal Radiol 2000;29(10):555–62.

31. Guo Y, Cai YQ, Cai ZL, et al. Differentiation of clinically benign and malignant breast lesions using diffusion-weighted imaging. J Magn Reson Imaging 2002;16(2):172–8.

32. Gauvain KM, McKinstry RC, Mukherjee P, et al. Evaluating pediatric brain tumor cellularity with diffusion-tensor imaging. AJR Am J Roentgenol 2001;177(2): 449–54.

33. Sugahara T, Korogi Y, Kochi M, et al. Usefulness of diffusion-weighted MRI with echo-planar technique in the evaluation of cellularity in gliomas. J Magn Reson Imaging 1999;9(1):53–60.

34. Lang P, Wendland MF, Saeed M, et al. Osteogenic sarcoma: noninvasive in vivo assessment of tumor necrosis with diffusion-weighted MR imaging. Radiology 1998;206(1):227–35.

35. Maeda M, Matsumine A, Kato H, et al. Soft-tissue tumors evaluated by line-scan diffusion-weighted imaging: influence of myxoid matrix on the apparent diffusion coefficient. J Magn Reson Imaging 2007; 25(6):1199–204.

36. Van Rijswijk CS, Kunz P, Hogendoorn PC, et al. Diffusion-weighted MRI in the characterization of soft-tissue tumors. J Magn Reson Imaging 2002;15(3):302–7.

37. Roth Y, Tichler T, Kostenich G, et al. High-b-value diffusion-weighted MR imaging for pretreatment prediction and early monitoring of tumor response to therapy in mice. Radiology 2004;232(3):685–92.

38. Ragab Y, Emad Y, Gheita T, et al. Differentiation of osteoporotic and neoplastic vertebral fractures by chemical shift (in-phase and out-of phase) MR imaging. Eur J Radiol 2009;72(1):125–33.

39. Erly WK, Oh ES, Outwater EK. The utility of in-phase/opposed-phase imaging in differentiating malignancy from acute benign compression fractures of the spine. AJNR Am J Neuroradiol 2006;27(6):1183–8.

40. Hwang S, Panicek DM. Magnetic resonance imaging of bone marrow in oncology, Part 2. Skeletal Radiol 2007;36:1017–27.

41. Zajick DC Jr, Morrison WB, Schweitzer ME, et al. Benign and malignant processes: normal values and differentiation with chemical shift MR imaging in vertebral marrow. Radiology 2005;237(2):590–6.

42. Chai JW, Hong SH, Choi JY, et al. Radiologic diagnosis of osteoid osteoma: from simple to challenging findings. Radiographics 2010;30(3):737–49.

43. Nogués P, Martí-Bonmatí L, Aparisi F, et al. MR imaging assessment of juxta cortical edema in osteoid osteoma in 28 patients. Eur Radiol 1998; 8(2):236–8.

44. Liu PT, Kujak JL, Roberts CC, et al. The vascular groove sign: a new CT finding associated with osteoid osteomas. AJR Am J Roentgenol 2011; 196(1):168–73.

45. Davies M, Cassar-Pullicino VN, Davies AM, et al. The diagnostic accuracy of MR imaging in osteoid osteoma. Skeletal Radiol 2002;31(10):559–69.

46. Assoun J, Richardi G, Railhac JJ, et al. Osteoid osteoma: MR imaging versus CT. Radiology 1994; 191(1):217–23.

47. Ilaslan H, Sundaram M. Advances in musculoskeletal tumor imaging. Orthop Clin North Am 2006; 37(3):375–91.

48. Nagata S, Nishimura H, Uchida M, et al. Diffusion-weighted imaging of soft tissue tumors: usefulness of the apparent diffusion coefficient for differential diagnosis. Radiat Med 2008;26(5):287–95.

49. Sah PL, Sharma R, Kandpal H, et al. In vivo proton spectroscopy of giant cell tumor of the bone. Am J Roentgenol 2008;190(2):133–9.

50. Dinauer PA, Brixey CJ, Moncur JT, et al. Pathologic and MR imaging features of benign fibrous soft-tissue tumors in adults. Radiographics 2007;27(1): 173–87.

51. Lee JC, Thomas JM, Phillips S, et al. Aggressive fibromatosis: MRI features with pathologic correlation. AJR Am J Roentgenol 2006;186(1):247–54.

52. Kransdorf MJ, Murphey MD. Imaging of soft tissue tumors. In: Mc Allister L, Barrett K, editors. Imaging of soft tissue tumors. 2nd edition. Philadelphia: Lippincott Williams & Wilkins; 2006. p. 38–79.

53. Harish S, Chiavaras MM, Kotnis N, et al. MR imaging of skeletal soft tissue infection: utility of diffusion-weighted imaging in detecting abscess formation. Skeletal Radiol 2011;40(3):285–94.

54. Nakayama T, Yoshimitsu K, Irie H, et al. Usefulness of the calculated apparent diffusion coefficient value in the differential diagnosis of retroperitoneal masses. J Magn Reson Imaging 2004;20:735–42.

55. Chang SC, Lai PH, Chen WL, et al. Diffusion-weighted MRI features of brain abscess and cystic or necrotic brain tumors: comparison with conventional MRI. Clin Imaging 2002;26(4):227–36.

56. Oka K, Yakushiji T, Sato H, et al. Ability of diffusion-weighted imaging for the differential diagnosis between chronic expanding hematomas and malignant soft tissue tumors. J Magn Reson Imaging 2008;28(5):1195–200.

57. Sumi M, Ichikawa Y, Nakamura T. Diagnostic ability of apparent diffusion coefficients for lymphomas and carcinomas in the pharynx. Eur Radiol 2007; 17:2631–7.

58. King AD, Ahuja AT, Yeung DK, et al. Malignant cervical lymphadenopathy: diagnostic accuracy of diffusion-weighted MR imaging. Radiology 2007; 245:806–13.

59. Toh CH, Castillo M, Wong AM, et al. Primary cerebral lymphoma and glioblastoma multiforme: differences in diffusion characteristics evaluated with diffusion tensor imaging. AJNR Am J Neuroradiol 2008;29: 471–5.

60. Lin C, Luciani A, Itti E, et al. Whole-body diffusion-weighted magnetic resonance imaging with apparent diffusion coefficient mapping for staging patients with diffuse large B-cell lymphoma. Eur Radiol 2010;20(8):2027–38.

61. Nagata S, Nishimura H, Uchida M, et al. Usefulness of diffusion-weighted MRI in differentiating benign from malignant musculoskeletal tumors. Nippon Igaku Hoshasen Gakkai Zasshi 2005;65(1):30–6.

62. Sundaram M, Baran G, Merenda G, et al. Myxoid liposarcoma: magnetic resonance imaging appearances with clinical and histological correlation. Skeletal Radiol 1990;19(5):359–62.

63. Focacci C, Lattanzi R, Iadeluca ML, et al. Nuclear medicine in primary bone tumors. Eur J Radiol 1998;27(Suppl 1):S123–31.

64. Geirnaerdt MJ, Hogendoorn PC, Bloem JL, et al. Cartilaginous tumors: fast contrast-enhanced MR imaging. Radiology 2000;214(2):539–46.

65. Brisse H, Ollivier L, Edeline V, et al. Imaging of malignant tumours of the long bones in children: monitoring response to neoadjuvant chemotherapy and preoperative assessment. Pediatr Radiol 2004; 34(8):595–605.

66. Hayashida Y, Yakushiji T, Awai K, et al. Monitoring therapeutic responses of primary bone tumors by diffusion-weighted image: initial results. Eur Radiol 2006;16(12):2637–43.

67. Holscher HC, Bloem JL, Vanel D, et al. Osteosarcoma: chemotherapy-induced changes at MR imaging. Radiology 1992;182(3):839–44.

68. Uhl M, Saueressig U, Koehler G, et al. Evaluation of tumour necrosis during chemotherapy with diffusion-weighted MR imaging: preliminary results in osteosarcomas. Pediatr Radiol 2006;36(12): 1306–11.

69. Uhl M, Saueressig U, van Buiren M, et al. Osteosarcoma: preliminary results of in vivo assessment of tumor necrosis after chemotherapy with diffusion- and perfusion-weighted magnetic resonance imaging. Invest Radiol 2006;41:618–23.

70. Dudeck O, Zeile M, Pink D, et al. Diffusion-weighted magnetic resonance imaging allows monitoring of anticancer treatment effects in patients with soft-tissue sarcomas. J Magn Reson Imaging 2008;5: 1109–13.

71. Oka K, Yakushiji T, Sato H, et al. The value of diffusion-weighted imaging for monitoring the chemotherapeutic response of osteosarcoma: a comparison between average apparent diffusion coefficient and minimum apparent diffusion coefficient. Skeletal Radiol 2010;39(2):141–6.

72. Stejskal EO, Tanner JE. Spin diffusion measurements: spin-echo in the presence of a time dependent field gradient. J Chem Phys 1965;42:288–92.

73. Goudarzi B, Kishimoto R, Komatsu S, et al. Detection of bone metastases using diffusion weighted magnetic resonance imaging: comparison with (11)C methionine PET and bone scintigraphy. Magn Reson Imaging 2010;28(3):372–9.

74. Chen WT, Shih TT, Chen RC, et al. Blood perfusion of vertebral lesions evaluated with gadolinium-enhanced dynamic MRI: in comparison with compression fracture and metastasis. J Magn Reson Imaging 2002;15:308–14.

75. Padhani AR, Khan AA. Diffusion-weighted (DW) and dynamic contrast-enhanced (DCE) magnetic resonance imaging (MRI) for monitoring anticancer therapy. Target Oncol 2010;5(1):39–52.

76. Padhani AR, Liu G, Koh DM, et al. Diffusion-weighted magnetic resonance imaging as a cancer biomarker: consensus and recommendations. Neoplasia 2009;11(2):102–25.

77. Kwee TC, Takahara T, Klomp DW, et al. Cancer imaging: novel concepts in clinical magnetic resonance imaging. J Intern Med 2010;268(2):120–32.

78. Moffat BA, Hall DE, Stojanovska J, et al. Diffusion imaging for evaluation of tumor therapies in preclinical animal models. MAGMA 2004;17(3–6):249–59.

79. Thoeny HC, De Keyzer F, Chen F, et al. Diffusion-weighted MR imaging in monitoring the effect of a vascular targeting agent on rhabdomyosarcoma in rats. Radiology 2005;234(3):756–64.

80. Baur A, Huber A, Arbogast S, et al. Diffusion-weighted imaging of tumor recurrencies and post-therapeutical soft-tissue changes in humans. Eur Radiol 2001;11(5):828–33.

81. Bley TA, Wieben O, Uhl M. Diffusion-weighted MR imaging in musculoskeletal radiology: applications in trauma, tumors, and inflammation. Magn Reson Imaging Clin N Am 2009;17(2):263–75.

Index

United States Postal Service

Statement of Ownership, Management, and Circulation
(All Periodicals Publications Except Requestor Publications)

1. Publication Title	2. Publication Number	3. Filing Date
Radiologic Clinics of North America	5 9 6 - 5 1 0	9/16/11

4. Issue Frequency	5. Number of Issues Published Annually	6. Annual Subscription Price
Jan, Mar, May, Jul, Sep, Nov	6	$386.00

7. Complete Mailing Address of Known Office of Publication (Not printer) (Street, city, county, state, and ZIP+4®)

Elsevier Inc.
360 Park Avenue South
New York, NY 10010-1710

Contact Person
Stephen Bushing
Telephone (Include area code)
215-239-3688

8. Complete Mailing Address of Headquarters or General Business Office of Publisher (Not printer)

Elsevier Inc., 360 Park Avenue South, New York, NY 10010-1710

9. Full Names and Complete Mailing Addresses of Publisher, Editor, and Managing Editor (Do not leave blank)

Publisher (Name and complete mailing address)

Kim Murphy, Elsevier, Inc., 1600 John F. Kennedy Blvd. Suite 1800, Philadelphia, PA 19103-2899

Editor (Name and complete mailing address)

Barton Dudlick, Elsevier, Inc., 1600 John F. Kennedy Blvd. Suite 1800, Philadelphia, PA 19103-2899

Managing Editor (Name and complete mailing address)

Barton Dudlick, Elsevier, Inc., 1600 John F. Kennedy Blvd. Suite 1800, Philadelphia, PA 19103-2899

10. Owner (Do not leave blank. If the publication is owned by a corporation, give the name and address of the corporation immediately followed by the names and addresses of all stockholders owning or holding 1 percent or more of the total amount of stock. If not owned by a corporation, give the names and addresses of the individual owners. If owned by a partnership or other unincorporated firm, give its name and address as well as those of each individual owner. If the publication is published by a nonprofit organization, give its name and address.)

Full Name	Complete Mailing Address
Wholly owned subsidiary of	4520 East-West Highway
Reed/Elsevier, US holdings	Bethesda, MD 20814

11. Known Bondholders, Mortgagees, and Other Security Holders Owning or Holding 1 Percent or More of Total Amount of Bonds, Mortgages, or Other Securities. If none, check box   ☐ None

Full Name	Complete Mailing Address
N/A	

12. Tax Status (For completion by nonprofit organizations authorized to mail at nonprofit rates) (Check one)
The purpose, function, and nonprofit status of this organization and the exempt status for federal income tax purposes:
☐ Has Not Changed During Preceding 12 Months
☐ Has Changed During Preceding 12 Months (Publisher must submit explanation of change with this statement)

PS Form 3526, September 2007 (Page 1 of 3 (Instructions Page 3)) PSN 7530-01-000-9931 **PRIVACY NOTICE**: See our Privacy policy in www.usps.com

---

13. Publication Title	14. Issue Date for Circulation Data Below
Radiologic Clinics of North America	July 2011

15. Extent and Nature of Circulation			Average No. Copies Each Issue During Preceding 12 Months	No. Copies of Single Issue Published Nearest to Filing Date
a. Total Number of Copies (Net press run)			4901	4674
b. Paid Circulation (By Mail and Outside the Mail)	(1)	Mailed Outside-County Paid Subscriptions Stated on PS Form 3541. (Include paid distribution above nominal rate, advertiser's proof copies, and exchange copies)	2109	2007
	(2)	Mailed In-County Paid Subscriptions Stated on PS Form 3541 (Include paid distribution above nominal rate, advertiser's proof copies, and exchange copies)		
	(3)	Paid Distribution Outside the Mails Including Sales Through Dealers and Carriers, Street Vendors, Counter Sales, and Other Paid Distribution Outside USPS®	1026	1035
	(4)	Paid Distribution by Other Classes Mailed Through the USPS (e.g. First-Class Mail®)		
c. Total Paid Distribution (Sum of 15b (1), (2), (3), and (4))			3135	3042
d. Free or Nominal Rate Distribution (By Mail and Outside the Mail)	(1)	Free or Nominal Rate Outside-County Copies Included on PS Form 3541	142	98
	(2)	Free or Nominal Rate In-County Copies Included on PS Form 3541		
	(3)	Free or Nominal Rate Copies Mailed at Other Classes Through the USPS (e.g. First-Class Mail)		
	(4)	Free or Nominal Rate Distribution Outside the Mail (Carriers or other means)		
e. Total Free or Nominal Rate Distribution (Sum of 15d (1), (2), (3) and (4))			142	98
f. Total Distribution (Sum of 15c and 15e)			3277	3140
g. Copies not Distributed (See instructions to publishers #4 (page #3))			1624	1534
h. Total (Sum of 15f and g)			4901	4674
i. Percent Paid (15c divided by 15f times 100)			95.67%	96.88%

16. Publication of Statement of Ownership

If the publication is a general publication, publication of this statement is required   Will be printed ☐ Publication not required
in the November 2011 issue of this publication.

17. Signature and Title of Editor, Publisher, Business Manager, or Owner

Stephen R. Bushey   Date September 16, 2011

Stephen R. Bushing –Inventory Distribution Coordinator

I certify that all information furnished on this form is true and complete. I understand that anyone who furnishes false or misleading information on this form or who omits material or information requested on the form may be subject to criminal sanctions (including fines and imprisonment) and/or civil sanctions (including civil penalties).

PS Form 3526, September 2007 (Page 2 of 3)

Moving?

Make sure your subscription moves with you!

To notify us of your new address, find your **Clinics Account Number** (located on your mailing label above your name), and contact customer service at:

Email: journalscustomerservice-usa@elsevier.com

800-654-2452 (subscribers in the U.S. & Canada)
314-447-8871 (subscribers outside of the U.S. & Canada)

Fax number: 314-447-8029

Elsevier Health Sciences Division
Subscription Customer Service
3251 Riverport Lane
Maryland Heights, MO 63043

*To ensure uninterrupted delivery of your subscription, please notify us at least 4 weeks in advance of move.